MW00846356

# Musculoskeletal Imaging

Rotations in Radiology

Volume 1

# Musculoskeletal Imaging

**Edited by**

**Mihra S. Taljanovic, MD, PhD, FACR**

Professor, Radiology and Orthopaedic Surgery
Director of Musculoskeletal Imaging Research and Development
Department of Medical Imaging
The University of Arizona, College of Medicine
Banner University Medical Center
Tucson, Arizona

**Imran M. Omar, MD**

Associate Professor of Radiology
Chief, Musculoskeletal Radiology
Department of Radiology
Northwestern Memorial Hospital
Northwestern University Feinberg School of Medicine
Chicago, Illinois

**Kevin B. Hoover, MD, PhD**

Associate Professor
Director of Musculoskeletal Imaging and Intervention
Department of Radiology
Virginia Commonwealth University
Richmond, Virginia

**Tyson S. Chadaz, MD**

Assistant Professor of Radiology
Associate Program Director, Diagnostic Radiology Residency
Department of Medical Imaging
The University of Arizona, College of Medicine
Banner University Medical Center
Tucson, Arizona

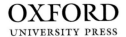

OXFORD
UNIVERSITY PRESS

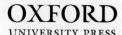

Oxford University Press is a department of the University of Oxford. It furthers
the University's objective of excellence in research, scholarship, and education
by publishing worldwide. Oxford is a registered trade mark of Oxford University
Press in the UK and certain other countries.

Published in the United States of America by Oxford University Press
198 Madison Avenue, New York, NY 10016, United States of America.

© Oxford University Press 2019

All rights reserved. No part of this publication may be reproduced, stored in
a retrieval system, or transmitted, in any form or by any means, without the
prior permission in writing of Oxford University Press, or as expressly permitted
by law, by license, or under terms agreed with the appropriate reproduction
rights organization. Inquiries concerning reproduction outside the scope of the
above should be sent to the Rights Department, Oxford University Press, at the
address above.

You must not circulate this work in any other form
and you must impose this same condition on any acquirer.

Library of Congress Control Number: 2018060177

ISBN 978-0-19-093816-1

9 8 7 6 5 4 3 2 1

Printed by Sheridan Books, Inc., United States of America

# Foreword

Musculoskeletal radiology as a subspecialty encompasses all modalities and disease categories; it is difficult to master its many facets. Furthermore, it is challenging to create a text that succinctly yet comprehensively covers the subject. Rotations in Radiology, Musculoskeletal Imaging, edited by Drs. Taljanovic, Omar, Hoover and Chadaz achieves this goal. The contents accurately represent the series title: a clinical rotation in musculoskeletal radiology encompasses a vast array of diagnoses and techniques, with training led by a trusted mentor. Together the trainer and trainee embark on an educational adventure! The editors have captured this experience, organizing an amazing collection of authors, all internationally recognized experts in their field. Cutting-edge information is presented, along with the basics on all aspects of musculoskeletal radiology. Key points, bulleted lists and diagrams facilitate quick reference. Treatment options are included to provide additional insight. Each anatomic area is featured in a separate chapter with space dedicated to ultrasound techniques. Imaging features of trauma and sports injuries is presented as well as common and atypical infections, metabolic disease and hematopoietic disorders. A large section on musculoskeletal neoplasms is included. Techniques for common musculoskeletal procedures including arthrography of various joints are reviewed. Rounding out the text are chapters on relatively uncommon musculoskeletal diseases. This book is a must for the practitioner who would like to improve their musculoskeletal knowledge and skills—it is like sitting next to the experts.

— William B. Morrison, MD

# Contents

# Contributors

**Sonia Airaldi, MD**
Radiologia III—DISSAL
University of Genoa
Genoa, Italy

**Nabeel Anwar, MD**
Rush University Medical Center
Chicago, Illinois

**Remide Arkun, MD**
Professor of Radiology
Ege University Medical School
Bornova, Izmir, Turkey

**Laura W. Bancroft, MD, FACR**
Professor of Radiology and Educational Chair of Radiology
University of Central Florida College of Medicine
Chief of Musculoskeletal Radiology
Florida Hospital
Orlando, Florida

**Noam Belkind, MD**
Clinical Assistant Professor of Radiology
University of Arizona College of Medicine - Phoenix
Carl T Hayden VA Medical Center
Phoenix, Arizona

**Eléonore Blondieux, MD, PhD**
Associate Professor of Radiology
Faculté de Médecine, Sorbonne Université, Paris 06
Assistance Publique des Hôpitaux de Paris
Hôpital Armand-Trousseau
Paris, France

**Kevin J. Blount, MD**
Assistant Professor of Radiology
Northwestern University Feinberg School of Medicine
Chicago, Illinois

**David Brandel, MD**
Department of Radiology
University of Michigan Health System
Ann Arbor, Michigan

**Tyson S. Chadaz, MD**
Assistant Professor of Radiology
Associate Program Director, Diagnostic Radiology Residency
Department of Medical Imaging
The University of Arizona, College of Medicine
Banner University Medical Center
Tucson, Arizona

**Andrew L. Chiang, MD**
Assistant Professor of Radiology and Orthopedics
Medical Director, Musculoskeletal Imaging
Department of Radiology
Loyola University Medical Center
Maywood, Illinois

**Abhijit Datir, MD, FRCR**
Assistant Professor of Radiology
Emory University School of Medicine
Atlanta, Georgia

**Matthew DelGiudice, MD**
Musculoskeletal Radiologist
East Valley Diagnostic Imaging
Phoenix, Arizona

**Vishal Desai, MD**
Assistant Professor of Radiology
Musculoskeletal Division
Thomas Jefferson University
Philadelphia, Pennsylvania

**Swati Deshmukh, MD**
Assistant Professor of Radiology
Northwestern University Feinberg School of Medicine
Chicago, Illinois

**Girish Gandikota, MBBS, FRCS, FRCR, RMSK**
Professor of Radiology
Department of Radiology
University of Michigan Health System
Ann Arbor, Michigan

**Ankur Garg, MD, MBA**
Assistant Professor of Radiology
Northwestern University Feinberg School of Medicine
Chicago, Illinois

**Dorothy L. Gilbertson-Dahdal, MD, MS**
Professor of Radiology
Vice-Chair Education & Program Director, Diagnostic
Radiology Residency
Pediatrics Medical Director
Department of Medical Imaging
The University of Arizona, College of Medicine
Banner University Medical Center
Tucson, Arizona

**Lana H. Gimber, MD, MPH**
Adjunct Assistant Professor of Radiology
Department of Medical Imaging
The University of Arizona, College of Medicine
Banner-University Medical Center
Tucson, Arizona

**James F. Griffith, MD, FRCR**
Professor
Department of Imaging and Interventional Radiology
The Chinese University of Hong Kong
Hong Kong, China

**Ali Guermazi, MD, PhD**
Professor of Radiology & Medicine
Boston University School of Medicine
Boston, Massachusetts

**Peter J. Haar, MD, PhD**
Assistant Professor of Radiology
VCU Health
Virginia Commonwealth University
Richmond, Virginia

**Daichi Hayashi, MD, PhD**
Assistant Professor of Radiology
Stony Brook University School of Medicine
Stony Brook, New York
Research Assistant Professor of Radiology
Boston University School of Medicine
Boston, Massachusetts

**Kevin B. Hoover, MD, PhD**
Associate Professor of Radiology
Director of Musculoskeletal Imaging
and Intervention
VCU Health
Virginia Commonwealth University
Richmond, Virginia

**Tim B. Hunter, MD, MSc**
Emeritus Professor of Radiology
Department of Medical Imaging
The University of Arizona, College of Medicine
Banner University Medical Center
Tucson, Arizona

**Apostolos H. Karantanas, MD, PhD**
Professor of Radiology
University of Crete
Heraklion, Greece
Chairman, department of Medical Imaging
Heraklion University Hospital
Head - Hybrid Imaging, ICS - FORTH
Heraklion, Greece

**Kiran Khursid, MD**
Research Associate
Department of Trauma
and Emergency Radiology
Vancouver General Hospital
Vancouver, British Columbia, Canada

**Benjamin D. Levine, MD**
Associate Professor of Radiology
UCLA Health
Los Angeles, California

**Laurie M. Lomasney, MD**
Professor of Radiology and Orthopedics
Medical Director, Musculoskeletal Imaging
Loyola University Medical Center
Maywood, Illinois

**Robert Lopez-Ben, MD**
Clinical Adjunct Professor
University of North Carolina School of Medicine
Charlotte Radiology
Charlotte, North Carolina

**Winnie A. Mar, MD**
Associate Professor of Radiology
University of Illinois Hospital and Health Sciences Center
Chicago, Illinois

**Carlo Martinoli, MD**
Associate Professor of Radiology
Radiologia III—DISSAL
University of Genoa
Genoa, Italy

**Stephanie McCann, MD**
Radiology Resident, Class of 2017
Department of Radiology
University of Chicago School of Medicine
Chicago, Illinois

**John Meyer, DO**
Assistant Professor, Department of Diagnostic Radiology
and Nuclear Medicine, Rush Medical College
Vice Chair, Department of Radiology
Director, Division of Body Imaging, Department of
Diagnostic Radiology and Nuclear Medicine
Rush University Medical Center
Chicago, Illinois

**Yoav Morag, MD**
Associate Professor of Radiology
Musculoskeletal Imaging Division
University of Michigan Health System
Ann Arbor, Michigan

**Peter L. Munk, MDCM, FRCPC, FSIR**
Professor of Radiology, Orthopedics and Palliative Care
University of British Columbia
Skeletal Imaging Section Head
Vancouver General Hospital
Vancouver, British Columbia, Canada

**Michael O'Keeffe, MB Bch, BAO, MRCSI, FFRRCSI**
Assistant Professor of Radiology
University of Toronto
Staff Radiologist Dept. of Emergency &Trauma Radiology
Sunnybrook Health Sciences Centre
Toronto, Ontario, Canada

**Imran M. Omar, MD**
Associate Professor of Radiology
Chief, Musculoskeletal Radiology
Northwestern Memorial Hospital
Northwestern University Feinberg School of Medicine
Chicago, Illinois

**Pavan Parasu, MD**
Radiology Resident
University of Illinois at Chicago
Department of Radiology
Chicago, Illinois

**Wilfred C. G. Peh, MBBS, MD, FRCP (Glasg), FRCP (Edin), FRCR**
Senior Consultant and Head, Department of Diagnostic Radiology
Khoo Teck Puat Hospital
Clinical Professor
Yong Loo Lin School of Medicine
National University of Singapore
Republic of Singapore

**Jack Porrino, MD**
Associate Professor of Radiology
Yale School of Medicine
New Haven, Connecticut

**Paul J. Read, MD**
Clinical Assistant Professor of Radiology
Sidney Kimmel Medical College
Thomas Jefferson University Hospitals
Philadelphia, Pennsylvania

**Frank W. Roemer, MD**
Professor of Radiology
University of Erlangen-Nuremberg
Erlangen, Germany
Adjunct Associate Professor of Radiology
Boston University School of Medicine
Boston, Massachusetts

**Jonathan D. Samet, MD**
Assistant Professor of Radiology
Section Head, Musculoskeletal Imaging
Ann & Robert H. Lurie Children's Hospital of Chicago
Northwestern University Feinberg School of Medicine
Chicago, Illinois

**Leanne L. Seeger, MD, FACR**
Professor of Radiology and Orthopedic Surgery
Chief, Musculoskeletal Imaging
UCLA Health System
Los Angeles, California

**Sumer N. Shikhare, MBBS, DNB, MMed, FRCR**
Consultant
Department of Diagnostic Radiology
Khoo Teck Puat Hospital
Republic of Singapore

**Albert Song, MD**
Associate Professor of Musculoskeletal Imaging
Program Director Diagnostic Radiology Residency
Loyola University Medical Center
Maywood, Illinois

**G. Scott Stacy, MD**
Professor of Radiology
Section Chief, Musculoskeletal Radiology
The University of Chicago Medicine
Chicago, Illinois

**Kathryn J. Stevens, MD**
Associate Professor of Radiology and Orthopaedic Surgery (by courtesy)
Stanford University Medical Center
Stanford, California

**Mihra S. Taljanovic, MD, PhD, FACR**
Professor, Radiology and Orthopaedic Surgery
Director of Musculoskeletal Imaging Research and Development
The University of Arizona, College of Medicine
Banner University Medical Center
Tucson, Arizona

**Stephen Thomas, MD**
Associate Professor of Radiology
University of Chicago School of Medicine
Chicago, Illinois

**Josephina A. Vossen MD, PhD**
Assistant Professor of Radiology
VCU Health
Virginia Commonwealth University
Richmond, Virginia

**Alvin R. Wyatt II, MD**
Department of Radiology
University of Washington
Seattle, Washington

**Corrie M. Yablon, MD**
Clinical Associate Professor of Radiology
Fellowship Director, Musculoskeletal Imaging
University of Michigan Health System
Ann Arbor, Michigan

**Federico Zaottini, MD**
Radiologia III—DISSAL
University of Genoa
Genoa, Italy

**Adam C. Zoga, MD**
Professor of Radiology
Vice Chair for Clinical Practice
Director of Musculoskeletal MRI
Musculoskeletal Fellowship Program Director
Thomas Jefferson University
Philadelphia, Pennsylvania

# Trauma

Section One

Trauma

1

# Spine

Edited by Imran M. Omar

# CHAPTER 1

# Introduction to Fractures

Swati Deshmukh

## Introduction

Bone is designed to resist forces from 3 main vectors: *compression, traction*, and *shear*. The Wolff law states that bone adapts proportionally to the stresses that are placed on it. If bone undergoes chronic low-grade stress, for example, the cortex may thicken in response; however, if bone is underused, such as in immobilized patients, the cortex may thin and the patient may develop disuse osteoporosis. As a result of the Wolff law, bone is typically able to withstand stresses that occur over a long enough period. However, any one of these vector forces can result in a fracture when applied with sufficient energy on a bone in the axial or appendicular skeleton, particularly if the force occurs suddenly such that the bone has not had enough time to adapt. Common mechanisms of osseous injury include axial loading and compression, avulsion, distraction, bending and torsion, or a combination of these pure force vectors. Both direct forces (eg, gunshot wound) and indirect forces (eg, twisting injury) can result in fracture. The integrity of the overlying skin defines whether a fracture is closed (intact skin) or open (penetrated skin either because of the cause of injury itself or as a result of a fracture fragment). Imaging plays a key role in the initial diagnosis of a fracture as well as for follow-up assessment of fracture healing.

## Pathophysiology

Fracture healing requires an optimal biological and mechanical environment. There are 3 essential steps in the bone healing process: *inflammation, repair*, and *remodeling*.

*Inflammation* starts at the moment of injury and extends to 3 to 4 days after injury. The fracture acutely disrupts medullary vessels leading to blood extravasation and hematoma and clot formation. This results in release of growth factors, which stimulate angiogenesis and bone formation. Subsequently, there is infiltration of mesenchymal cells that begin to differentiate. Intramembranous bone formation on periosteum provides an early scaffold for endochondral bone. In addition, phagocytes from extraosseous blood supply remove necrotic bone, leading to resorption of the margins of the bone fragments. Radiographically, this appears as widening of the fracture gap. It should be noted that bone fragments must initially be closely apposed to one another in order to instigate the healing cascade. If the gap between the fracture fragments is too wide, there may be failure of fracture healing.

*Repair* involves granulation tissue that matures into connective tissue as mesenchymal cells differentiate into osteoblasts or chondrocytes. Initially, external *soft* callus forms, typically at 3 weeks. As the soft callus matures, it undergoes mineralization, leading to formation of *hard* callus, which begins at the fracture site and progresses centripetally. Endochondral bone formation eventually leads to bony bridging. Although bone union is expected at the end of the repair phase, the bone geometry is still inadequate to sustain high-impact stress.

*Remodeling* is the final phase of fracture healing in which osteoclasts and osteoblasts function to strengthen the bone as explained by the Wolff law. At the end of these processes, the bone should achieve normal tensile strength.

## Common Terminology

The goal of radiologic interpretation in fracture imaging is to accurately identify and describe fracture morphology and orientation as well as any potential complicating factors. There are several characteristics that should be assessed when describing fractures on imaging studies. A thorough report should include as many applicable characteristics as possible.

- Orientation of the fracture line (Figure 1.1)
  - *Transverse fractures* occur along the short axis of the bone. These are often the result of tensile forces on the bone.
  - *Longitudinal (vertical) fractures* are oriented along the long axis of the bone.
  - *Oblique fractures* are angled with respect to the long and short axes of the bone.
  - *Spiral fractures* are the result of rotational forces around the surface of the bone.
  - *Distraction* occurs when there is abnormal widening between fracture fragments. This may indicate intervening tissue that could prevent the fracture fragments from healing appropriately.
  - *Impacted fractures* are the result of axial loading in which osseous fragments are driven into one another. This can result in shortening of the bone and angular deformities.
- Number of fracture fragments
  - *Simple fractures* involve 1 fracture line resulting in 2 fracture fragments.
  - *Comminuted fractures* have more than 1 fracture line and more than 2 fracture fragments.
  - *Segmental fractures* occur when there are a least 2 fractures in the same bone leading to at least 3 fracture fragments.

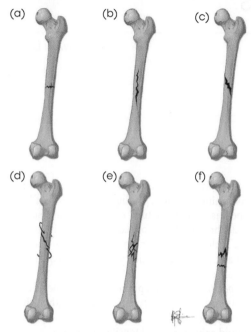

**Figure 1.1.** Illustration demonstrating fracture orientation types. (A) transverse fracture, (B) longitudinal fracture, (C) oblique fracture, (D) spiral fracture, (E) comminuted fracture, and (F) segmental fracture. Artistic credit: Sonja Eagle.

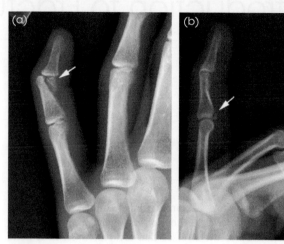

**Figure 1.2.** Intraarticular fracture in a 36-year-old woman with deformity of the distal interphalangeal joint of the fifth digit after boxing injury. Oblique (A) and lateral (B) radiographs demonstrate an oblique fracture of the middle phalanx of the fifth digit (*arrow*) extending into the distal interphalangeal joint as well as an oblique volar plate fracture at the base of the middle phalanx of the fifth digit (*arrow*) extending into the proximal interphalangeal joint. Both fracture lines are therefore intraarticular.

- Relationship of fracture fragment to native bone
  - *Nondisplaced fractures* (eg, stress fracture) are those in which there is no migration of the fracture fragments with respect to one another.
  - *Displacement* refers to the relative position of one fracture fragment from another. Typically, the position of the more distal fragment is reported with respect to the more proximal one. Radiologists conventionally discuss the degree of displacement as a percentage of shaft width of the bone or as minimal, mild, moderate, or complete.
  - *Angulated fractures* occur when there is abnormal rotation of an osseous fragment. This can be described in the report by indicating the direction the distal fragment is pointed, or noting the direction the apex of the fracture is pointing. Therefore, when describing angulation, it is important to describe whether this is based on the direction of the apex or distal fracture fragment. For example, in the case of a Colles fracture in the wrist, the fracture could be described with "apex-volar" angulation or "distal fragment-dorsal" angulation.
  - *Bayonet (overlapped) fractures* are often the result of muscular contraction and can lead to posttraumatic deformity, such as limb shortening. Thus, overlapping fracture fragments are important to note on imaging studies.
- Articular involvement (Figures 1.2 and 1.3)
  - *Intraarticular* involvement occurs when the fracture line extends to the articular surface of a bone. This can result in articular surface irregularity and/or cartilage injury, which can lead to accelerated cartilage loss and posttraumatic osteoarthritis (OA). As a result, the imaging report should document whether the fracture extends to the articular surface as well as the degree of articular surface depression.
  - *Extraarticular fractures* are those in which the fracture line does not extend to the articular surface.
  - *Associated joint subluxation or frank dislocation* can occur in the setting of either intra- or extraarticular fractures and should be noted.
- Degree of cortical disruption
  - *Complete fractures* are those with circumferential cortical disruption that result in 2 or more separate osseous fragments.
  - *Incomplete fractures* result when only a portion of the cortex is fractured, and there is only 1, partially disrupted osseous structure. These are more common in younger children, in whom the bone is relatively elastic. Common examples of incomplete fractures are *greenstick* or *buckle* fractures.
- Quality of native bone
  - *Pathologic fractures* occur in the setting of abnormal bone, most commonly when there is underlying neoplasm, but they can also occur in the setting of bone infection and metabolic and other diseases.
  - *Insufficiency fractures* are a subtype of pathologic fractures that occur when the bone is demineralized.

## Complications

There are a number of complications following fracture of bone that can lead to significant morbidity for patients, such as delayed union, nonunion, malunion, osteomyelitis, osteonecrosis (ON), and occasionally chronic regional pain syndrome. Failure of fracture healing includes delayed union and nonunion and may require surgical intervention. A number of risk factors have been noted to impact fracture healing,

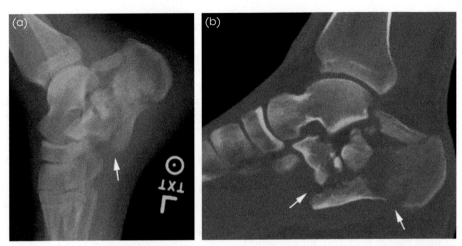

**Figure 1.3.** Intraarticular comminuted fracture in a 23-year-old man presenting after a fall. Lateral radiograph (*A*) and sagittal CT reformatted image (*B*) demonstrate an intraarticular comminuted fracture of the calcaneus (*arrows*) with multiple bone fragments.

including advanced age, diabetes, smoking, nutritional deficiency, antiinflammatory medications, regional infections, excessive soft tissue injury, and compartment syndrome.

*Delayed union* is defined as insufficient healing response to a fracture within the time frame that it would be expected to heal. For example, a paucity of bridging trabeculae and marginal callus across a distal radial fracture at more than 8 weeks (usually at least 3 months) following trauma would indicate delayed healing. Longer bones such as the tibia may require as long as 6 months to heal normally. Nonunion is defined as a lack of healing response at any time point far beyond the expected time frame for healing (Figure 1.4). Thus, in many cases, a lack of healing response at 6 months after the initial injury is concerning for nonunion. Serial imaging studies may be performed to assess the state of fracture repair. Nonunion may be classified as either *hypertrophic* nonunion, in which there is abundant nonbridging callus caused by suboptimal mechanical stability, or as *atrophic* nonunion, in which there is no or minimal callus formation.

Malunion occurs when the fracture heals with a posttraumatic deformity that impacts the normal biomechanics of the bone and adjacent joints. This may include abnormal angulation or limb shortening. Some mild deformities are tolerated well, such as dorsal or volar angular deformities in the distal radius, whereas others, such as medial or lateral angulation in the tibia, may be poorly tolerated and can lead to chronic pain and early onset OA.

Posttraumatic osteomyelitis may develop in the setting of open fractures or after placement of fixation hardware. Osteomyelitis generally manifests a few days following inoculation. The imaging findings of osteomyelitis are further described in Chapter 86, "Osteomyelitis of the Long and Flat Bones."

Fractures of bones with tenuous vascular supply may result in ON. Common examples are transverse fractures of the proximal pole of the scaphoid bone and femoral subcapital fractures. ON may eventually lead to collapse of the bone, followed by OA. In many patients sustaining these injuries,

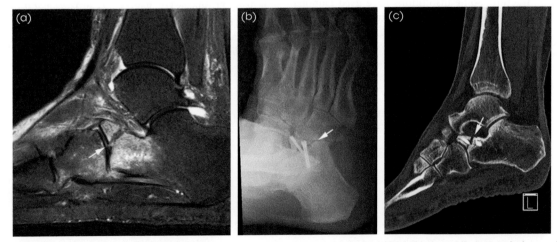

**Figure 1.4.** Fracture nonunion in a 48-year-old woman with ankle and foot pain. Sagittal STIR MR image (*A*) demonstrates a minimally displaced fracture of the anterior process of the calcaneus (*arrow*) with surrounding BME. The patient underwent screw fixation of the fracture. Oblique radiograph (*B*) and sagittal reformatted CT image (*C*) 1 year later demonstrate persistent nonunion of the fracture with no evidence of osseous bridging or callus formation (*arrows*).

serial radiography is performed to detect early signs of ON. In some cases, magnetic resonance imaging (MRI) may be helpful to detect ON at an even earlier stage. The imaging findings of ON are further described in Chapter 115, "Osteonecroses and Osteochondroses."

### Imaging Strategy

- Radiographs are typically the first-line imaging study to evaluate for a suspected fracture, to determine alignment of bones and orthopedic hardware and for follow-up assessment of fracture healing.
- Computed tomography (CT) scanning may be used to describe complex or subtle fractures, such as calcaneal fractures, fractures in which radiography may not provide sufficient detail to help determine treatment (eg, tibial plateau fractures), for assessment of fracture healing or potential nonunion, and to detect complications of orthopedic hardware, such as subtle hardware fracture or findings of loosening or infection.
- MRI is excellent for detection of subtle nondisplaced fractures, to detect fracture complications, such as ON or infection, and to assess the integrity of soft tissue structures such as ligaments and tendons. T1-weighted (T1W) pulse sequences without fat saturation are useful to look for fracture lines, which are usually linear or curvilinear and dark compared to the bright marrow signal. T2-weighted (T2W), proton density (PD), and short tau inversion recovery (STIR) fat-saturated, fluid-sensitive sequences are helpful to look for bone marrow edema (BME), which appears bright. Occasionally, these sequences can highlight low-signal intensity fracture lines as well. Finally, both MRI and CT scanning can be helpful to look for underlying pathology in the setting of pathologic fracture.
- Ultrasound (US) occasionally can be used to look for radiographically occult fractures of superficial bones. Following acute trauma, such as injury to a rib, a fracture may appear as a focal discontinuity of the superficial cortex of a bone on US. In subacute and chronic cases, echogenic callus material may form at the site of the fracture. Some institutions have used Doppler US to detect vascularity at the fracture sites in order to assess the potential for healing in instances of delayed union.

## Treatment Options

The goal of fracture treatment is to ensure mechanical stability and proper alignment to allow for optimal healing and function. Many fractures can be treated nonoperatively if they are stable and would not be expected to result in significant dysfunction or other morbidity. For fractures requiring surgical intervention, numerous devices and hardware options exist.

- Conservative treatment uses external slings, splints, casts, and braces.
- External fixation employs external devices for open fractures or fractures with significant associated soft tissue injury.
- Internal fixation uses wires, pins, screws, plates, intramedullary nails or rods, and staples.
- Bone defects are treated with autogenous bone grafts, allografts, and bone graft substitutes.
- Infected fractures are treated with antibiotic beads.
- Bone morphogenic proteins are used to promote fracture healing.

## Key Points

- Fractures can be characterized on the basis of orientation of the fracture line, number of fracture fragments, relationship of the fracture fragments to native bone, articular involvement, degree of cortical disruption, and quality of native bone.
- The pattern of fracture healing involves 3 stages: inflammation, repair, and remodeling.
- Failure of fracture repair (eg, nonunion) can have severe morbidity consequences and may require surgical intervention.

### References

1. Kostenuik P, Mirza FM. Fracture healing physiology and the quest for therapies for delayed healing and nonunion. *J Orthop Res.* 2017;35:213–223.
2. Pope TL, Bloem HL, Beltran J, et al. *Musculoskeletal Imaging.* 2nd ed. Philadelphia, PA: Elsevier Saunders; 2015.
3. Taljanovic MS, Jones MD, Ruth JT, et al. Fracture fixation. *Radiographics.* 2003;23:1569–1590.

# CHAPTER 2

# Cervical Spine Trauma

Paul J. Read

## Introduction

Approximately 2.4% of patients experiencing blunt trauma suffer cervical spine injuries. C2 is the most commonly involved level (24%), followed by C6 and C7 (39.3% combined). Cervical spine traumatic injuries are categorized by mechanism of injury, stability, and location. The most common mechanisms of injury in the cervical spine are *hyperflexion, hyperextension*, and *axial compression*, and these mechanisms often result in predictable radiographic abnormalities. Furthermore, injuries can be divided into those that are *stable*, or those in which the bone fragments do not significantly shift with physiologic loads, and those that are *unstable*, or those in which the bone fragments can significantly move with respect to one another. Denis described a "three column model," which divides the spine into anterior, middle, and posterior columns:

- The anterior column consists of the anterior longitudinal ligament (ALL) and the anterior two-thirds of the vertebral body and intervertebral disc.
- The middle column is composed of the posterior one-third of the vertebral bodies and intervertebral discs along with the posterior longitudinal ligament (PLL).
- The posterior column is made up of the pedicles, lateral masses, facet joints, and remaining posterior arch, as well as the ligamentum flavum and posterior supporting ligaments.

Disruption of 2 or more columns result in unstable injuries.

## Basic Anatomy

The cervical spine consists of 7 vertebral bodies, along with the intervertebral discs and supporting ligaments and muscles. These structures help to protect and stabilize the spinal cord, cervical nerve roots, and vertebral arteries. The first 2 vertebral bodies are unique in their shape. The first vertebral body, called *C1* or the *atlas*, is a bony ring that forms plane and pivot joints with the elongated anterior process of C2, often called the *axis*. Associated ligamentous complexes provide stability during flexion, extension, and rotation. The C3-C7 vertebral morphologies more closely resemble the thoracic and lumbar vertebrae, and consist of cylindrical bodies, transverse foramina, transverse processes, pedicles, lateral masses, facets, and spinous processes (Figure 2.1)

Multiple ligaments help to provide and maintain anatomic alignment of the vertebral bodies. The ALL originates from the anterior arch of C1, extends inferiorly to attach at the sacrum, and is tightly adherent to the vertebral bodies and discs. The PLL originates at C2, attaches inferiorly to the sacrum, and is tightly adherent to the annulus of the discs. However, it is only loosely attached to the vertebrae. The posterior ligamentous complex (PLC) consists of the ligamentum flavum, facet joint capsules, and interspinous and supraspinous ligaments. Intervertebral discs are positioned between the vertebral bodies, helping to maintain alignment and provide shock absorption. They are composed of collagen and organized as a central nucleus pulposus and peripheral annulus fibrosus.

## Imaging Strategy

The first question regarding utilization of imaging in the setting of cervical spine trauma is whether imaging is warranted. According to the National Emergency X-Radiography Utilization Study (NEXUS), cervical spine imaging is warranted unless there is no focal neurologic deficit, no midline spinal tenderness, no alteration in level of consciousness, no distracting injury, and the patient is not intoxicated.

Standard spine radiographic series include anterior-posterior (AP), lateral, and AP open-mouth (odontoid) views in the neutral position. The lateral radiograph should include all the cervical vertebrae as well as the cervicothoracic junction, particularly in cases of trauma. If the cervicothoracic junction cannot be adequately seen because of overlap with the shoulders, a swimmer's view can also be obtained to assess alignment at the cervicothoracic junction. Often the easiest and quickest imaging study to obtain on initial presentation of cervical spine trauma is radiography, and the most important view to obtain is the lateral projection, because it allows for fast identification of injury and classification by mechanism. Approximately 85-90% of injuries are seen on lateral radiographs. In addition to assessment for fracture, it is crucial to assess for underlying ligamentous injury and instability by evaluating 4 parallel lines (Figure 2.2):

1. Anterior vertebral line
2. Posterior vertebral line
3. Spinolaminar line
4. Posterior spinous line

Additional features to assess include vertebral body height, prevertebral soft tissue swelling (>4 mm at C3, and >22 mm at C6), and widening of the predental interval between the odontoid process and the anterior C1 arch (>3 mm in adults). Any abnormality such as *spondylolisthesis*, which is abnormal displacement of one vertebral body with respect to an adjacent vertebral body, deformity of the spinal lines, or focal kyphosis

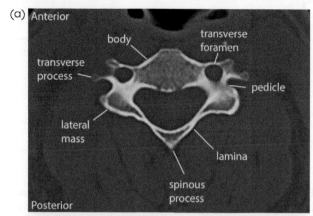

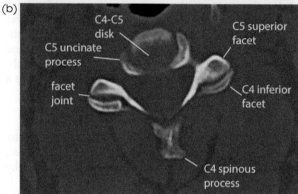

**Figure 2.1.** Normal anatomy of the cervical spine. (*A*) Axial CT of the C4 vertebra shows the anatomic segments of a cervical vertebra. (*B*) Axial CT of the C4-C5 disc space level demonstrates the uncovertebral joints between adjacent vertebral bodies and the facet joints.

on radiography is highly suspicious for underlying injury and should prompt advanced imaging.

In the setting of trauma, the AP radiograph is obtained if there is no unstable injury seen on lateral radiographs, and this projection is helpful to assess the vertebral body heights, the lateral contours of the lateral masses, and the uncovertebral joints (Luschka joints). The lower 5 cervical vertebrae are usually well seen. The mandible, however, may obscure the upper cervical vertebrae, and an AP open-mouth view, centered at the C2 level is necessary to assess the upper cervical vertebrae.

For cases in which there is no documented unstable injury, but there is a suspected soft tissue injury that can lead to instability, lateral views of the cervical spine in flexion and extension may be obtained. Usually, these are obtained several days after the initial injury to allow swelling to subside. The difference in the positions of adjacent vertebral bodies is assessed by measuring the distance between lines drawn along the posterior vertebral body cortices. There is great variability in this distance, which can measure up to 3.5 mm in normal subjects.

The choice of further imaging modality depends on the results of initial imaging as well as clinical concern for additional soft tissue trauma, such as spinal cord, ligamentous, or vascular injuries. The American College of Radiology (ACR) has developed guidelines that help steer clinicians and radiologists to the best first choices for a number of scenarios. For example, in the setting of suspected cervical spine trauma

without myelopathy, the guidelines recommend cervical spine CT with 3-plane reconstructions as the best first test. If myelopathy is present, CT and MRI are indicated. If vascular injury is suspected, CT combined with CT or MR angiography is recommended.

## Patterns of Injury

### Flexion Injuries

Flexion injuries usually result in simple anterior vertebral body compression fractures, PLC sprains, interfacetal dislocations, flexion teardrop injuries, and clay shoveler's fractures. This mechanism results in compression along the anterior column and distraction along the posterior column and PLC. The pattern of injuries depends on the location of the site of the fulcrum. A fulcrum anterior to the spine can lead to significant injury of the PLC without vertebral body injury, whereas a more posterior fulcrum can result in significant vertebral body trauma without PLC injury. Injury to all 3 columns can result in significant instability and subluxation of the vertebral bodies.

### Posterior Ligament Complex Sprain
- *Pathophysiology*
  - Hyperflexion injuries can lead to sprains of the PLC that can range from mild to severe. By themselves, PLC sprains are stable. However, if they include disruption of the PLL and the posterior disc annulus, they can become unstable and lead to anterolisthesis. These injuries can be subtle on initial radiographs, and delayed diagnosis can lead to pain, instability, and neurological deficit.
- *Imaging findings*
  - Radiography
    - Localized kyphosis
    - Possible widening of the interspinous processes on AP and lateral radiographs
    - Anteriorly displaced inferior articulating facet of the lateral mass of the involved upper cervical vertebra compared with the superior facet of the level below it
    - Possible anterior subluxation without fracture
  - MRI
    - Posterior paraspinal edema on fluid-sensitive sequences with possible ligamentous and/or cord injury
- *Treatment options*
  - For isolated flexion sprains, often a period of immobilization with a collar is sufficient to allow adequate healing.

### Unilateral and Bilateral Interfacetal Dislocations
- *Pathophysiology*
  - Extreme flexion leads to one or both facets being *jumped*, resulting in traumatic spondylolisthesis and often instability. The posterior ligaments are completely disrupted, along with the intervertebral disc and often the ALL. In unilateral interfacetal dislocation (UID), there is significant disruption of one of the interfacetal

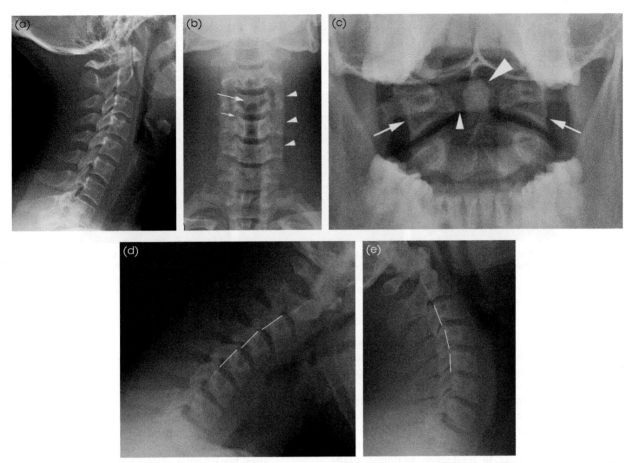

**Figure 2.2.** Normal radiographic appearance of the cervical spine. (*A*) Lateral radiograph depicts the 7 cervical vertebrae as well as the cervicothoracic junction and shows the anterior (*solid white line*), posterior (*dashed white line*), spinolaminar (*solid black line*), and posterior spinal (*dashed black line*) arcs, which all maintain smooth contours. The alignment is anatomic without fracture. The predental and prevertebral soft tissues are normal. (*B*) AP radiograph shows the lower 5 vertebrae. The upper vertebral bodies are poorly seen because of overlap with the mandible and occiput. The vertebral bodies are normal in height. The *longer arrow* indicates the C4 spinous process, whereas the *shorter arrow* points to the right uncinate process of C5. This articulates with the C4 vertebral body to form the uncovertebral joint, or joint of Luschka. The *arrowheads* are directed toward the lateral masses of C4, C5, and C6. In patients without vertebral abnormalities, the lateral cortical margin formed by these joints is smooth, continuous, and regularly undulating. (*C*) AP open-mouth image demonstrates the normal appearance of the dens and the lateral masses of the C1 vertebra. The *arrows* point to the C1 lateral masses. The lateral cortical margins on each side are aligned with the lateral margins of C2. The *longer arrowhead* indicates the peg-shaped odontoid process. In a true AP projection, the distances between the lateral margins of the odontoid and the adjacent C1 lateral masses should be equal. When the posterior arch of C1 (*shorter arrowhead*) crosses the base of the odontoid process, it can create a mach effect on the image that can simulate a type II odontoid fracture. (*D*) Lateral flexed radiograph of the cervical spine in a 23-year-old man with persistent neck pain following trauma shows normal alignment of the vertebrae. Lines drawn along the posterior margins of the C3, C4, and C5 vertebral bodies demonstrate a slight *stair-step* appearance. However, the distance of the step-off is less than 2 mm, and patients without vertebral abnormalities may demonstrate a step-off of less than 3.5 mm. (*E*) Lateral extended radiograph in the same patient shows no significant step-off based on lines drawn along the posterior margins of the C3-C5 vertebral bodies.

joints and much less injury to the other side, resulting in vertebral body rotation. Bilateral interfacetal dislocation (BID) is more severe because the interfacetal joints on both sides are significantly disrupted, resulting in an unstable injury often with cord injury.

- *Imaging findings* (Figure 2.3)
  - The lateral mass of the upper cervical vertebral body at the involved level is anteriorly subluxated and/or dislocated.
    - A *perched* vertebra refers to an incomplete interfacetal dislocation, in which the inferior facet of the lateral mass belonging to the involved superior vertebra sits on top of the superior facet of the lateral mass of the immediately inferior vertebra.

- A jumped facet occurs when there is complete anterior dislocation of the lateral mass of the involved superior vertebra compared the lateral mass of the immediately inferior vertebra.
- For UID, the degree of subluxation is usually less than 25% of the vertebral body AP width on lateral cervical spine radiographs.
- The vertebral body is rotated because the interfacetal joint on one side is disrupted and the involved superior lateral mass is significantly anteriorly subluxated or dislocated, while the contralateral joint is mildly subluxated.
- On AP radiographs, the spinous processes above the level of injury are laterally rotated compared with those below the level of injury.

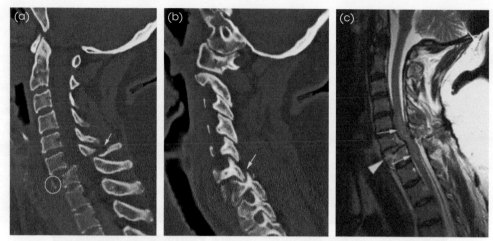

**Figure 2.3.** Combination flexion teardrop fracture with BID. (*A*) Sagittal CT images in a 58-year-old man after a fall from a ladder demonstrate anterolisthesis of C6 on C7 with a teardrop fracture fragment (*oval*) and C6 spinous process fracture (*arrow*). (*B*) The C6 facet (*arrow*) is jumped, or dislocated anteriorly and fixed in position, consistent with BID. (*C*) Sagittal T2W MR image shows extensive spinal cord injury with edema tracking several levels in both cranial and caudal directions (*arrows*). The *arrowhead* shows the level of injury at C6-C7 with anterolisthesis.

- For BID, the involved superior lateral masses on both sides are anteriorly dislocated or significantly subluxated. This produces anterolisthesis of greater than 25% of the AP vertebral body width.
- On AP radiographs, there is widening of the interspinous distance at the involved level.
- *Treatment options*
  - Interfacetal dislocations may initially require traction in order to reestablish anatomic alignment. For less severe UID (<25% anterolisthesis), a period of immobilization is typically adequate. For UID with more advanced anterolisthesis, the risk of delayed instability usually warrants subsequent surgical fixation. BID requires surgical fixation.

**Flexion Teardrop**
- *Pathophysiology*
  - Hyperflexion and compression result in 3-column disruption with focal kyphosis, anterior-inferior vertebral body fracture, and abnormal widening of the posterior stabilizing structures. These are unstable injuries, and spinal cord trauma is common (Figure 2.3).
- *Imaging findings*
  - Radiography
    - Kyphosis at the involved level
    - Triangular fracture fragment through the anterior-inferior corner of the upper involved cervical vertebral body
    - Spinal canal narrowing
    - Widened interspinous distances on AP and lateral radiographs
  - MRI
    - Disruption of the ALL, PLC, and intervertebral disc
    - Spinal cord impingement and edema and/or hemorrhage
    - Epidural hematoma
- *Treatment options*
  - Flexion teardrop-hyperflexion and compression requires surgical stabilization.

**Clay Shoveler's Fracture**
An example of clay shoveler's fracture is shown in Figure 2.4.

- *Pathophysiology*
  - Spinous process fracture related to interspinous ligament avulsion because of strong muscular contraction that occurs between C6 and T1, which results from hyperflexion against resistance (ie, clay). These fractures are stable.
- *Radiographic findings*
  - Usually obliquely oriented fracture line through the spinous process, perpendicular to the interspinous ligament
- *Treatment options*
  - Clay shoveler's fractures are usually conservatively treated with rest and nonsteroidal antiinflammatory drugs (NSAIDs).

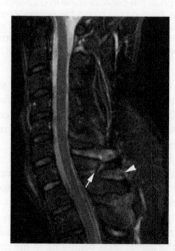

**Figure 2.4.** Clay shoveler's fracture. Sagittal T2W image in a 25-year-old man after a motor vehicle collision shows an avulsion fracture (*arrow*) of the C6 spinous process. There is a disruption of the interspinous ligament (arrowhead).

## Extension Injuries

Extension injuries are divided into hangman's fractures, extension teardrop fractures, and fractures through the posterior arch of C1. In general, extension injuries are more severe than trauma associated with hyperflexion. Similar to flexion injuries, the pattern of extension fractures depends on the location of the fulcrum. A more anterior fulcrum produces fractures of the posterior arches of the vertebrae, while a more posterior fulcrum can lead to distraction injuries of the ALL and extension teardrop injuries.

### Hangman's Fracture
- *Pathophysiology*
  - Hangman's fractures are the most common extension fracture and involve both C2 pars interarticularis. This occurs in the setting of sudden forced hyperextension and is an unstable injury although spinal cord injury is uncommon because the canal is capacious at this level (Figure 2.5).
- *Imaging findings*
  - This is best seen on lateral radiographs as a lucent cleft through the C2 pars interarticularis.
  - If the fracture involves the transverse foramina, consider angiography to evaluate vertebral artery injury.
- *Treatment options*
  - Hangman's fractures are typically treated with surgical fixation.

### Extension Teardrop
- *Pathophysiology*
  - Avulsion of the ALL during hyperextension results in fracture of an anterior-inferior vertebral body. Spinal cord injury may result because of compression by the ligamentum flavum. This injury is stable with flexion but unstable in extension. They are often seen after diving accidents and more commonly involve the lower cervical vertebrae. Extension teardrop injuries are not generally as severe as flexion teardrop injuries.

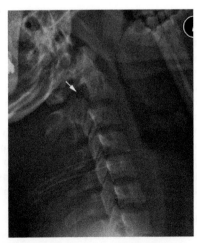

**Figure 2.5.** Hangman's fracture. Lateral radiograph of the cervical spine in a 23-year-old woman after a fall shows nondisplaced fractures (*arrow*) through the pars interarticularis of the C2 vertebral body.

- *Imaging findings*
  - Characteristic triangular anterior-inferior vertebral body fracture
- *Treatment options*
  - Extension teardrop injuries are often treated for a period with either hard collar or halo fixation. If subsequent evaluation raises concern for instability, permanent fixation may be considered.

## Axial Loading Injury

Axial loading injuries include Jefferson fracture, burst fracture of the lower cervical vertebrae and lateral mass (pillar) fractures. Axial loading injuries are usually the result of diving injuries, falls and motor vehicle collisions in which the head impacts the roof of the vehicle. Burst fractures in the cervical spine inferior to C1 have a similar mechanism as those in the thoracolumbar spine, and burst fractures will be discussed as a group in the chapter on thoracolumbar spinal trauma.

### Jefferson Fracture
- *Pathophysiology*
  - A Jefferson fracture is a C1 burst fracture extending through the anterior and posterior arches. The C1 bone fragments are displaced away from the spinal cord, and there is a low risk of spinal cord injury.
- *Imaging findings* (Figure 2.6)
  - Typically, on AP odontoid view, there is bilateral lateral subluxation of the C1 lateral masses relative to C2.
  - A posterior C1 arch fracture is seen on lateral radiograph.
  - CT is necessary to confirm diagnosis and detect additional findings.
- *Treatment options*
  - Jefferson burst fractures isolated to one side of the ring are typically only treated nonoperatively. Bilateral anterior and/or posterior fractures usually require surgical fixation.

### Odontoid Fracture
- *Pathophysiology*
  - The C2 vertebral body superior process articulates with C1 and is called the *odontoid process* or *dens*. Odontoid fractures are commonly seen in younger patients following motor vehicle accidents, or in patients older than 65 years of age who experience falls. Although the mechanism of injury is not well known, they may be caused by flexion and/or extension and rotation. Additionally, they may be stable or unstable depending on the location of the fracture line. There are 3 types:
    - Type I—odontoid tip avulsion (very rare)
    - Type II (high dens fracture)—fracture at the base of the odontoid process
    - Type III (low dens fracture)—fracture extending into the C2 body
  - Type II and most type III fractures are unstable.
- *Imaging findings*
  - Type I fractures may resemble an os odontoideum, which is a corticated ossification in the same location. There is some debate whether the os odontoideum represents a developmental variant or a chronic, unfused fracture, usually occurring early in life. Acute fractures will not be completely corticated, although

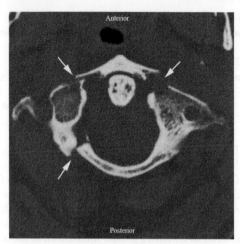

**Figure 2.6.** Jefferson fracture. Axial CT image of the cervical spine in a 38-year-old man taken after he dove into the shallow end of a pool shows fractures (*arrows*) through the anterior and right posterior arches of C1.

- CT is advised for further assessment as these fractures are often associated with other cervical spine or maxillofacial fractures.
- *Treatment options*
  - Unstable odontoid fractures typically require surgical fixation.

### Atlantooccipital Dissociation

- *Pathophysiology*
  - High-energy trauma can result in disruption of the ligamentous complex at the cervical spine–occipital junction. These injuries are usually immediately fatal because of brainstem injury.
- *Imaging findings* (Figure 2.7)
  - Widening of the basion-dens and atlantodental intervals can be seen if imaging is performed.

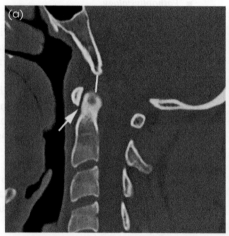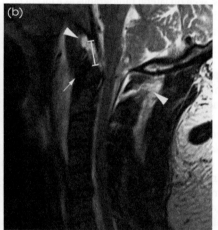

**Figure 2.7.** Atlantooccipital dissociation. (*A*) Sagittal CT reformatted midline image of the cervical spine shows the normal basion-dens interval (*white line*), which should be taken from the inferior tip of the basion to the proximal tip of the odontoid process. On CT, the maximum distance is 8.5 mm. The *arrow* indicates the atlantodental interval, which is taken between the posterior margin of the anterior C1 arch and the anterior surface of the odontoid process. In adults without vertebral abnormalities, this should be less than 3 mm and is usually less than 2 mm. In children, this should be less than 5 mm. (*B*) Sagittal T2W image in a 52-year-old woman following high-energy trauma shows abnormal atlantodental relationship (*arrow*) and widening of the basion-dens interval (*bracket*) with extensive anterior and posterior soft tissue edema (*arrowheads*) related to ligamentous disruption.

CT may be needed to adequately characterize the osseous fragment.

- Type II fractures present as transverse fracture lines through the base of the odontoid process. They are best seen on an AP open-mouth view. On this view, the posterior arch of C1 may produce a mach line that mimics a fracture.
- Type III fractures are also best seen on an AP open-mouth view. They appear as curvilinear fracture lines from one C2 superior articulating facet to the other that extends into the C2 vertebral body.
- Disruption of the radiographic oval-shaped ring along the C2 vertebral body is seen on lateral radiographs and is referred to as the *axis ring*.
- If there is posterior displacement of the inferior C2 vertebral body fragment, it may produce a widened appearance of the vertebral body on a lateral radiograph (*fat vertebral body sign*).

### Key Points

- Cervical spine traumas are classified by mechanism of injury, the most common of which are hyperflexion, hyperextension, axial loading, and rotational forces.
- The mechanism of injury can be helpful in predicting patterns of injuries seen on imaging studies.
- Additionally, the cervical spine has been divided into 3 columns: anterior, middle, and posterior. Injuries to only 1 of the columns is generally considered stable, while injury to more than 1 column is considered unstable.
- The lateral radiograph is the most helpful initial projection in most patients, and the vast majority of fractures can be seen on this view.
- CT is much more sensitive in detecting cervical spine fractures, and imagers must have a low threshold for recommending CT in patients with suspected cervical spine injuries.

- MRI is most useful in detecting associated soft tissue injuries, such as spinal cord trauma, or injuries to the supporting ligaments, muscles, and intervertebral discs.
- Conventional or CT angiography should be considered when there is concern for vertebral artery injuries.

**Recommended Reading**

Mirvis SE, Harris JH. *The Radiology of Acute Cervical Spine Trauma*. 3rd. sub-ed. Philadelphia: Lippincott Williams & Wilkins; 1996.

**References**

1. Daffner RH, Hackney DB. ACR Appropriateness criteria on suspected spine trauma. *J Am Coll Radiol*. 2007;4(11):762–775.
2. Denis F. The three column spine and its significance in the classification of acute thoracolumbar spinal injuries. *Spine*. 1983;8(8):817–831.
3. Goldberg W, Mueller C, Panacek E, et al. Distribution and patterns of blunt traumatic cervical spine injury. *Ann Emerg Med*. 2001;38(1):17–21.
4. Hoffman JR, Wolfson AB Todd K, et al. Selective cervical spine radiography in blunt trauma: methodology of the National Emergency X-Radiography Utilization Study (NEXUS). *Ann Emerg Med*. 1998;32(4):461–469.

# Traumatic Injuries of the Thoracolumbar Spine

Andrew L. Chiang and  Laurie M. Lomasney

## Introduction

Approximately 50% of all vertebral fractures involve the thoracolumbar spine. One of the most feared complications of these fractures is neurologic compromise, which has been reported in anywhere from 19 to 50% of patients with thoracolumbar spine fractures who report to a level 1 trauma center. Delays in diagnosing these fractures can lead to a significantly increased incidence of neurologic deficits. Several mechanisms of injury, including *compression, flexion-distraction*, and *axial loading*, are commonly seen in these patients. Although mechanisms of injury to the thoracolumbar spine are uncommonly the result of single-force vectors, categorization of the fracture patterns by predominant force facilitates description of expected fracture patterns.

## Basic Anatomy

The thoracolumbar spine provides support to the body, particularly while standing erect and walking upright, while allowing movements such as flexion, extension, and rotation of the trunk. The vertebrae form the walls of the spinal canal and protect the spinal cord and the segmental nerve roots before they exit the central canal. The thoracic spine generally consists of 12 segments that articulate with the ribs at the costovertebral and costotransverse junctions. They are made of the vertebral bodies, the pedicles, the laminae with superior and inferior articular processes, and the transverse processes (Figure 3.1A). The more inferior vertebral bodies are progressively larger, and there is a normal mild kyphosis of the thoracic spine that measures between 20 and 40 degrees.

In contrast to the thoracic spine, the lumbar vertebral segments usually lack articulations with ribs. The lumbar spine, however, is usually comprised of 5 levels but can be made of 4 to 6 vertebrae. Occasionally, the lowest lumbar vertebral body has features that resemble the upper sacrum, called *sacralization,* with enlargement of the transverse processes that can articulate or partially fuse with the upper margin of the sacral ala (Figure 3.1B). Vertebral body height increases at successive levels of the lumbar spine. The lumbar spine normally has a mild lordosis, approximately 20-45 degrees.

Similar to the cervical spine, the thoracolumbar vertebrae are separated by the intervertebral discs, which are made of a central nucleus pulposus, and a peripheral annulus fibrosus, which help to cushion the spine during axial loading. The vertebrae are connected anteriorly by the ALL and posteriorly by the PLL, which extend inferiorly from C2 to the sacrum.

## Imaging Strategy and Classifications of Injuries

Radiographs represent the initial imaging test of choice in the setting of trauma and are generally the primary imaging modality. However, complete characterization frequently requires the use of cross-sectional imaging, CT more commonly than MRI. Thin-section axial CT images can be reformatted into other planes without the need for additional radiation exposure. Selection of a secondary imaging modality is partly based on radiographic imaging findings and partly on a clinical scenario that includes the concern for associated soft tissue injuries.

Actual classification of fracture patterns may be derived from anatomical patterns (reflected on imaging). The Denis classification divides the spine into 3 parallel vertical columns, and structural stability is dependent on preservation of 2 columns. The anterior column consists of the anterior two-thirds of the vertebral body; the middle column includes the posterior aspect of the vertebral body and the pedicles and is integral to stability; finally, the posterior column consists of the facet articulations, laminae, and spinous processes (Figure 3.2).

This system is easily applied to cross-sectional imaging, and is somewhat useful for prediction of axial stability, but is limited in its utility for guiding management.

Conversely, the Thoracolumbar Injury Classification and Severity Score (TLICS) incorporates elements of anatomical fracture pattern as well as neurologic status. Points are accrued based on fracture type, PLC involvement, and neurologic symptoms (Box 3.1). Morphologic descriptions parallel the descriptors for the Denis system, but the integrity of the posterior stabilizing ligaments is also considered. A greater number of points are awarded based on the degree of neurologic deficit, which is divided into no neurologic deficit, incomplete deficit, or complete deficit. This grading system more effectively directs clinical management and is more commonly applied by clinical services.

- TLICS scores of 3 or lower generally indicate conservative management.
- TLICS score of 4 can either be treated operatively or nonoperatively.
- TLICS scores of 5 or greater may indicate surgical management.

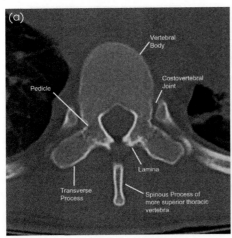 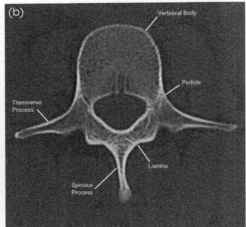

**Figure 3.1.** Normal vertebral anatomy in the thoracic and lumbar spine. (*A*) Axial CT of a mid-thoracic vertebral body shows the normal anatomic segments as well as the articulation with paired ribs. (*B*) Axial CT of a mid-lumbar vertebral body demonstrates the normal anatomic segments.

## Patterns of Injury

### Compression

#### Pathophysiology and Clinical Presentation

Compression injuries are the most common pattern of thoracolumbar spine fractures and are the result of truncal flexion on an anterior vertebral fulcrum, with anterior vertebral compression and loss of anterior vertebral height. The height of the posterior vertebral body is preserved and the spinal canal is intact (Denis = anterior column; TLICS usually <3). It most commonly results in one endplate failure, predominantly the superior endplate of the vertebral body at the inferior aspect of the fulcrum, and occurs most commonly at T4-T5, followed by the thoracolumbar junction. Torus fractures are seen in skeletally immature patients with buckling of the central portion of the vertebra anteriorly. Depending on forces applied, there may be multiple sequential compression fractures.

### Imaging Findings

Imaging findings are shown in Figures 3.3 and 3.4.

- Radiography
  - AP and lateral views of the thoracolumbar spine are generally sufficient to diagnose these fractures.
  - The interpretative report should include which endplate is affected and the approximate percentage of height loss.
    - One commonly used scoring system to classify osteoporotic vertebral fractures is the *Genant semiquantitative scoring system*, which assesses the fracture morphology (simple wedge, bicondylar, or crush fracture) and the degree of vertebral body height loss (mild, moderate, severe).
  - If possible, acute fractures should be distinguished from chronic ones, although this may be difficult in the absence of prior imaging.

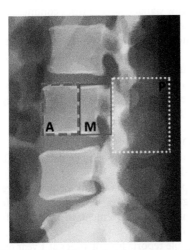

**Figure 3.2.** *Denis classification:* Lateral radiograph of the lumbar spine shows demarcations of the 3 columns in the Denis classification system including anterior (A; *red dashed line*), middle (M; *blue solid line*), and posterior (P; *yellow dashed line*).

---

**Box 3.1.** Thoracolumbar Injury Classification and Severity Score (TLICS)

- Morphology
  - Compression fracture (1 point)
  - Burst fracture (2 points)
  - Translational/rotational injury (3 points)
  - Distraction injury (4 points)
- Posterior ligamentous complex integrity
  - Intact (0 points)
  - Suspected or indeterminate injury (2 points)
  - Definite injury (3 points)
- Neurologic involvement
  - Intact (0 points)
  - Nerve root injury (2 points)
  - Incomplete spinal cord/conus medullaris injury (3 points)
  - Complete spinal cord/conus medullaris injury (2 points)
  - Cauda equina injury (3 points)

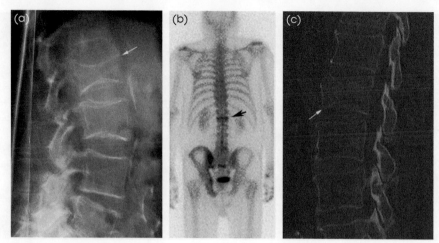

**Figure 3.3.** Compression fracture. (*A*) Lateral radiograph of the lumbar spine in a 78-year-old man shows acute superior endplate fracture of L1 (*arrow*) with loss of one-third of the vertebral body height. The posterior wall (*arrow*) of L1 is intact. (*B*) Posterior view of whole body bone scan shows abnormal tracer accumulation at L2 vertebra (*arrow*), confirming an acute fracture. (*C*) Sagittal reformatted CT image confirms the integrity of the posterior vertebral wall of the L1 vertebral body, diagnostic of a simple compression fracture. This image also confirms involvement of the inferior endplate (*arrow*).

- Acute fractures usually have acute angular margins at the anterior vertebral wall, in contrast to the rounded margins often seen in chronic fractures.
- Although vertebral sclerosis can be seen more often with chronic fractures, it is not always an accurate determinant in assessing fracture age. Occasionally, impacted bone can simulate sclerosis.
- Degenerative-type findings at the endplate, including osteophytosis, support chronicity.
- Nuclear imaging
  - A bone scan lacks specificity for diagnosing compression fracture, although single-photon emission computed tomography (SPECT)/CT enhances morphologic characterization.
  - A bone scan is predominantly useful for characterizing acute versus chronic fracture patterns. Especially in the setting of acute back pain and multiple compression levels, a bone scan can define the acute levels potentially contributing to symptoms, with relatively increased radiotracer distribution compared to the remaining bony skeleton.
- CT
  - CT is used as a secondary imaging modality for confirmation of compression patterns and for potential differentiation of acute versus chronic time course.
  - Coronal and sagittal reformations derived from noncontrast axial images are routine and confirm the integrity of the posterior vertebral body wall and posterior elements as well as marginal bony structures.
- MRI
  - Axial and sagittal imaging, with predominantly T1W and fluid-sensitive sequences, is routine.
  - MR imaging is useful for differentiation of acute versus chronic fracture, as well as for excluding underlying processes.
  - Chronic fractures have bland imaging features with marrow signal characteristics commensurate with regional vertebrae.
  - Acute fractures, however, show irregular low T1 signals with heterogeneous ill-defined high T2 signals (Figure 3.5).
  - Intravenous contrast is used selectively to exclude underlying pathologies including malignancy and discitis.

**Treatment Options**
- Thoracolumbosacral spinal orthosis (TLSO) and analgesia
- Kyphoplasty, which is useful for pain not responsive to bracing or for fractures with rapid progression
  - Immediate improvement in pain and function per most studies
  - Variable reports for outcomes at 1 year or more
- Posterior fusion
  - Kyphosis greater than 30 degrees
  - Compression more than 50%

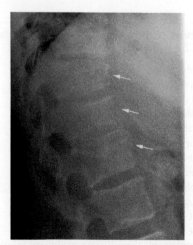

**Figure 3.4.** Sequential compression fractures. Lateral radiograph centered at the thoracolumbar spine in a 25-year-old man shows sequential acute compression fractures of T11, T12, and L1 (*arrows*) with buckling of the anterior vertebral body cortices.

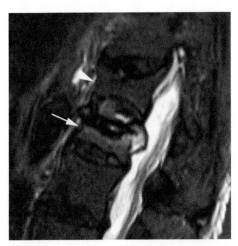

**Figure 3.5.** Acute and chronic compression fractures. Sagittal STIR MR image in an 88-year-old woman shows compression fractures at L1 and L2. The high STIR signal at L2 (*arrow*) supports the conclusion of a more acute fracture. The low STIR signal at L1 (*arrowhead*) supports chronicity.

## Burst Fractures

### Pathophysiology and Clinical Presentation

Burst fractures also result from flexion forces (caused by high-energy blunt trauma or a fall), but the fulcrum is more posterior and there is also an axial load. They result in compression of the posterior vertebral body in addition to the anterior column. Forces released inferiorly to the level of the basivertebral foramen result in a dominant posterior fragment in 50% of cases that can be displaced into the canal, and a sagittally oriented fracture through the remaining vertebral body. Most of these fractures occur at L1 or L2, and neurologic sequelae at these levels are common, resulting in conus medullaris or cauda equina injuries in two-thirds of cases. Neurologic injury is even more common in thoracic burst fractures as a result of its narrower canal. Because of the high-energy forces in these cases, coincident visceral and extremity injuries, such as calcaneal fractures, are common.

### Imaging Findings

Refer to Figure 3.6.

- Radiography
  - Lateral supine radiographs usually show the characteristic findings of loss of anterior vertebral body height and protrusion of the posterior vertebral wall. Up to 25% of fractures may be misconstrued as simple compression fractures. On the AP view, 80% of cases will also show widening of the interpediculate distance 4 mm greater than the same distance at the adjacent, intact levels.

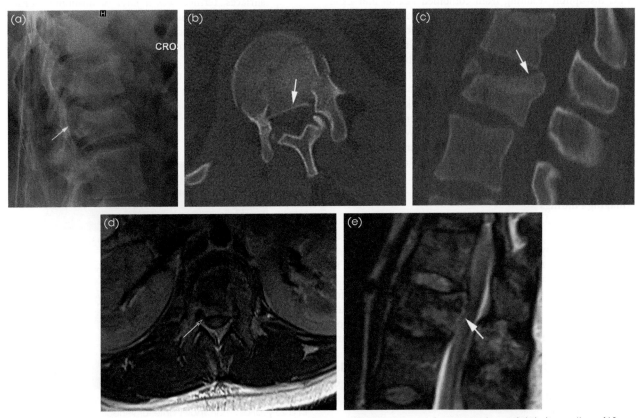

**Figure 3.6.** Burst fracture. (*A*) Lateral radiograph of the lumbar spine in a 25-year-old man shows superior endplate impaction of L1, with protrusion of the superior aspect of the posterior vertebral wall. Axial CT image (*B*) and sagittal reformatted image (*C*) confirm anterior vertebral compression with posterior displacement of a dominant posterior wall fragment (*arrows*) and marked narrowing of the bony canal. The posterior facet articulations are intact. Axial (*D*) and sagittal (*E*) T2 weighted (T2W) MR images also show retropulsion of the bone fragment into the canal (*arrows*), with direct impingement on the thecal sac.

- Asymmetrical force may result in eccentric posterior wall fragment displacement or asymmetrical loss of vertebral body height.
- CT
  - CT with sagittal and coronal reformatted imaging is valuable for detection of fragment displacement, anterior compression, fracture of the facet articulations, and widening of the interpediculate distance.
- MRI
  - MRI more accurately characterizes spinal canal contents as well as root impingement or transection. Especially if the patient is neurologically intact, MRI can be used to assess the PLC for injury, and thus directly assess stability.

**Treatment Options**

- Bracing is performed when there is no neurologic compromise and good bone stock, and can result in accelerated ambulation.
- Surgical indications
  - If there is incomplete deficit, anterior decompression and/or posterior stabilization are performed.
  - If there is complete deficit, posterior stabilization is preferred.

**Flexion-Distraction**
**Pathophysiology and Clinical Presentation**
Flexion-distraction (F-D) injuries are highly unstable, with PLC disruption resulting from combined flexion and axial forces centered on the middle column and an additional distraction force posteriorly. There may be additional shear or rotational forces. In the classic injury pattern, there are severe anterior compression deformities (greater than 50% height loss) and transverse laminae and spinous process fractures. Often, there is a large triangular fragment originating from the anterior superior vertebral body. Focal kyphosis is typical. Injuries are most common in the upper thoracic spine followed by the thoracolumbar junction. With large force mechanisms and unstable bony injuries, neurologic deficit is common, occurring in approximately 60-70% of injuries at the thoracolumbar junction.

**Imaging Findings**
Refer to Figures 3.7 and 3.8.

- Radiography
  - AP and cross-table lateral radiographs are essential to initial evaluation.
  - Radiographs should be carefully scrutinized for fractures and facet pathology rather than just malalignment because post trauma immobilization on a trauma board may result in partial or even complete reduction.
  - Anteriorly, there is displacement of a triangular fragment from the anterior superior endplate of the caudal vertebra, with subjacent compression of the body.
  - Posteriorly, there are either fractures of the associated articular facets, or anterior subluxation or perching of the cephalad vertebral facets. A rotational force may result in asymmetrical facet injury patterns.

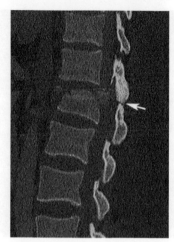

**Figure 3.7.** Flexion-distraction injury. Sagittal reformatted CT image in a 39-year-old woman shows abnormal uncovering of the superior articular facet of L2 with perched inferior articular facet of L1 (*arrow*) from distraction, and L2 compression fracture from flexion.

- CT
  - Axial images depict the fractures of the facet articular processes and pedicles.
  - *Naked facet sign* is an abnormal facet uncovering seen in the case of facet subluxation.
  - *Reverse hamburger sign* is reversal of the articular surfaces, termed *locked facet* (a misnomer considering the highly unstable pattern of injury).
  - Compression fracture of the vertebral body is noted, with classical anterior triangular vertebral body bone fragment.
  - Kyphosis is most easily seen on the sagittal images, and the facet articulations can be further inspected.

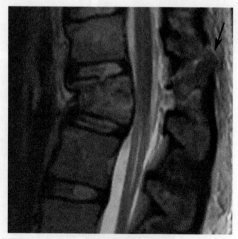

**Figure 3.8.** Flexion-distraction injury. Sagittal T2W MR image in a 23-year-old man shows anterior vertebral body loss of height with BME and posterior bowing of the posterior vertebral body cortex, consistent with an acute burst fracture. The retropulsed bone effaces the anterior thecal sac. In addition, there is disruption of the supraspinous ligament (*arrow*) as a component of PLC injury.

- Coronal reformatted images evaluate alignment following more complex shear and lateral forces.
- MRI
  - Bony findings will also be noted on MRI examinations. In addition, the direct effects of the fractures/malalignment on the spinal canal as well as PLC injury can be assessed.

## Treatment Options

- Open reduction and fixation, possibly with canal debridement
  - Potential reduction in permanent neurologic sequelae
  - Restoration of stability of the axial column, regardless of neurologic outcome

## Chance Fractures
### Pathophysiology and Clinical Presentation

Chance fractures are a subcategory of F-D injuries, with disruption of all 3 columns from compressive and distraction forces. However, the fulcrum of the flexion force is redistributed anterior to the vertebral column. Following rapid deceleration and acute flexion of the body at the waist, as historically seen with wearing a lap belt at the waist, there is propagation of disruptive forces from the posterior elements anteriorly through the vertebral body. These injuries are preferentially located at the thoracolumbar junction. Classically, there is a horizontal fracture plane through the spinous process into the pedicles, with minimal or no anterior wedging of the vertebral body. Although Chance fractures are highly unstable, neurologic deficit is present in only approximately 30% of cases, which is less than that seen in other patterns of F-D injuries. More significantly, there may be contiguous levels of bone injury or even noncontiguous levels of injury. In addition, up to 50% of patients will have acute visceral injuries.

## Imaging Findings
Refer to Figures 3.9 and 3.10.

- Radiography
  - Supine AP and lateral radiographs provide initial identification and basic characterization, including transverse fracture planes through the spinous process and pedicles (well depicted on AP imaging).
  - Focal kyphosis with distraction of the spinous process fracture is seen on the lateral view.
  - Anterior vertebral compression may be minimal.
- CT
  - CT imaging is essential to surgical planning.
  - The fracture planes and/or ligamentous disruption (with better visualization of horizontal planes) are further clarified.
  - Malalignment, usually kyphosis, is confirmed on sagittal images.
  - Because significant visceral injuries are common in patients with Chance fractures, CT imaging of the abdomen and pelvis is routinely completed, and spine imaging can be derived from preexisting data sets.

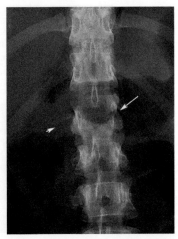

**Figure 3.9.** Chance fracture. Coned-down AP radiograph centered at the thoracolumbar junction in a 26-year-old man shows a horizontal fracture plane (*white arrow*) with global increase in size of the left L1 pedicle in a Chance fracture. Note also an oblique fracture of the right L1 transverse process (*black arrow*), indicative of more complex fracture pattern than a simple transverse process fracture.

- MRI
  - Superior to CT for defining ligamentous injury, MRI provides crucial information for the injuries that are predominantly or entirely soft tissue, including those to the PLC.
  - Contiguous and noncontiguous bony injuries can be identified.

## Treatment Options
- Bracing in extension, if reduction can be maintained, is used with relatively lengthy immobilization. High compliance is required.
- Surgical fixation with posterior construct may be helpful to restore alignment and decompress the spinal canal if necessary.

## Transverse Process Fracture
### Pathophysiology and Clinical Presentation

Transverse process fractures are commonly part of a more complex fracture pattern, especially when occurring in the thoracic spine; a horizontal fracture plane is especially suspicious. Alternatively, these fractures can result from a direct impact (blunt force or penetrating injury) or eccentric paraspinal muscle contraction. They are more common in the lumbar spine and are usually oriented vertically. Frequently, there are multiple sequential transverse process fractures.

## Imaging Findings
Refer to Figures 3.11 and 3.12.

- Radiography
  - Many factors contribute to poor visualization including bowel content, osteoporosis, and overlying artifacts.
  - A scoliotic curve may be present, either ipsilateral concave if the patient is splinting, or ipsilateral convex if there is quadratus lumborum deficiency and/or disruption.

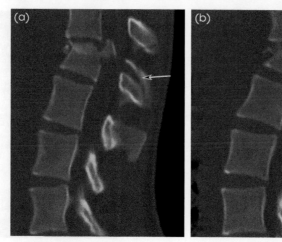

**Figure 3.10.** Chance fracture. Sagittal reformatted CT images in the midline (*A*) and through the left pedicle (*B*) of L1 in a 16-year-old girl show the classic horizontal fracture planes (*arrows*) through the spinous process and pedicle in a Chance fracture. There is a burst fracture of the vertebral body as well, with anterior vertebral body compression and a retropulsed fragment. Incidental note is made of an additional T12 spinous process fracture.

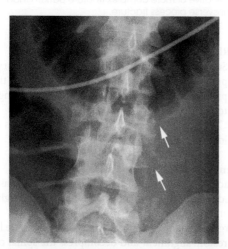

**Figure 3.11.** Transverse process fracture. AP radiograph of the lumbar spine shows acute, minimally displaced fractures of left L3 and L4 transverse processes (*arrows*) as well as an L3 compression fracture.

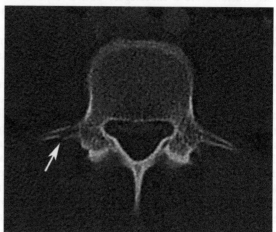

**Figure 3.12.** Transverse process fracture. Axial CT image in a 31-year-old man shows acute, minimally displaced fracture of a right transverse process (*arrow*).

- Fractures often have disrupted trabeculae and are frequently displaced. These features help differentiate them from unfused ossification centers, which are well-formed, corticated ossicles and uncommon.
- CT
  - More extensive osseous injury or additional malalignment can be evaluated.
  - There is an up to 20% incidence of visceral injury, such as hepatic and splenic laceration, in the setting of transverse process fractures. CT of the abdomen and pelvis is routinely completed, which also allows survey examination of the lumbar spine (or dedicated reformations in 3 planes if desired).

**Treatment Options**

- Bracing, pain control for isolated fractures

**Key Points**

- Compression fractures are the most common pattern of thoracolumbar spine fractures. They are often isolated to one level, but it is important to scrutinize images for sequential fractures.
- Burst fractures are 2-column fractures that include the posterior vertebral wall, and may be stable or unstable. There is a high incidence of neurologic deficit, and these injuries have higher TLICS scores than compression fractures.
- F-D injuries are highly unstable with a high frequency of partial and complete neurologic deficits, and imaging can underestimate the pattern of malalignment because of the reducible nature.
- Chance fractures are a version of F-D injury at the thoracolumbar junction with classic imaging findings of horizontal cleavage planes through spinous process and pedicles. Significant visceral injuries should be anticipated.
- Isolated transverse process fractures have a relatively high association with visceral injuries.

**Recommended Reading**

Denis F. The three column spine and its significance in the classification of acute thoracolumbar spinal injuries. *Spine* 1983;8(8):817–31.

Khurana B, Sheehan SE, Sodickson A, et al. Traumatic thoracolumbar spine injuries: what the spine surgeon wants to know. *Radiographics* 2013;33(7):2031–46.

**References**

1. Chance GQ. Note on type of flexion fractures of the spine. *Br J Radiol.* 1948;21:452.
2. Dalbayrak S, Yaman O, Yulmaz T. Current and future surgery strategies for spinal cord injuries. *World J Orthop.* 2015;6(1):34–41.
3. Denis F. The three column spine and its significance in the classification of acute thoracolumbar spinal injuries. *Spine* 1983;8(8):817–31.
4. Groves CJ, Cassar-Pullicino VN, Tins BJ, et al. Chance-type flexion-distraction injuries of the thoracolumbar spine: MR imaging characteristics. *Radiology* 2005;236:601–608.
5. Khurana B, Sheehan SE, Sodickson A, et al. Traumatic thoracolumbar spine injuries: what the spine surgeon wants to know. *Radiographics.* 2013;33(7):2031–46.
6. Mirza SK, Mirza AJ, Chapman JR, Anderson PA. Classifications of thoracic and lumbar fractures: rationale and supporting data. *J Am Acad Orthop Surg.* 2002;10:364–77.
7. Patel AA, Vaccaro AR. Thoracolumbar spine trauma classification. *J Am Acad Orthop Surg.* 2010;18:63–71.
8. Rajasekaran S. Thoracolumbar burst fractures without neurological deficit: the role for conservative management. *Eur Spine J.* 2010;19:S40–47.
9. Rogers L. Chapter 13: the spine. In: *Radiology of Skeletal Trauma.* 2nd ed. New York, NY: Churchill Livingstone; 1992:521–76.
10. Sweis O, Lomasney LM, Demos TC, et al. Chance fracture. *Orthopedics* 2011;34(12):925, 1011–14.
11. Whang PG, Vaccaro AR. Thoracolumbar fracture: posterior instrumentation using distraction and ligamentotaxis reduction. *J Am Acad Orthop Surg.* 2007;15:695–701.
12. Wong CC, McGirt MJ. Compression fractures: a review of management and multimodal therapy. *J Multidiscip Healthc.* 2013;6:205–14.

# CHAPTER 4

# Spine Trauma with Preexisting Conditions

Andrew L. Chiang and Laurie M. Lomasney

## Introduction

A number of conditions predispose the spine to significant injury in the setting of low-energy trauma. Some processes, such as osteoporosis and neoplasms, weaken the bone, whereas others, such as ankylosing spondylitis and diffuse idiopathic skeletal hyperostosis, make the spine more rigid and thus less able to withstand minor forces. Because imaging plays a critical role in the characterization of fracture patterns and underlying disease, imaging data provide information crucial to management of the mechanical destabilization as well as the underlying condition. This chapter focuses on fracture of the spine in the setting of underlying pathology. In addition, an overview of strategies for conservative and surgical management will be reviewed.

## Patterns of Injury

### Osteoporosis
**Pathophysiology and Clinical Presentation**
Fractures in the osteoporotic spine can occur in the setting of acute trauma or without defining event. These fractures usually involve the endplate, and have an eccentric or wedge configuration. The fractures can be stable or can cause sufficient structural compromise to result in progressive deformities.

**Imaging Findings**
Refer to Figure 4.1 and 3.5 in Chapter 3, "Traumatic Injuries of the Thoracolumbar Spine."

- Radiography
  - Imaging appearance is similar to that seen in acute fractures in normally mineralized vertebrae. However, characterizing the acuity of the injury can be problematic on radiographs because of reduced radiographic density and potentially increased overlying artifacts such as gastrointestinal contents or cardiopulmonary disease.
  - Findings that may suggest alternative underlying process, such as malignancy, must be excluded.
  - Any suspicious finding, such as local or regional bone destruction or paraspinal soft tissue mass, should prompt further investigation.
- Nuclear imaging
  - A whole body bone scan may assess the acuity of compression fractures. Particularly in the setting of multiple fractures and when considering vertebroplasty, defining the most likely symptomatic level(s) allows focused interventional plans.

- Assessment of the skeleton outside the affected level(s) is useful to determine the probability of an alternative underlying diagnosis, such as metastasis.
- Dual-energy x-ray absorptiometry (DXA) scan
  - This is a valuable tool for assessment of osteoporosis. By stratifying the patient's risk category, medical management can be optimized.
- CT
  - Application of CT for this category of compression fractures is similar to that for compression fractures in the normally mineralized skeleton.
- MRI
  - When there is confounding history, such as known primary malignancy or multiple involved segments of indeterminate acuity, MRI can exclude potential underlying pathology as well as identify imaging findings such as BME, which suggest acuity and thus the most likely symptomatic level(s).

**Treatment Options**
- Bracing, pain control, and medical therapy for osteoporosis can potentially reduce subsequent events related to osteoporosis.
- Vertebral augmentation (vertebroplasty or kyphoplasty) stabilizes weakened vertebrae, preventing further collapse; for symptomatic lesions refractory to conservative measures, targeted therapy is used.
  - Augmentation is controversial, with some evidence suggesting local stabilization of the vertebral body on which the vertebroplasty is performed, but secondary destabilization of the adjacent superior and/or inferior vertebral bodies.
  - It can be used to stabilize vertebrae at risk for fracture.
  - Augmentation is used to stabilize painful metastases and myelomatous lesions or hemangiomas
  - Contraindications include untreated coagulopathy, discitis and/or osteomyelitis, and presence of a posterior cortical defect, such as burst fractures with retropulsed fragment.
- Surgical fusion is excellent for regional stabilization, but has the potential for marginal destabilization of vertebrae above and below the unfused level(s).
  - Indicated in patients with severe, progressive pain and neurologic deficit that does not respond to medical management and progressive deformity
  - Increasing risk factors for surgery in potentially elderly population
  - Does not manage systemic issue

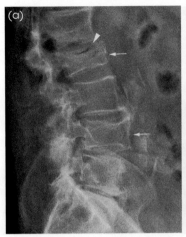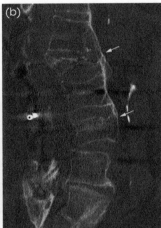

**Figure 4.1.** Osteoporotic compression fracture. (*A*) Lateral radiograph of the lumbar spine in 57-year-old man shows osteoporosis. There are superior endplate compression fractures of the lumbar spine at L2 and L4 (*arrows*). There is near-vertebra plana of the L2 level with intravertebral vacuum phenomenon (*arrowhead*), highly suggestive of an osteoporotic compression fracture. (*B*) Sagittal reformatted CT image redemonstrates the fractures (*arrows*) and shows significant osteopenia and accentuation of vertical trabeculae caused by osteoporosis. Prominent anterior ossifications may indicate underlying diffuse idiopathic skeletal hyperostosis (DISH).

## Metastasis and Myeloma
### Pathophysiology and Clinical Presentation

Marrow replacement by metastases or myeloma may destabilize the bone, which may result in compression and burst fractures. The same forces that might result in minor injury in the intact skeleton may cause a more severe injury in bone that is weakened by marrow infiltration. Spinal metastases occur in approximately 40% of patients with cancer. The thoracic spine is most commonly involved with spinal metastases and accounts for 70% of cases. The lumbar spine is the next most commonly involved spinal segment. Initial tumoral deposits most commonly occur at the posterior vertebral body as this is the location of the basivertebral plexus. Management of spinal metastasis with pathologic fracture is challenging, given the need to manage the loss of structural integrity and the underlying malignant and potentially progressive lesion. A classification proposed by Tomita et al. bases treatment on considerations including aggressiveness of primary tumor, presence of visceral metastases, and extent of bony metastases.

### Imaging Findings
Refer to Figure 4.2.

- Radiography
  - Radiography may identify the actual fracture as well as the underlying lesion. Screening assessment of the adjacent vertebrae can identify multiple levels of involvement, supporting diagnosis of underlying metastasis and/or myeloma.
  - Additional levels at risk for pathologic fracture may be seen.
  - Radiography is the modality most often used for follow-up imaging.
- CT
  - Used to characterize bony pathology and soft tissue abnormalities especially in the lumbar spine

- Intravenous contrast makes soft tissue components, including epidural tumor, more conspicuous.
- MRI
  - Generally, MRI with and without intravenous contrast of the entire spinal segment (cervical, thoracic, and/or lumbar) is completed.
  - Precontrast images show abnormal low or intermediate T1 signal abnormalities that contrast to the expected high T1 signal of normal adult fatty marrow.
  - Individual lesions frequently have high T2 signal (more conspicuous on fat-suppressed sequences), although T2 signal may be reduced in some specific diagnoses, such as myeloma, or in densely osteoblastic lesions.
  - Most metastatic lesions show contrast enhancement, which may be rimlike, heterogeneous, or homogeneous. Particularly if intervention (surgery or radiation) at one level is contemplated, the entire spine should be scanned to identify unknown levels of involvement.

### Treatment Options
- Bracing, pain management, systemic therapy
- Surgical decompression for neurologically impaired, fusion (especially for lesions less responsive to radiotherapy), and/or external beam radiation therapy or systemic therapy
- Radio-kyphoplasty
- Radiofrequency tumoral ablation
- Vertebroplasty for restoration of structural stability

## Rigid Spine—Ankylosing Spondylitis and Diffuse Idiopathic Skeletal Hyperostosis
### Pathophysiology and Clinical Presentation

Despite the hyperostosis in ankylosing spondylitis (AS) and diffuse idiopathic skeletal hyperostosis (DISH), the induced rigidity predisposes the spine to fracture. Furthermore, with the development of a focal level of motion in an otherwise rigid spine, non-bony union is a common complication. There is

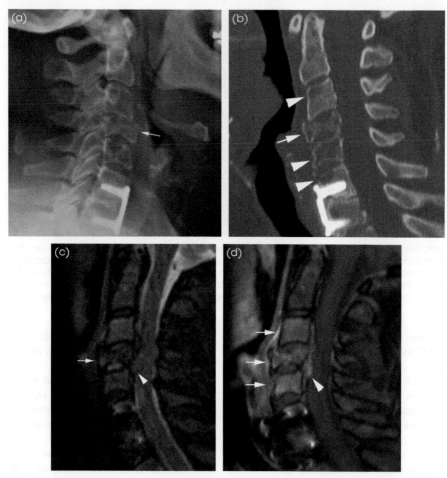

**Figure 4.2.** Pathologic burst fracture. (*A*) Lateral radiograph of the cervical spine in a 54-year-old woman with history of colon carcinoma and neck pain. There is a compression fracture of the C4 vertebral body (*arrow*) with mild posterior vertebral body wall bowing into the canal, suggesting a burst fracture. The endplates are ill-defined, concerning for an underlying pathologic fracture. (*B*) Sagittal reformatted CT image confirms a burst fracture of C4 with underlying bone destruction (*arrow*). Additional lytic lesions in the C3, C5, and C6 vertebral bodies (*arrowheads*) are also noted. (*C*) Sagittal T2W MR image confirms burst fracture at C4 (*arrow*) with clearer depiction of spinal canal narrowing (*arrowhead*). Note mildly increased signal in the C3 and C5 vertebral bodies. (*D*) Sagittal T1W MR image better shows multiple additional enhancing metastases (*arrows*) with enhancing epidural mass contributing to canal compromise (*arrowhead*).

direct correlation between the number of fused segments and potential for long-term instability. With continued motion at a single level, increasing instability or hypertrophic non-bony union is likely. Both of these scenarios are associated with development of new neurologic deficits or progression of existing deficits. Fractures of the rigid spine are considered high risk with a mortality of approximately 18% in the 3-month interval after fracture. Multiple cofactors contribute to this, including increased patient age, obesity, and aortitis in cases of inflammatory spondyloarthropathy.

For greater detail regarding these conditions, see Chapter 32, "Ankylosing Spondylitis" and Chapter 48, "Diffuse Idiopathic Skeletal Hyperostosis" (for a comparison between AS and DISH, see Table 48.2). There are a number of clinical and imaging features, however, which can be helpful for distinguishing between AS and DISH. Patients with AS tend to be younger than 40 years at initial presentation, human leukocyte antigen B27 (HLA-B27) positive on serology, and present with inflammatory back and sacroiliac pain and stiffness. Conversely, those with DISH often present when they are

older than 50 years. They tend to be asymptomatic or have mild thoracolumbar pain and restricted range of motion. Patients with AS present with periarticular erosions of the sacroiliac joints and pubic symphysis, and uniform narrowing of the hip joints. Additionally, enthesophytes with erosions are common. Patients with DISH tend to have bulkier osseous enthesopathy without erosions. Osseous bridging of the sacroiliac joints involves the superior, ligamentous portion only, and there is osseous bridging of the pubic symphysis without erosions. Spinous manifestations in patients with AS include thin, linear syndesmophytes that form along the periphery of the annulus fibrosus, and erosions of the anterior corners of the vertebral bodies are associated with osteitis, leading to a *squared* appearance of the vertebra on lateral imaging and sclerosis of the vertebral body corners (ie, *shiny corner sign*). This is commonly associated with interspinous process ossification (ie, *dagger sign*) and erosion of the costovertebral joints. In patients with DISH, vertebral enthesophytes tend to be bulkier and much more frequently involve the ALL and PLL, layering along the length of the vertebral body.

**Imaging Findings**
Refer to Figure 4.3.

- Radiography
  - Diagnose underlying spondyloarthropathy (either AS or DISH) and displaced fractures.
  - Most fractures occur in the axial plane, frequently involving the peripheral bridging syndesmophyte or ankylosed ligament and the disc space, traversing posteriorly through the facets and laminae (more common in AS).
  - The fused spinal segment may undergo sufficient demineralization such that the fracture plane goes through the vertebral body with sparing of the relatively fortified bridging ossification (more common in DISH).
  - Extension force results in anterior gaping at the fracture site, enhancing visualization of the injury.
  - Fractures can be completely reduced by supine positioning. Further, osteoporosis seen in many elderly patients or considerable overlying artifact, such as pulmonary fibrosis, aortic calcifications, and postural limitations, may also reduce visibility of fractures.
  - Because of the challenge of diagnosis on radiography, and because the patient may not identify the change in the pattern of pain, the diagnosis may be delayed ("the fatal pause").
  - Concerning clinical symptomatology, such as pain out of proportion to imaging findings or neurologic deficits, should prompt additional imaging.
- CT
  - A 3-plane CT better characterizes fractures seen on radiographs and may be essential for diagnosis when radiographs fail to detect the fracture.
  - Sagittal reformatted images are often best at showing discontinuity of the anterior vertebral wall or bridging intervertebral ossification.
  - CT is also extremely beneficial for assessment of healing in cases with progressive radiologic abnormalities or ongoing pain or other symptoms.
- MRI
  - MRI is frequently indicated in cases with new or progressive neurologic deficits.
  - Important soft tissue findings that may be associated with neurologic compromise, such as epidural hematoma, are readily depicted. This is more pertinent in injuries of the thoracic spine.
  - Radiographically occult coincident vertebral injuries will also be evident.

**Treatment Options**
- TLSO is recommended but is less effective for high thoracic lesions.
- Surgical management is controversial, with greater risks of complication in elderly populations.
- A combined AP surgical approach results in the greatest stability, although the isolated posterior approach may achieve sufficient stability.

**Key Points**
- Osteoporotic compression fractures can occur with or without inciting events, although exclusion of underlying alternative pathologies is essential.
- Imaging patterns of osteoporotic fractures parallel compression fractures in the well-mineralized skeleton.
- Management of neoplastic lesions associated with thoracolumbar spine fractures cannot be initiated without identification of the underlying lesion.
- Imaging of neoplastic lesions may include assessment of regional effects and survey for extent of involvement of the axial skeleton, and intravenous contrast administration is usually indicated for both CT and MRI.

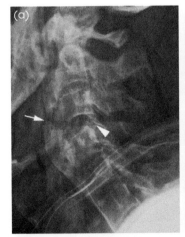 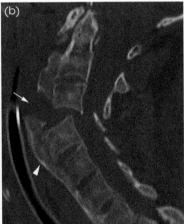

**Figure 4.3.** Acute fracture in DISH. (*A*) Lateral radiograph of the cervical spine in a 62-year-old man who had a low-impact fall shows an acute fracture through the anterior-inferior C3 vertebral body (*arrow*) and retrolisthesis of C3 on C4 (*arrowhead*) in this spine with dense bridging bone from DISH. (*B*) Sagittal reformatted CT image confirms an axially oriented fracture through the C3 anterior-inferior vertebral body with anterior gaping of the disc level (*arrow*), typical of an extension injury. There is significant bridging ossification along the ALL (*arrowhead*).

- Rigidity of the thoracolumbar spine in the setting of AS and DISH places patients at increased risk for fractures, especially after extension forces.
- Neurologic sequelae in patients with spinal fractures in the setting of AS and DISH are common.
- Radiographs may be insufficient for diagnosis because of reduced bone density, postural limitations, and coincident imaging findings and/or artifacts obscuring detail.
- CT is often critical for diagnosis, especially in radiographically occult fractures.

## Recommended Reading

Singh K, Samartzis D, Vaccaro AR, et al. Current concepts in the management of metastatic spinal disease. *J Bone Joint Surg Br*. 2006;8:434–42.

Talijanovic MS, Hunter TB, Wisneski RF, et al. Imaging characteristics of diffuse idiopathic skeletal hyperostosis with an emphasis on acute spinal fractures: review. *AJR Am J Roentgenol* 2009;193:s10–19.

Olivieri I, D'Angelo S, Palazzi C, Padula A, Mader R, Khan MA. Diffuse idiopathic skeletal hyperostosis: differentiation from ankylosing spondylitis. *Curr Rheumatol Rep*. 2009 Oct;11(5):321–28.

## References

1. Kondo KL. Osteoporotic compression fractures and vertebral augmentation. *Semin Intervent Radiol*. 2008;25:413–24.
2. Masala S, Roselli M, Massari F, et al. Radiofrequency heat ablation and vertebroplasty in the treatment of neoplastic vertebral body fracture. *Anticancer Res*. 2004;24:3129–34.
3. Matthews M, Bolesta MJ. Treatment of spinal fractures in ankylosing spondylitis. *Orthopedics* 2013;36:e1203–208.
4. Singh K, Samartzis D, Vaccaro AR, et al. Current concepts in the management of metastatic spinal disease. *J Bone Joint Surg Br*. 2006;88:434–42.
5. Talijanovic MS, Hunter TB, Wisneski RF, et al. Imaging characteristics of diffuse idiopathic skeletal hyperostosis with an emphasis on acute spinal fractures: review. *AJR Am J Roentgenol* 2009;193:s10–19.
6. Tomita K, Kawahara N, Kobayashi T, et al. Surgical strategy for spinal metastases. *Spine* 2001;26:298–306.
7. Vogler JB, Murphy WA. Diffuse marrow diseases. In: Berquist T, ed. *MRI of the Musculoskeletal System*. 5th ed. Philadelphia, PA: Lippincott Williams and Wilkins; 2006:948–1005.
8. Westerveld LA, Verlaan JJ, Oner FC. Spine fractures in patients with ankylosing spinal disorders: a systematic review of the literature on treatment, neurological status and complications. *Eur Spine J*. 2009;18:145–56.

# CHAPTER 5

# Sacral Fractures

Kevin J. Blount

## Introduction

Sacral fractures typically occur either in the setting of high-speed trauma or elderly patients with osteopenia and resultant insufficiency injury. Fractures of the sacrum are present in 45% of all pelvic fractures. Because of the high association of sacral fractures with neurologic injury, familiarity with the imaging and classification of sacral fractures is critical to determine appropriate management. The purpose of this chapter is to outline the approach to imaging of sacral fractures with specific attention to the anatomic factors that influence fracture classification and treatment.

### Basic Anatomy

The sacrum is composed of 5 vertebrae, which fuse during adulthood. Its function is to transfer load from the spinal column to the pelvis and hips. Multiple ligaments are critical for stabilizing the pelvic ring and sacrum. These include

- The *ALL* and *PLL* course along the anterior and posterior margins of the sacral vertebral bodies.
- Each sacroiliac (SI) joint is stabilized by 3 main ligaments, which are the *anterior sacroiliac, interosseous sacroiliac,* and *posterior sacroiliac ligaments.* The lumbosacral and iliolumbar ligaments also add to posterior stability.
- The *sacrospinous* and *sacrotuberous ligaments* stabilize the pelvic floor.

The coccyx is a small, triangular shaped bone that forms the inferior tip of the spine. It is formed by the fusion of 3-5 rudimentary vertebral segments and attaches to the distal tip of the sacrum via a fibrocartilaginous disc, called the *sacrococcygeal disc.*

The sacral canal contains the sacral and coccygeal nerve roots, the thecal sac, and the filum terminale. The lumbosacral plexus is formed by contributions from L4, L5, and S1-S4, and tracks along the posterolateral wall of the sacrum and pelvic cavity. The common iliac, internal iliac, and external iliac arteries course near the anterior sacrum. The sigmoid colon and rectum are also positioned anterior to the sacrum and are at risk for injury with sacral fracture.

## Patterns of Injury

### Pathophysiology and Clinical Presentation

Traumatic sacral fractures usually occur as a result of lateral compressive forces on the pelvis or vertical shear injuries. Those occurring as a result of lateral compression tend to be stable. Conversely, those that occur as a result of shear forces are generally unstable. U-shaped fractures can result from axial loading injuries. Sacral fractures can result in traction injury or nerve transection, depending on the nature of the injury. Of patients with sacral fractures, 15-40% will present with a neurologic deficit. The S1 and S2 nerve roots are larger in size relative to their respective neural foramina compared to S3 and S4, and are therefore at higher risk of injury. The sacral dorsal root ganglia are located medial and superior to their respective neural foramina. Transverse sacral fractures have been associated with cauda equina compression.

Patients with sacral stress fractures often present with low back and possibly gluteal pain, and tenderness to palpation on physical examination. Because of the mixed sclerosis and lucency caused by fracturing and callus formation, insufficiency fractures can resemble aggressive lesions, such as metastases. Occasionally, healing sacral fractures can produce anterior sacral alar periosteal edema that can irritate the exiting sacral nerve roots and produce radiculopathy.

Coccygeal injuries usually occur by direct trauma, such as falling in a seated position, or during childbirth. Patients present with localized pain and tenderness over the coccyx that worsens with prolonged sitting.

### Classification

The location and pattern of sacral fracture has implications with regards to stability and management. There are multiple classification systems in existence. The appropriate classification depends on the type of fracture:

- Denis classification (Figure 5.1 and Box 5.1)
  - For fractures confined to the sacrum only
  - Divides the sacrum into 3 zones
  - Denis zone III fractures have been further subclassified by Roy-Camille et al and Strange-Vognsen and Lebech (Figure 5.2 and Box 5.2)
- Isler classification (Figure 5.3 and Box 5.3)
  - For fractures that involve the sacrum and lumbosacral junction, typically in the setting of high-energy trauma are classified using this system.
  - Classification is based on the location of the fracture relative to the L5-S1 facet.
  - Bilateral type III fractures may be classified as *lumbosacral dissociation.*
- Transverse sacral fractures (Figure 5.4)
  - Relatively uncommon, accounting for less than 5% of all sacral fractures
  - A variation of type III Denis fracture because the fracture lines traverse the spinal canal

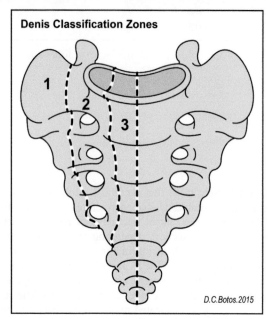

**Denis Classification Zones**

D.C.Botos.2015

**Figure 5.1.** Denis classification of sacral fractures.

- Can be described by the letter of the alphabet that the fracture lines resemble, such as H, U, λ (lambda), and T
  - Have high incidence of neurologic dysfunction or nerve injury

### Imaging Strategy

- Sacral fractures are often not visualized on routine AP pelvis radiographs because of the inclination of the sacrum. Only 30% of sacral fractures are visualized on radiography.
- CT protocol using thin axial sections at 1 or 2 mm intervals with sagittal and coronal reconstructions is diagnostic for most sacral fractures, particularly in the setting of acute trauma.
- MRI is the gold standard for detection of sacral insufficiency fractures with sensitivity approaching 100%.

---

**Box 5.1.** Denis Classification of Sacral Fractures

- Zone I—lateral to the neural foramina
  - The most common pattern of Denis fracture (50% of sacral fractures)
  - Rare nerve injury to the L5 nerve root or sciatic nerve (6% of cases)
- Zone II—through the neural foramina
  - The second most common fracture pattern (34% of sacral fractures)
  - Can be stable or unstable; 28% result in nerve injury to L5, S1, or S2, which may cause bladder and/or bowel dysfunction or sciatic nerve injury
  - Highly unstable if shear component
- Zone III—medial to the neural foramina and involve the spinal canal
  - Have the highest rate of neurologic deficits (60% of patients), commonly resulting in bowel, bladder, and/or sexual dysfunction

---

### Imaging Findings

- Radiography
  - Inlet and outlet radiographs of the pelvis can be helpful.
    - The inlet view allows for better visualization of the sacral spinal canal.
    - The outlet view provides a true AP view of the sacrum.
  - Lateral view of the sacrum is helpful to evaluate alignment in the sagittal plane, however, osseous detail is limited by overlying soft tissue.
  - Stress fractures can mimic metastases. However, fractures tend to have a linear morphology with vertical or horizontal orientations.
  - On plain radiographs, important findings may heighten suspicion for sacral fracture:
    - L4 or L5 transverse process fractures
    - Disruption of the anterior pelvic ring
    - Disruption of the anterior superior sacral foraminal lines, also known as sacral arcuate lines
    - In the setting of insufficiency fracture, linear bands of sclerosis along the neural foramina resembling the letter "H"
  - Coccygeal injuries are best detected on lateral radiographs. They often occur at the sacrococcygeal junction, and there may be anterior or posterior displacement of the coccyx with respect to the distal sacrum. Angulation may also be seen; however, this may also be developmental (Figure 5.5). Coccygeal fractures may be difficult to detect unless there is displacement.
- CT (Figure 5.6)
  - Recommended measurements
    - On axial images, measure AP fracture displacement, horizontal displacement, canal occlusion, and foraminal encroachment.
    - On sagittal images, measure AP translation and kyphotic angulation.
      - Additionally, sagittal reformatted images can be helpful for looking for horizontal fracture lines and for sacral canal narrowing.
    - On coronal images, measure vertical sacral fracture displacement.
- MRI (Figure 5.7)
  - Most sacral insufficiency fractures demonstrate both BME on fluid-sensitive sequences and a low signal intensity fracture line on T1W and often fluid-sensitive sequences. However, a discrete fracture line is absent in 7% of cases.
  - MRI is also indicated for further evaluation of any sacral fracture when neural compromise is suspected and can define areas of neural compression better than CT because of superior soft tissue detail.
  - MRI can be helpful to detect nondisplaced coccygeal injuries (Figure 5.5). Injuries to the sacrococcygeal junction may demonstrate bright signal in the fibrocartilaginous disc with surrounding soft tissue edema on fluid-sensitive sequences. Coccygeal contusions and fractures may demonstrate BME on fluid-sensitive sequences. Occasionally, fracture lines may be visible on T1W imaging although the bone may be too small to detect these fracture line well.

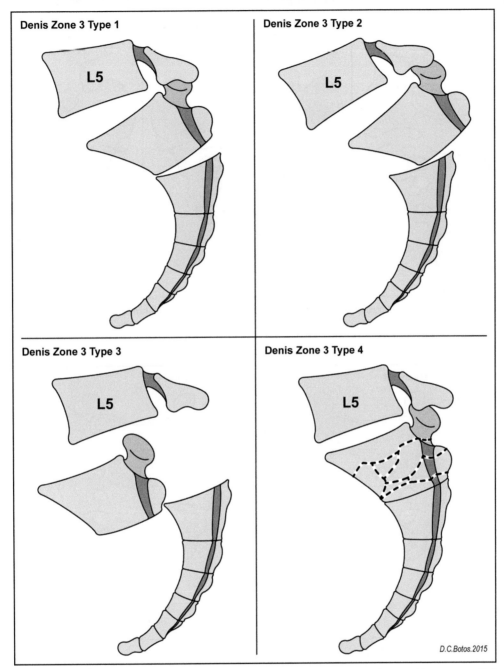

Denis Zone 3 Type 1

L5

Denis Zone 3 Type 2

L5

Denis Zone 3 Type 3

L5

Denis Zone 3 Type 4

L5

D.C.Botos.2015

**Figure 5.2.** Subclassification of Denis zone III fractures as described by Roy-Camille et al and Strange-Vognsen and Lebech.

- Nuclear imaging
  - Technetium-99 bone scan may be helpful for detection of insufficiency fractures in elderly patients, with a sensitivity of 96% in this setting, and uptake

at the fracture site that has a linear or curvilinear morphology.
- The *H-sign* on nuclear medicine studies resulting from vertical fracture lines through both sacral ala, and horizontal fracture through the mid-sacrum, is characteristic of sacral insufficiency fracture. Many patients only demonstrate incomplete H's, with partial or complete absence of one or more of the fracture limbs.

**Treatment Options**
- Sacral fractures are often defined as stable or unstable.
  - Unstable fractures shift or change position with physiologic loads.

---

**Box 5.2.** Strange-Vognsen and Lebech Subclassification of Denis Classification

- Type 1—flexion fracture with anterior angulation
- Type 2—flexion fracture with anterior angulation and posterior displacement of the upper sacral fracture fragment
- Type 3—extension fractures with anterior translation and inferior migration of the upper sacral segment
- Type 4—comminuted fracture of the upper sacral segment caused by axial impaction

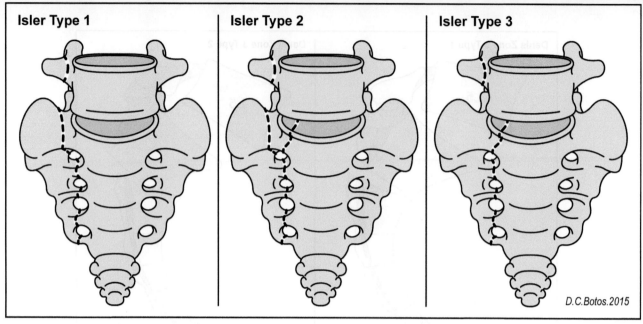

**Figure 5.3.** Isler classification of sacral fractures, for fractures involving the lumbosacral junction and sacrum.

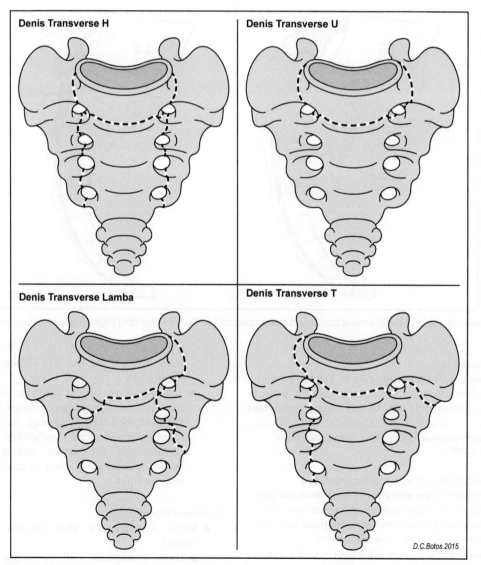

**Figure 5.4.** Descriptive classifications of transverse sacral fractures.

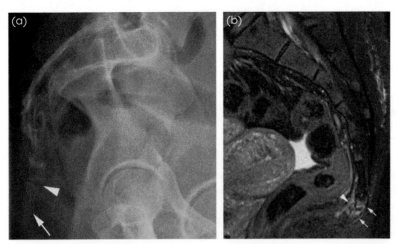

**Figure 5.5.** Coccygeal injuries. (*A*) Lateral sacral radiograph in 33-year-old woman with coccygeal region pain following childbirth demonstrates mild posterior angulation of the coccyx at the sacrococcygeal junction (*arrow*) and widening of the anterior disc space (*arrowhead*). Although this can be developmental, the patient had significant tenderness in this area. (*B*) Sagittal T2W FS MR image of the coccygeal region in a 36-year-old woman with regional pain and tenderness after direct trauma reveals BME in the second and third coccygeal levels surrounding the intervertebral disc (*arrows*) with anterior soft tissue edema (*arrowhead*), consistent with additional soft tissue injury at this level. No coccygeal displacement or angulation is seen.

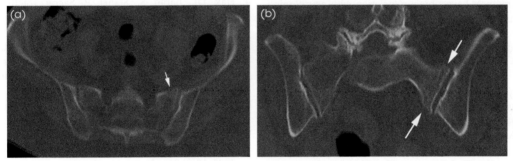

**Figure 5.6.** Lateral sacral alar fracture. A 76-year-old woman with left hip pain after a fall. (*A*) Axial CT image of the pelvis shows subtle buckling of the anterior cortex of the lateral left sacral ala (*arrow*), lateral to the neural foramina. This is better seen on a coronal reformatted image (*B*) and represents an example of a zone I fracture according to the Denis classification (*between white arrows*).

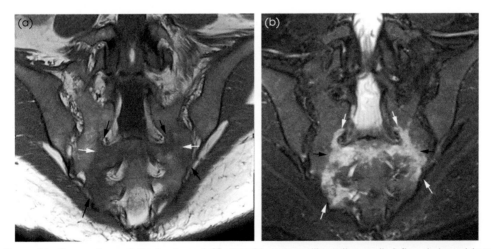

**Figure 5.7.** Radiographically occult sacral alar fractures. A 29-year-old woman with posttraumatic left posterior pelvic pain. Coronal oblique T1W (A) and STIR (B) MR images of the pelvis show vertically oriented sacral alar fractures (between vertically-oriented opposing arrows) through the neural foramina (Denis classification zone II). The fracture lines are less conspicuous on the T1W image. However, the associated BME seen on the STIR sequence makes these findings much more conspicuous. Additionally, there is horizontally oriented BME bridging the right and left sacral alae at the S3 level (between opposing horizontally-oriented arrows), which likely represents additional stress response. The fracture was not visible on prior radiographs (not shown).

**Box 5.3.** Isler Classification System of Sacral Fractures

- Type I—fractures lateral to the L5-S1 facet, unlikely to result in lumbosacral instability but can impair stability of the pelvic ring
- Type II—fractures through the L5-S1 facet
- Type III—fractures medial to the L5-S1 facet, usually associated with significant instability

- Instability is usually associated with disruption of the SI joints, tear of the sacrospinous or sacrotuberous ligaments, or vertical fractures.
- Surgical intervention is indicated in the setting of unstable fractures, neurologic deficit, or severe misalignment.
- Stable, nondisplaced sacral fractures without disruption of the pelvic ring or involvement of the lumbosacral junction are usually managed nonoperatively.

## Key Points
- Sacral fractures have a high association with neurologic injury and therefore require appropriate classification to determine management.
- Thin section CT with sagittal and coronal reconstructions or MRI are preferred imaging methods for fracture detection and classification. Bone scan is also highly sensitive, particularly in the setting of elderly patients with insufficiency injury. Sacral fractures are often not visualized on routine AP pelvis radiographs.
- The Denis classification is used for fractures confined to the sacrum and divides the sacrum into 3 zones relative to the sacral neural foramina. The Isler classification is utilized for fractures involving the sacrum and lumbosacral junction, depending on involvement of the L5-S1 facets.

- Stable fractures are usually managed nonoperatively. Unstable fractures, fractures with neurologic deficit, and fractures with severe malalignment usually require surgical intervention.

## Recommended Reading
White JH, Hague C, Nicolaou S, et al. Imaging of sacral fractures. *Clin Radiol.* 2003 Dec;58(12):914–21.

Lyders EM, Whitlow CT, Baker MD, Morris PP. Imaging and treatment of sacral insufficiency fractures. *AJNR Am J Neuroradiol.* 2010 Feb;31(2):201–10.

## References
1. Isler B. Lumbosacral lesions associated with pelvic ring injuries. *J Orthop Trauma.* 1990;4(1):1–6.
2. Bydon M, Fredrickson V, De la Garza-Ramos R, et al. Sacral fractures. *Neurosurg Focus.* 2014;37(1):E12.
3. Denis F, Davis S, Comfort T. Sacral fractures: an important problem. Retrospective analysis of 236 cases. *Clin Orthop Relat Res.* 1988 Feb;227:67–81.
4. Hak DJ, Baran S, Stahel P. Sacral fractures: current strategies in diagnosis and management. *Orthopedics.* 2009 Oct;32(10).
5. Kuklo TR, Potter BK, Ludwig SC, et al. Radiographic measurement techniques for sacral fractures consensus statement of the Spine Trauma Study Group. *Spine* 2006 Apr 20;31(9):1047–55.
6. Mehta S, Auerbach JD, Born CT, Chin KR. Sacral fractures. *J Am Acad Orthop Surg.* 2006 Nov;14(12):656–65.
7. Roy-Camille R, Saillant G, Gagna G, Mazel C. Transverse fracture of the upper sacrum: Suicidal jumper's fracture. *Spine.* 1985; 10(9):838–45.
8. Strange-Vognsen HH, Lebech A. An unusual type of fracture in the upper sacrum. *J Orthop Trauma.* 1991;5(2):200–203.

# 2

# Rib Cage and Upper Extremity

Edited by Mihra S. Taljanovic and Tyson S. Chadaz

# CHAPTER 6

# Rib Trauma

Michael O'Keeffe, Kiran Khursid, Peter L. Munk, and Mihra S. Taljanovic

## Basic Anatomy and Mechanism of Injury

### Basic Anatomy

The ribs are 12 sets of paired bones that form the protective cage around the thoracic organs. They articulate with the vertebral column posteriorly and terminate anteriorly as costal cartilage (Figure 6.1). During chest expansion, the rib cage moves to permit lung inflation. Rib morphology can be described as typical or atypical. Typical ribs have 2 articulating facets, one of which articulates with the corresponding vertebra, and the other of which articulates with the vertebra above (Figure 6.2). Additionally, they directly attach onto the anterior rib cage. Ribs 3-10 are considered typical and have a wedge-shaped head that contains the articulating facets, a neck, and a body. Conversely, the first, second, eleventh, and 12th ribs are considered atypical. The first and second ribs each articulate with only 1 thoracic vertebra, T1 and T2 respectively. The 11th and 12th ribs are considered atypical because they do not extend to the anterior aspect of the rib cage and appear as incomplete ribs.

The ribs can also be classified as true and false ribs:

- True ribs include the first 7 pairs and are called *sternal ribs*, because they directly attach anteriorly on to the sternum.
- *False ribs* are the lower 5 pairs that do not directly connect to the sternum.
  - Ribs 8-10 attach to the costal cartilage superior to them.

- Ribs 11 and 12 have no anterior attachment and are therefore called *floating ribs*.

### Mechanism of Injury

Blunt chest trauma is a common cause of rib injury. This injury can vary in severity from minor contusion or isolated rib fracture to severe crush injuries of both hemithoraces with multiple displaced fractures, leading to respiratory compromise. Ribs usually fracture at the point of impact or posteriorly, where their anatomy renders them structurally weakest.

Flail chest occurs when 3 or more contiguous ribs are fractured in 2 or more places, separating a segment that is free-floating and moves independently. Flail chest is a serious condition that can lead to long-term disability and even death. Clinically the *flail segment* can demonstrate paradoxical movement during respiration, that is, indrawing on inspiration and moving outward on expiration. Consequently, the flail segment does not contribute to normal lung expansion during breathing (Figure 6.3A).

## Imaging Strategy

Radiography is the mainstay of initial investigation for potential rib fractures. Dedicated frontal and oblique rib views can be helpful in these cases. Displaced fractures can often be readily identified, however, nondisplaced fractures may be radiographically occult. However, the increased availability

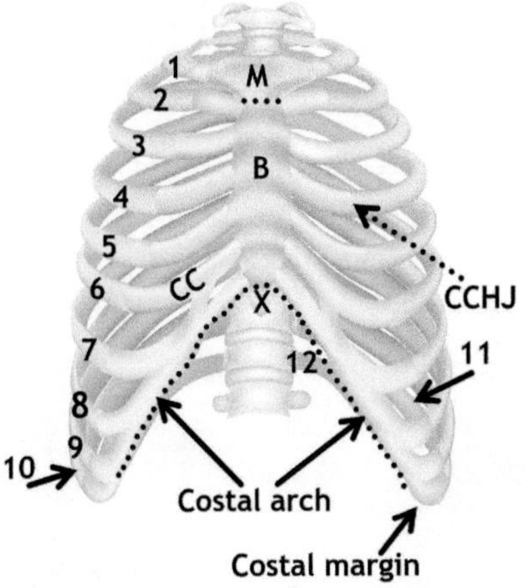

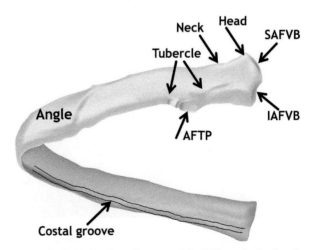

**Figure 6.1.** Artist drawing of a normal rib cage. CC = costal cartilage; CCHJ = costochondral junction; M = manubrium, B = sternal body; X = xiphoid process.

**Figure 6.2.** Artist drawing of a normal rib. AFTP = articular facet for the transverse process; SAFVB = superior articular facet for the vertebral body; IAFVB = inferior articular facet for the vertebral body.

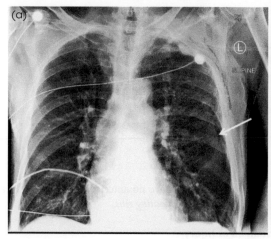 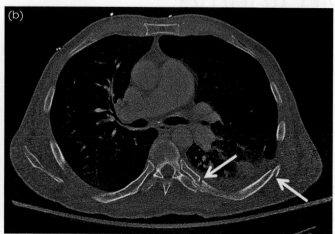

**Figure 6.3.** Flail chest in a trauma patient. (*A*) Posterior-anterior (PA) chest radiograph demonstrates multiple segmental left-sided rib fractures in more than 3 contiguous ribs in keeping with a flail segment, which are better seen on the subsequent CT study. Note associated pneumothorax (*arrow*). (*B*) Axial CT image of the chest in the same patient shows a segmental left rib fracture (*arrows*).

of multidetector CT in the acute trauma setting has substantially increased detection rates and has provided invaluable information, not only for demonstrating the distribution of rib fractures (Figure 6.3B), but also for evaluating injury to underlying structures such as lung parenchyma and upper abdominal organs. Incidentally, rib fractures may be detected on nuclear studies. However, in acute rib fractures, bone scan may be false negative for 2 days in younger patients and up to 2 weeks in older patients.

### Imaging Findings
- Radiography is the primary imaging modality (Figure 6.3A).
- CT offers increased diagnostic accuracy, especially for nondisplaced fractures (Figure 6.3B).
- US used in a focused examination may show cortical step-off in acute fractures (Figure 118.21A) and callus formation

with healing fractures (Figure 118.21B) and may also detect cartilaginous fractures. The imaging findings often correspond to point tenderness on graded compression.
- MRI is not routinely used, but is most useful in evaluation of rib cartilage and costochondral junction injuries.

### Mimics and Pathologic Fractures
- Incidental findings in the ribs on radiography and cross-sectional imaging are extremely common.
- Findings include but are not limited to fibrous dysplasia, multiple myeloma, and metastatic disease. These entities are addressed in other chapters and are susceptible to pathologic fractures (Figure 6.4).

### Treatment Options
- Nondisplaced rib fractures are treated conservatively.
- Operative management of flail segments includes open reduction and internal fixation as demonstrated in Figure 6.5.

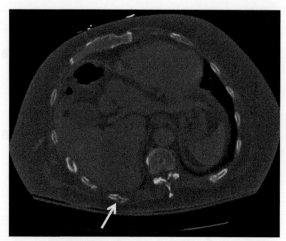

**Figure 6.4.** Pathologic rib fracture in a patient with multiple myeloma. Axial CT image of the chest shows a pathologic fracture of the posterior aspect of the right 10th rib (*arrow*) with an underlying osteolytic lesion. Note the mottled appearance and additional scattered small osteolytic lesions throughout the skeletal structures in keeping with multiple myeloma.

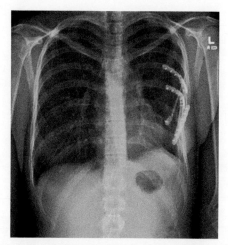

**Figure 6.5.** Postoperative flail chest. Postoperative PA radiograph of the chest demonstrates 3 plates and multiple screw fixation of the flail segment of the left ribs.

## Key Points

- There are a variety of rib morphologies as described, with 8 typical and 4 atypical ribs.
- Rib trauma takes many forms, ranging from nondisplaced fractures to multiple comminuted fractures and flail segments.
- CT examination is increasingly used for the identification of rib fractures and preoperative planning for thoracic wall reconstruction following trauma.
- Nontraumatic rib lesions may often be incidental findings on chest radiography and may be susceptible to pathologic fractures.

## Recommended Reading

Talbot BS, Gange CP, Chaturvedi A, Klionsky N, Hobbs SK, Chaturvedi C. Traumatic rib injury: Patterns, imaging pitfalls, complications, and treatment. *Radiographics*. 2017;37:628–51.

## References

1. Bhavnagri SJ, Mohammed TL. When and how to image a suspected broken rib. *Cleve Clin J Med*. 2009;76(5):309–14.
2. Oikonomou A, Prassopoulos P. CT imaging of blunt chest trauma. *Insights Imaging*. 2011;2(3):281–95.
3. Shweiki E, Klena J, Wood GC, Indeck M. Assessing the true risk of abdominal solid organ injury in hospitalized rib fracture patients. *J Trauma*. 2001 Apr. 50(4):684–8.
4. Traub M, Stevenson M, McEvoy S, et al. The use of chest computed tomography versus chest X-ray in patients with major blunt trauma. *Injury*. 2007 Jan. 38(1):43–47.

# CHAPTER 7

# Sternum Trauma

Michael O'Keeffe, Kiran Khursid, Peter L. Munk, and Mihra S. Taljanovic

## Basic Anatomy and Mechanism of Injury

### Basic Anatomy

The sternum or *breastbone* is a flat bone located in the anterior center of the chest. The sternum along with the ribs and vertebrae form the thoracic cage, which protects the thoracic organs and vessels. The sternum has a convex anterior surface and concave posterior border. The adult sternum is approximately 17 cm long and is comprised of 3 parts (see Figure 6.1 in Chapter 6, "Rib Trauma").

The manubrium is the broad upper part of the sternum. Its upper border forms the suprasternal notch that can be felt between the medical aspects of the clavicles. The lower border of the manubrium is covered by a thin layer of cartilage that articulates with the body of the sternum. The body is the largest of the 3 segments. Its flattened surface provides attachment for the pectoralis major and the origin for the transversus thoracis muscles, which arise from both sides of the lower sternal body. The xiphoid process is the pointed inferior end of the sternum.

The manubrium articulates with the clavicles at the clavicular notches and the first costal cartilages forming the right and left sternoclavicular joints. The second costal cartilages articulate with the sternum at the sternal angle. The first 7 costal cartilages join with the sternum forming the sternocostal joints.

### Mechanism of Injury

Sternal fractures are generally associated with direct blunt trauma, most commonly in motor vehicle accidents. Vigorous cardiopulmonary resuscitation (CPR) can also lead to sternal fracture, particularly at the xiphoid process. Associated injuries occur in up to 50% of cases, often because of the force of impact related to the fracture. These include rib fractures, mediastinal hematomas, aortic injuries, and pulmonary contusion. The manubrium and the body of the sternum are the most common sites of fracture. Insufficiency fractures can also occur, particularly in the elderly and kyphotic patient with decreased bone density.

### Imaging Strategy

Radiological assessment of sternal fractures traditionally involved dedicated sternal radiographs (Figure 7.1). However, these, particularly the oblique view, have a relatively low sensitivity for nondisplaced fractures.

CT examination has surpassed radiography in the assessment of sternal fractures and, more crucially, the diagnosis of secondary findings (Figure 7.2).

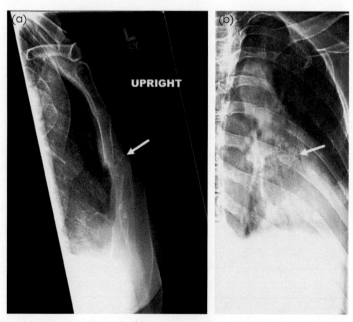

**Figure 7.1.** Sternal body fracture. (*A*) Lateral radiograph of the sternum shows a healing displaced sternal body fracture (*arrow*). (*B*) Oblique radiograph of the sternum in the same patient is of limited utility with sternal body fracture poorly seen (*arrow*).

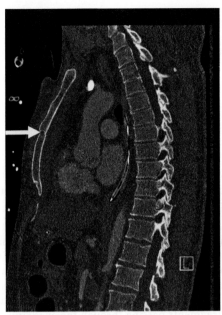

**Figure 7.2.** Mildly displaced sternal body fracture. Reformatted sagittal CT image demonstrates a mildly displaced fracture of the sternal body (*arrow*).

MRI is a superb imaging modality in detecting occult sternal fractures, including the relatively rare stress fractures, as well as pathologic fractures associated with malignancies, osteomyelitis, or metabolic bone diseases. Occult sternal fractures may also be detected on nuclear studies.

## Imaging Findings
- Radiography—fractures are often best detected in the lateral projection, and oblique projections are of limited use (Figure 7.1).

- CT is the imaging modality of choice for occult and displaced fractures and provides excellent evaluation of associated mediastinal injuries (Figure 7.2).
- MRI is reserved for occult and pathologic fractures and provides valuable information of associated muscular and sternocostal injuries.
- Nuclear studies are rarely performed.

## Treatment Options
- Uncomplicated sternal fractures usually respond well to conservative management.
- Surgical fixation is uncommon and generally reserved for more complex fractures.

## Key Points
- Sternal fractures are often associated with severe direct blunt chest trauma such as that acquired in motor vehicle accidents.
- Significant mortality may be associated with displaced sternal fractures because of aortic, cardiac, or pulmonary injury.
- CT examination is the gold standard for radiological diagnosis of sternal injury. It has superior sensitivity to radiography and is valuable in diagnosing serious associated injuries.

### References
1. Bar I, Friedman T, Rudis E, Shargal Y, Friedman M, Elami A. Isolated sternal fracture—a benign condition? *Isr Med Assoc J.* 2003;5(2):105–106.
2. Huggett JM, Roszler MH. CT findings of sternal fracture. *Injury.* 1998;29(8):623–26.
3. Restrepo CS, Martinez S, Lemos DF, et al. Imaging appearances of the sternum and sternoclavicular joints. *Radiographics.* 2009;29(3):839–59.

# CHAPTER 8

# Clavicle Trauma

Michael O'Keeffe, Kiran Khursid, Peter L. Munk, and Mihra S. Taljanovic

## Basic Anatomy and Mechanism of Injury

### Basic Anatomy

Fractures of the clavicle are a common injury in many age groups. The clavicle is the first bone to begin ossification (approximately the fifth week of gestation), and it continues to develop into early adulthood with completion of ossification at approximately 21 years (Figure 8.1).

### Mechanism of Injury

The frequent rate of injury to the clavicle at various age groups is likely caused by early ossification and its superficial anatomical location. Interestingly, the clavicle is the only long bone in the human body with a horizontal trajectory.

Causes of injury include direct impact caused by direct fall or blow to the shoulder, seen in sports such as rugby or motor vehicle collision. Injury from indirect trauma is less common and usually is because of a fall on an outstretched arm. The clavicle is the most commonly fractured bone in infants and is often seen as a result of complicated deliveries.

The midshaft of the clavicle is the most common site of fractures (see Allman classification). This is the thinnest part of the bone, and the region with the least protection from overlying musculature and ligaments.

The *Allman classification* scheme assigns groups according to the site of clavicle fracture:

- Group 1 fractures are middle third injuries; 80% of cases.
- Group 2 fractures are lateral third injuries; 12-15% of cases.

- Group 3 fractures are medial third injuries; less than 5% of cases.

Clinical features of clavicle fractures include pain and swelling over the fracture site and reduced range of motion of the shoulder on the same side. There may be a visible protrusion of the displaced fracture fragments, *tenting* of the skin surface, or, less commonly, an open fracture with fracture fragments passing through the overlying skin.

Additional complications of clavicle fracture can include disruption of the sternoclavicular or acromioclavicular joints, or pneumothorax caused by injury of the adjacent lung apex. Fractures of the clavicle often heal with prominent initial callus formation and subsequent remodeling. However, nonunion of clavicle fractures may occur and can be related to the degree of comminution or displacement of the initial fracture and the age of the patient.

## Imaging Strategy

Dedicated clavicle radiographs are the mainstay of diagnosis. A frontal AP view and a 15- to 45-degree cephalic tilt view are the standard two imaging projections (Figure 8.2). CT and MRI may be helpful in evaluation of pathologic and complex fractures, but are generally not routinely performed.

### Imaging Findings

- Fractures of the clavicle are often displaced because of elevation of the medial fragment from the unopposed action

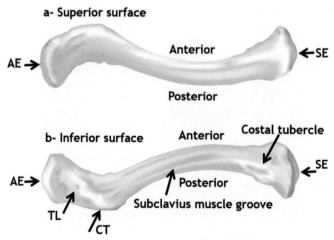

**Figure 8.1.** Artist drawings of the normal clavicle. (*A*) Superior surface and (*B*) inferior surface drawings of the clavicle show normal anatomic structures. AE = acromial end; SE = sternal end; TL = trapezoid (ligament) line; CT = conoid (ligament) tubercle.

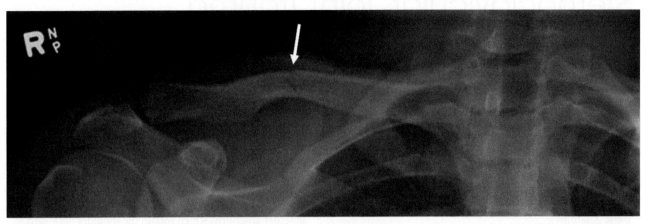

**Figure 8.2.** Nondisplaced clavicle midshaft fracture. Radiograph of the clavicle demonstrates a nondiplaced fracture of the midshaft (*arrow*).

of the sternocleidomastoid muscle and the downward traction of the upper limb on the lateral fragment (Figure 8.3). This propensity to displacement means that chest or AP shoulder radiographs are often sufficient for detecting clavicular fractures, particularly in the polytrauma setting.

## Treatment Options

- Usually, simple fractures with no displaced bone fragments can be managed conservatively with immobilization using a figure-of-eight sling for approximately 4-6 weeks, pain management, and physical therapy.
- Surgical management may be performed for displaced and complex fractures. Options include open reduction/internal fixation (ORIF) with plate and screws, hook plate and screws, or intramedullary nailing.
- Surgical management with ORIF and bone grafting may be required in patients with nonunited fractures.
- Because of the superficial location of the clavicle, the hardware may be removed in many cases after fracture healing to reduce irritation of the overlying skin and for a better cosmetic result.

### Key Points

- The superficial location of the clavicle renders it one of the most frequently fractured bones in the body at a variety of ages.
- Clavicle fractures are commonly displaced and treatment options vary from conservative management to operative techniques such as ORIF.
- Complications of clavicle fractures include pain, overlying swelling and distortion of shoulder anatomy, and nonunion.

### References

1. Assobhi JE. Reconstruction plate versus minimal invasive retrograde titanium elastic nail fixation for displaced midclavicular fractures. *J Orthop Traumatol.* 2011;12(4):185–92.
2. Bahk MS, Kuhn JE, Galatz LM, Connor PM, Williams GR Jr. Acromioclavicular and sternoclavicular injuries and clavicular, glenoid, and scapular fractures. *J Bone Joint Surg Am.* 2009;91(10):2492–510.
3. van der Meijden OA, Gaskill TR, Millett PJ. Treatment of clavicle fractures: current concepts review. *J Shoulder Elbow Surg.* 2012;21(3):423–29.

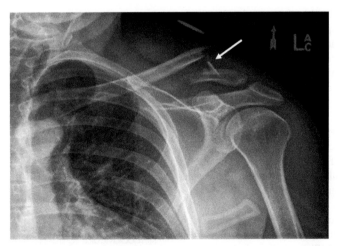

**Figure 8.3.** Displaced clavicular fracture. AP radiograph of the shoulder demonstrates a comminuted and displaced fracture of the distal clavicle (*arrow*) with superior displacement of the medial fragment. The displacement of the medial fragment is largely because of the action of sternocleidomastoid muscle.

# CHAPTER 9

# Sternoclavicular Joint Trauma

Michael O'Keeffe, Kiran Khursid, Peter L. Munk, and Mihra S. Taljanovic

## Basic Anatomy and Mechanism of Injury

### Basic Anatomy

The sternoclavicular joint is formed between the sternal end of the clavicle and the clavicular notch of the sternal manubrium, along with a small part of the first costal cartilage. The articular surface of the clavicle is much larger than of the sternum and is invested with a thicker layer of cartilage. This is a synovial joint divided into 2 portions by a fibrocartilage articular disc.

As approximately 50% of the medial end of the clavicle does not articulate with the manubrium, the sternoclavicular joint relies heavily on the joint capsule, which is strongest superiorly, and its adjacent ligaments for overall stability (Figure 9.1). These reinforcing ligaments include the

- *Anterior and posterior sternoclavicular ligaments*, which support the joint anteriorly and posteriorly
- *Interclavicular ligament*, which connects the sternal ends of the 2 clavicles to each other and to the superior part of the manubrium
- *Costoclavicular ligaments*, which are present laterally and connect the sternal end of the clavicle to the first costal cartilage

The sternoclavicular joint primarily allows the movement of the clavicle in AP and vertical planes which, along with minimal rotation, plays an important role in facilitating elevation, depression, and circumduction of the shoulder girdle.

### Mechanism of Injury

Direct or indirect force to the shoulder from mechanisms such as a motor vehicle collision, sporting injuries, or fall from a height can cause sternoclavicular joint injury. However, overall injury and dislocation rates are low when compared to more inherently unstable joints such as the shoulder or elbow.

There are 3 grades of sternoclavicular joint injury (Allman classification):

**Grade I:** Mild sprain of supporting ligaments without subsequent instability of the joint.

**Grade II:** Complete tear of the sternoclavicular ligaments and partial costoclavicular ligament injury. This results in subluxation of the sternoclavicular joint, either anterior or posterior.

**Grade III:** Complete rupture of the sternoclavicular and costoclavicular ligaments with resultant dislocation of the sternoclavicular joint (Figure 9.2).

Anterior dislocation (90% of the cases) is much more common than posterior and is often caused by a blow to the shoulder anteriorly, which rotates the shoulder backward.

There are 2 main mechanisms for posterior sternoclavicular joint dislocations: high-velocity posterior-lateral compressive force to the involved shoulder and direct force to the anterior-medial aspect of the clavicle, thus, causing the head of the clavicle to displace posteriorly.

Complications related to sternoclavicular joint injury are largely related to the mechanism of injury. Complications of anterior dislocation may be limited to mild discomfort and a cosmetic defect caused by asymmetry of both joints. Posterior dislocation may be associated with more severe complications such as aortic injury, mediastinal hematoma, tracheal injury, or pneumothorax.

## Imaging Strategy

Radiography is often inadequate for optimal evaluation of sternoclavicular joint injury as traditional radiographs in the trauma setting are limited to AP views. CT examination is the gold standard for assessment of dislocation and any potential injury to surrounding structures.

### Imaging Findings

- Radiography—dislocations and fractures are difficult to detect on limited AP views.
- CT is the imaging modality of choice for suspected dislocations (Figure 9.2) or displaced fracture and provides excellent evaluation of associated mediastinal injuries.

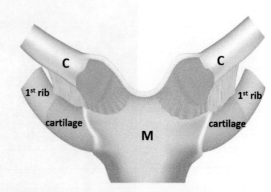

**Figure 9.1.** Artist drawing of the reinforcing sternoclavicular joint ligaments. Yellow = interclavicular ligament; Pink = anterior sternoclavicular ligament; Green = costoclavicular ligament; C = sternal end of the clavicle; M = manubrium.

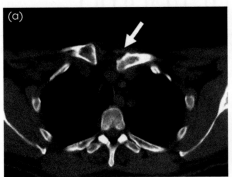 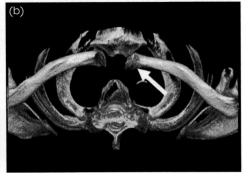

**Figure 9.2.** Left sternoclavicular joint posterior dislocation. (*A*) Axial CT image of the thorax demonstrates posterior dislocation of the left sternoclavicular joint (*arrow*) secondary to a grade III injury sustained while playing rugby. (*B*) Three-dimensional (3D) CT reformatted image confirms posterior dislocation of the left sternoclavicular joint (*arrow*).

- MRI is reserved for occult and pathologic fractures and provides valuable information of associated muscular and mediastinal injuries.
- Nuclear studies are rarely performed.

## Treatment Options
- Conservative management for low-grade injuries includes rest, immobilization, and analgesia.
- Higher-grade injuries often require surgical repair with open reduction and internal fixation.

## Key Points
- Sternoclavicular joint stability relies substantially on support from a dense joint capsule and surrounding ligaments.
- Sternoclavicular joint injury is relatively rare and ranges from sprains and partial tears of supporting ligaments to ligament rupture and joint dislocation.

- Anterior dislocation is more common. Although complications related to sternoclavicular joint injury are relatively rare, they can potentially be life threatening.
- Life-threatening injuries are more often associated with posterior dislocation.

## References
1. Lee JT, Campbell KJ, Michalski MP, et al. Surgical anatomy of the sternoclavicular joint: a qualitative and quantitative anatomical study. *J Bone Joint Surg Am*. 2014;96(19):e166.
2. Macdonald PB, Lapointe P. Acromioclavicular and sternoclavicular joint injuries. *Orthop Clin North Am*. 2008;39(4):535–45, viii.
3. Restrepo CS, Martinez S, Lemos DF, et al. Imaging appearances of the sternum and sternoclavicular joints. *Radiographics*. 2009;29(3):839–59.
4. Rogers LF, West OC. *Imaging Skeletal Trauma*. 4th ed. Philadelphia, PA: Elsevier; 2015.

# CHAPTER 10

# Acromioclavicular Joint Trauma

Michael O'Keeffe, Kiran Khursid, Peter L. Munk, and Mihra S. Taljanovic

## Basic Anatomy and Mechanism of Injury

### Basic Anatomy

The acromioclavicular (AC) joint is formed between the acromion process of the scapula and the lateral end of the clavicle. This is a synovial joint with an interposed fibrocartilaginous disc connecting the articulating surfaces.

Joint stability is provided by 3 ligaments:

1. The AC ligament consists of superior and inferior AC ligaments that supports the joint from above and below respectively.
2. The coracoacromial ligament is a strong triangular band that links the coracoid process to the acromion and forms a vault for protection of the head of humerus.
3. The coracoclavicular (CC) ligament comprises 2 ligaments, the medial coronoid and lateral trapezoid ligaments.

The AC joint contributes to the superior shoulder suspensory complex. This forms a biomechanical ring of bone and ligament that provides the normal anatomical relationship between the upper limb and the axial skeleton. The other components of the superior shoulder suspensory complex are the coracoid process, acromial process, coracoclavicular ligament, distal clavicle, and glenoid process.

### Mechanism of Injury

AC joint injuries are most common in active/athletic young adults. The most common among these is AC joint dislocation, seen mostly in contact sports such as rugby and football. The most common mechanism is fall on an outstretched arm.

Depending on the degree of separation of the acromion from the clavicle, the injury is divided into 6 types by the Rockwood classification:

**Type I:** Partially torn AC ligament. Clavicle not elevated relative to the acromion.
**Type II:** Complete tear of AC ligament with joint-space widening. Clavicle elevated but not above the superior border of the acromion (Figure 10.1).
**Type III:** Complete tear of AC and CC ligaments. Clavicle elevated above the level of the acromion, but coracoclavicular distance remains less than twice as normal (Figure 10.2).
**Type IV:** Lateral end of the clavicle is displaced posteriorly through the trapezius, which is best seen on axillary radiographs.

**Type V:** CC distance more than twice as normal with clavicle herniated through the deltotrapezial fascia, resulting in a subcutaneous distal clavicle (Figure 10.3).
**Type VI:** This is a rare injury with the distal clavicle lying either in a subacromial or subcoracoid position.

Any injury greater than type III involves disruption of the superior shoulder suspensory complex in 2 or more places and is often considered for surgical repair.

## Imaging Strategy

Radiographs (AP and 10- to 15-degree oblique with cephalad angulation) are the mainstay of initial radiological evaluation of the AC joint. Additional weight-bearing views may also be helpful with comparison views of the uninjured contralateral joint often advised. This is performed with weights ranging between 10 and 20 lb hanging from both wrists (Figure 10.4).

### Imaging Findings
- Radiography
  - Type 1 injuries may often demonstrate no abnormality on radiography or may only demonstrate minimal overlying soft tissue swelling.
  - Careful evaluation of the AC joint interval (normal = 5-8 mm) and the coracoclavicular distance (normal = 10-13 mm) is essential as these injuries may be subtle (Figure 10.1). Abnormal widening of either of these distances should raise concern for AC joint injury. (Figures 10.1 through 10.4))
  - The undersurface of the clavicle and the acromion also provide useful landmarks and should be aligned.
  - Look for asymmetry with the contralateral side on weight-bearing view (2 mm or more is considered abnormal).
- CT is generally not needed and may be performed on a case-by-case basis.
- MRI is useful in evaluation of occult fractures and ligamentous injuries. These injuries are frequently seen on routine shoulder MRI studies.

## Treatment Options
- Conservative for low-grade injuries
- CC ligament reconstruction in selected high-grade injuries; open reduction/internal fixation (ORIF) with associated distal clavicle fractures

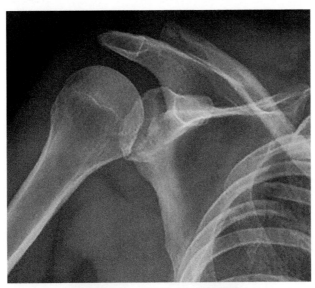

**Figure 10.1.** Subtle type II AC joint separation. AP radiograph demonstrates mild superior subluxation of the clavicle. Multiple displaced right-sided rib fractures are incidentally noted.

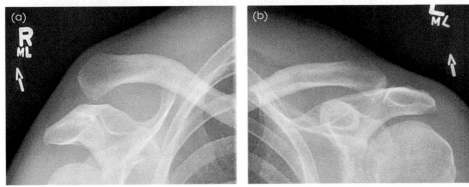

**Figure 10.2.** Type III AC joint separation. (*A*) AP radiograph of the right AC joint demonstrates superior dislocation of the clavicle above the acromion. (*B*) The normal contralateral left AC joint is well aligned.

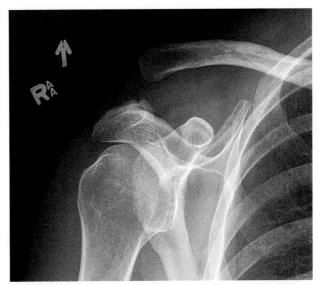

**Figure 10.3.** Type V AC joint separation. AP radiograph of the AC joint demonstrates severe superior dislocation of the lateral clavicle with the AC and CC intervals measuring above twice as normal.

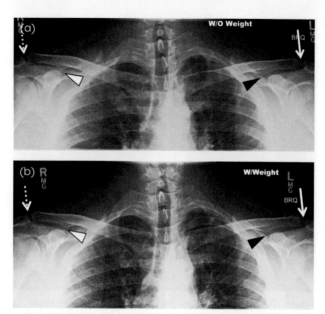

**Figure 10.4.** Normal alignment of the right AC joint and chronic type II left AC joint separation. AP radiographs of the bilateral AC joints (*A*) without weights and (*B*) with weights show normal width of the right AC joint (*dashed arrow*) and CC interval (*white arrowhead*), mild widening of the left AC joint (*arrow*) and normal width of the left CC interval (*black arrowhead*). There is no change in alignment in (*B*).

## Key Points

- The AC joint is frequently injured. Radiographs are usually sufficient in the evaluation of AC and CC intervals in the assessment of different types of AC joint injuries.
- The type of AC joint injury dictates the treatment plan. Higher-grade injuries often require surgical repair because of coexisting injuries to other elements of the superior shoulder suspensory ligament complex.

## References

1. Bishop JY, Kaeding C. Treatment of the acute traumatic acromioclavicular separation. *Sports Med Arthrosc.* 2006;14 (4):237–45.
2. Ha AS, Perscavage-Thomas JM, Tagoyolo GH. Acromioclavicular joint: the other joint in the shoulder. *AJR Am J Roentgenol.* 2014;202:375–85.
3. Renfree KJ, Wright TW. Anatomy and biomechanics of the acromioclavicular and sternoclavicular joints. *Clin Sports Med.* 2003;22(2):219–37.

# CHAPTER 11

# Scapula Trauma

Michael O'Keeffe, Kiran Khursid, Peter L. Munk, and Mihra S. Taljanovic

## Basic Anatomy and Mechanism of Injury

### Basic Anatomy

The scapula is a flattened, triangular bone that forms an essential component of the shoulder girdle (Figure 11.1). It articulates with the humerus at its glenoid fossa to form the glenohumeral joint. It also articulates with the clavicle at its acromion process to form the AC joint (see Chapter 10, "Acromioclavicular Joint Trauma" and Chapter 12, "Glenohumeral Joint Trauma"). The scapula forms a central component of the superior shoulder suspensory complex. This is a bone and soft tissue ring that forms the fundamental attachment of the upper limb to the trunk. The components of the superior shoulder suspensory complex are the coracoid, glenoid, and acromial processes of the scapula; the AC joint; coracoclavicular ligament; and distal clavicle.

### Mechanism of Injury

Trauma to the scapula can take many forms, ranging from simple, nondisplaced scapular body fractures to complex injuries such as scapulothoracic dissociation. The scapulothoracic dissociation is a severe injury to the shoulder girdle with disruption of the scapulothoracic articulation, which is formed by the convex surface of the posterior thoracic cage and the concave surface of the anterior scapula. It has a strong association with brachial plexus and vascular injuries.

Scapular fractures are generally uncommon, accounting for less than 1% of all fractures. However, they are often associated with high-energy trauma such as motor vehicle collisions. Thus, they are often associated with other injuries such as rib and clavicle fractures, pulmonary contusion, and brachial plexus injury.

Scapular fractures can be caused from direct or indirect trauma. Direct trauma can result from high-impact blunt trauma to the shoulder, seen in motor vehicle collisions or falls from a sufficient height. Indirect trauma is less common cause and includes falls on an outstretched arm, causing the humeral head to impact on the glenoid cavity.

Specific classifications are not routinely used for scapular fractures. Most of these fractures involve the scapular spine and body. In routine radiology practice, fractures of the scapula can be divided depending on their anatomical location to those involving the body, neck, glenoid, acromion/scapular spine, and coracoid. These fractures may be simple or comminuted and extraarticular or intraarticular. Scapular fractures are associated with a variable amount of displacement. All these findings should be addressed in the radiology report.

Ideberg classification of scapular fractures is as follows:

- Ia, anterior rim fracture; Ib, posterior rim fracture
- II, fracture through the glenoid exiting the scapula laterally
- III, fracture through the glenoid exiting the scapula superiorly
- IV, fracture through the glenoid exiting the scapula medially
- V and VI, combinations of I-IV with increasing degrees of comminution

Coracoid process fractures (7% of cases):

- Type I proximal to the coracoclavicular ligament.
- Type II distal to the coracoclavicular ligament.

Acromion process fractures (8% of the cases):

- Type I nondisplaced or minimally displaced.
- Type II displaced but not involving the subacromial space.
- Type III displaced with compromised subacromial space.

## Imaging Strategy

- Chest and shoulder radiographs may incidentally identify scapular fractures (Figure 11.2A).
- Dedicated scapular views including frontal and transscapular/lateral projections are usually subsequently performed (Figures 11.2B and 11.2C).
- CT examination with coronal, sagittal, and 3D reformatted images is the diagnostic gold standard in evaluation of scapular fractures. (Figure 11.3).

### Imaging Findings

- Any part of the scapula can be fractured. Anatomic location, degree of comminution, amount of displacement, articular extension into the glenohumeral joint, articular surface step-off, associated fractures, and thoracic injuries should be noted.
- CT examination is superior to radiographs in the evaluation of scapular fractures.

## Treatment Options

- Usually, simple fractures, with no displaced bone fragments can be managed conservatively with immobilization, pain relief, and physiotherapy.

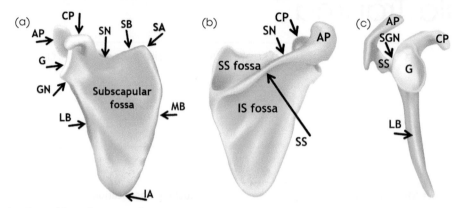

**Figure 11.1.** Artist drawings of the (A) anterior, (B) posterior, and (C) lateral aspects of the scapula show normal anatomic structures. AP = acromion process; CP = coracoid process; G = glenoid; GN = glenoid neck; IA = inferior angle; IS fossa = infraspinous fossa; LB = lateral border; MB = medial border; SA = superior angle; SB = superior border; SGN = spinoglenoid notch; SN = suprascapular notch; SS = scapular spine; SS fossa = supraspinous fossa.

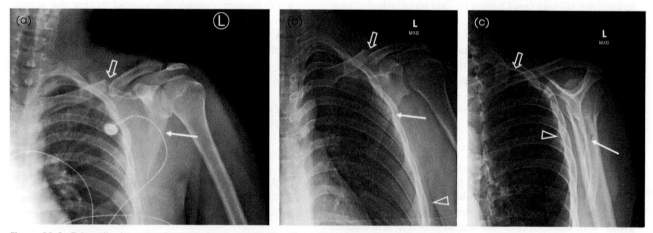

**Figure 11.2.** Extraarticular scapular body fracture. (A) AP radiograph of the left shoulder in a polytrauma patient status after a motor vehicle accident demonstrates a grossly nondisplaced extraarticular scapular body fracture (*arrow*). Note the associated displaced left mid clavicular shaft fracture (*open arrow*). Dedicated AP (B) and scapular Y (C) radiographs obtained 3 weeks later show healing scapular body (*arrow*) and clavicular midshaft (*open arrow*) fractures. Also note a healing left fifth rib fracture (*arrowhead*).

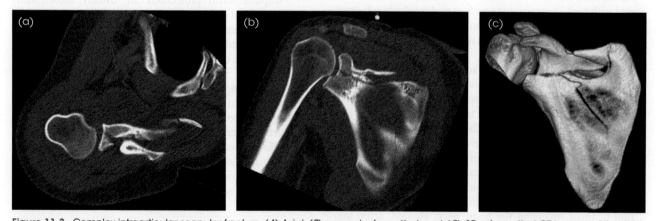

**Figure 11.3.** Complex intraarticular scapular fracture. (A) Axial, (B) coronal reformatted, and (C) 3D reformatted CT images of the right scapula demonstrate a complex comminuted fracture of the scapular body and glenoid extending into the glenohumeral joint with associated articular step-off at the glenoid articular surface.

- Surgical management is needed in injuries involving
  - Significantly displaced fractures of the glenoid neck and fossa
  - Disruption of the superior shoulder suspensory complex in which one or more elements of the scapula are significantly displaced

## Key Points

- The scapula forms a central component of the superior shoulder suspensory complex. This is an osseous and soft tissue ring that forms the fundamental connection between the upper limb and the trunk.
- Fractures of the scapula most commonly involve the body and spine. They are relatively uncommon, but are often associated with substantial trauma and additional injuries such as clavicle fracture, pulmonary contusion, or pneumothorax.
- Most scapular fractures are managed conservatively. However, comminuted fractures can involve injury to the superior shoulder suspensory complex and may require operative repair.
- Scapulothoracic dissociation occurs when there is severe injury to the shoulder girdle and disruption of the scapulothoracic articulation. It is often associated with significant vascular and brachial plexus injury.

## References

1. Baldwin KD, Ohman-Strickland P, Mehta S, Hume E. Scapula fractures: a marker for concomitant injury? A retrospective review of data in the National Trauma Database. *J Trauma.* 2008;65:430–35.
2. Cole PA, Freeman G, Dubin JR. Scapula fractures. *Curr Rev Musculoskelet Med.* 2013;6:79–87.

# CHAPTER 12

# Glenohumeral Joint Trauma

Michael O'Keeffe, Kiran Khursid, Peter L. Munk, and Mihra S. Taljanovic

## Basic Anatomy and Mechanism of Injury

### Basic Anatomy

The glenohumeral joint is formed by the articulation between the glenoid fossa of the scapula and the head of humerus. This is a multiaxial synovial ball and socket joint. Movements allowed at the glenohumeral joint include flexion; extension and 360-degree circumduction of the shoulder in the sagittal plane; abduction and adduction in the frontal plane; along with scapular protraction, retraction, elevation, and depression.

Only 25% of the humeral head fits in the glenoid fossa. This, along with the laxity of the joint capsule, makes it one of the most mobile joints in the body. However, this mobility comes at the cost of joint stability.

Stability of the glenohumeral joint is provided by the following:

- The glenoid labrum is a ring of cartilaginous fibers attached to the glenoid fossa making it deeper.
- The rotator cuff muscles, tendons, and ligaments include the supraspinatus, infraspinatus, teres minor, and subscapularis muscles and the glenohumeral ligaments. These structures support the joint anteriorly, superiorly, posteriorly, and inferiorly.

### Mechanism of Injury

The shoulder is one of the most frequently dislocated joints in the body. Injuries to the shoulder joint are a common sequela of trauma. These present with a wide variety of skeletal injury patterns. Injuries of the associated rotator cuff and labroligamentous structures are addressed in Chapter 104, "Internal Derangement of the Shoulder."

## Glenohumeral Joint Dislocations

### Types of Anterior and Inferior Glenohumeral Joint Dislocations

Anterior dislocation comprises approximately 95% of all glenohumeral joint dislocations and mostly occurs because of a direct blow to the shoulder or fall on an outstretched arm. The arm is typically abducted, extended, and externally rotated.

There are 4 main types of anterior dislocation of the shoulder:

1. Subcoracoid dislocation (anterior). In this type, the humeral head is displaced anterior and medial to the glenoid fossa, below the coracoid process of scapula (Figure 12.1). This is by far the most common type, with an occurrence of approximately 60% of all of the anterior dislocations. Findings include fixation of the greater tuberosity on the anterior glenoid rim while the neck of the scapula is elevated and shifted medially, resulting in the prominence of the tip of the scapula.

2. Subglenoid dislocation (anteroinferior). In this type, the humeral head is displaced anterior and inferior to the glenoid (Figure 12.2). As with subcoracoid dislocation, the humeral head also displaces medially. This dislocation comprises approximately 30% of the cases of anterior dislocations. These dislocations are associated with fractures of the greater tuberosity and/or anterior glenoid rim (bony Bankart lesion).

3. Subclavicular dislocation (anterior). In this rarer type of dislocation, the humeral head is displaced medially in relation to the coracoid, below the lower border of the clavicle. This along with true inferior dislocation comprises only approximately 4-10% of cases of anterior dislocations.

4. Luxatio erecta (Figure 12.3) or true inferior dislocation (0.5% of all shoulder dislocations). In this rare type, the humeral head is displaced inferior to the glenoid fossa and arm is fixed in abduction. Associated injuries include soft tissue trauma, fracture of the greater tuberosity and proximal humerus, and muscular avulsions.

The bony Bankart lesion is common with anterior dislocations and represents a fracture of the anterior inferior glenoid rim (Figure 12.4). Hill-Sachs injuries can also occur and represent posterosuperolateral humoral head impaction fractures because of impact of the humoral head on the anterior inferior glenoid (Figure 12.4).

The engaging Hill-Sachs lesion represents a defect of the humeral head that is large enough for the edge of the humeral head to drop over the anterior inferior glenoid rim during abduction and external rotation when the arm is at functional position.

Glenohumeral joint dislocations may be associated with rotator cuff injury, and the incidence of rotator cuff tendon injuries increases with patient's age. Conversely, younger patients have a lower rate of rotator cuff tendon injuries, but a higher redislocation rate.

### Posterior Glenohumeral Joint Dislocation

Posterior glenohumeral joint dislocations are rare, comprising 2-4% of all shoulder dislocations (Figure 12.5). They may be caused by violent muscle contractions such as those caused by

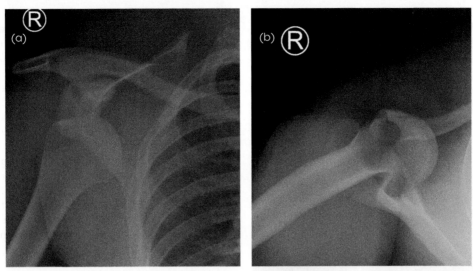

**Figure 12.1.** Subcoracoid anterior glenohumeral joint dislocation. (*A*) AP and (*B*) axillary radiographs of the right shoulder demonstrate anterior inferior dislocation of the humeral head from the glenoid fossa.

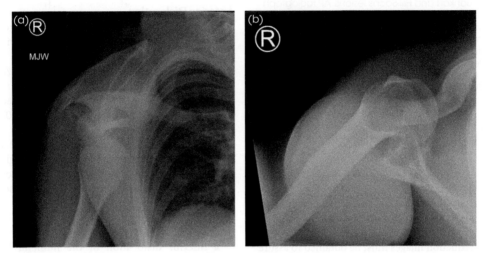

**Figure 12.2.** Subglenoid anterior glenohumeral joint dislocation. (*A*) AP and (*B*) axillary radiographs of the right shoulder demonstrate anterior inferior dislocation of the humeral head from the glenoid fossa, which is displaced anterior and inferior to the glenoid.

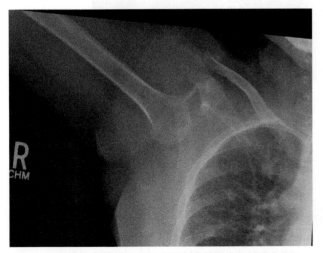

**Figure 12.3.** Luxatio erecta. AP radiograph of the left shoulder demonstrates inferior dislocation of the humeral head from the glenoid fossa with the arm fully abducted.

seizures or electrocution. The arm is typically adducted and internally rotated.

Fractures associated with posterior glenohumeral joint dislocation include the reverse bony Bankart lesion, which is a fracture of the posterior glenoid rim (Figure 12.6*A*); reverse Hill-Sachs lesion (Figures 12.6*A* and 12.6*B*), which is an impaction fracture at the anteromedial aspect of the humeral head; and sometimes lesser tuberosity fracture.

### Proximal Subluxation of the Humeral Head
With longstanding degenerative change and associated rotator cuff degeneration and tearing, the head of the humerus can migrate proximally. This is known as *pseudosubluxation* and can cause painful impingement symptoms when the subacromial space is narrowed (Figure 12.7).

### Inferior Subluxation of the Humeral Head
The humeral head is inferiorly positioned relative to the glenoid appearing to be subluxed when there is a large posttraumatic

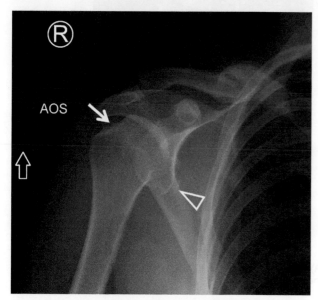

**Figure 12.4.** Bony Bankart and Hill-Sachs lesions. AP radiograph of the right shoulder after closed reduction of the anterior dislocation demonstrates a displaced mildly comminuted fracture of the anterior inferior glenoid rim consistent with a bony Bankart lesion (*arrowhead*) and impaction fracture at the posterosuperolateral aspect of the humeral head in keeping with a Hill-Sachs lesion (*arrow*). The glenohumeral joint is anatomically reduced.

hemarthrosis or lipohemarthrosis. This is also known as *inferior pseudosubluxation*.

## Imaging Strategy

- Imaging starts with dedicated shoulder radiographs that include AP views with external and internal rotation and axillary or scapular Y views.
- Post closed reduction images must be obtained to assure adequate reduction with anatomic alignment of the glenohumeral joint (Figures 12.4 and 12.6).

- CT examination may help in the evaluation of associated humeral head/tuberosity and glenoid rim fractures (Figure 12.8A–C) and with cases of engaging dislocation.
- CT examination is also helpful in preoperative planning in assessing the size of Hill-Sachs and bony Bankart lesions and the percent of glenoid bone loss.
- MRI is rarely needed for acute glenohumeral joint dislocations.
- MRI or magnetic resonance arthrography (MRA) (imaging modality of choice) are usually performed in the outpatient setting to evaluate for glenoid labral and capsular injuries, size of the Hill-Sachs lesion (Figure 12.8D) and size of the bony Bankart lesion (Figure 12.8E) with percent of glenoid involvement.

## Imaging Findings

### Anterior Dislocation

- The humeral head resides anterior to the glenohumeral joint (subcoracoid, subglenoid, subclavicular) (Figures 12.1 and 12.2).
- Hill-Sachs lesion (Figures 12.4, 12.8A and 12.8D). Impaction fracture at the posterosuperolateral aspect of the humeral head secondary to contact with the anterior glenoid rim, which is present in 80% of traumatic dislocations
- Bony Bankart lesion (Figures 12.4, 12.8B, 12.8C and 12.8E). Fracture of the anterior inferior glenoid, which is present in 49% of recurrent anterior dislocations
- Greater tuberosity fracture is usually seen in patients older than 50 years.

### Inferior Dislocation (Luxatio Erecta)

- Inferior dislocation of the humeral head from the glenoid fossa with arm fully abducted is shown in Figure 12.3.

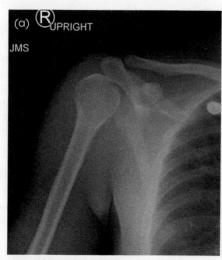
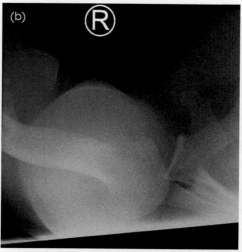

**Figure 12.5.** Posterior glenohumeral joint dislocation. (*A*) AP radiograph of the right shoulder demonstrates widening of the glenohumeral joint, which is held in fixed internal rotation. (*B*) Axillary radiograph of the same shoulder demonstrates posterior dislocation of the humeral head from the glenoid fossa.

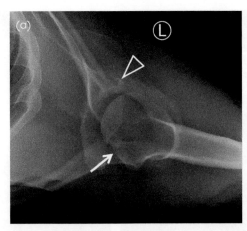
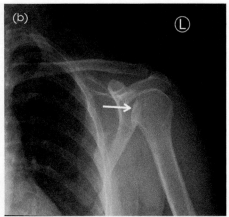

**Figure 12.6.** Reverse bony Bankart and reverse Hill-Sachs lesions. (*A*) Axillary radiograph of the left shoulder after closed reduction of the posterior glenohumeral joint dislocation demonstrates a small avulsed bone fragment off the posterior glenoid rim consistent with reverse bony Bankart lesion (*arrowhead*) and an impaction fracture at the anteromedial aspect of the humeral head in keeping with a reverse Hill-Sachs lesion (*arrow*). (*B*) AP radiograph of the same shoulder demonstrates a reverse Hill-Sachs lesion with a trough line sign at the anteromedial aspect of the humeral head (*arrow*).

## Posterior Dislocation

- Reverse Hill-Sachs lesion is an impaction fracture at the anteromedial aspect of the humeral head secondary to contact with the posterior glenoid rim (Figure 12.6).
- Trough line sign is seen on AP radiograph of the shoulder as a dense vertical line at the medial aspect of the humeral head representing an impaction fracture (reverse Hill-Sachs lesion) of the anteromedial humeral head (Figure 12.6*B*).
- Reverse bony Bankart lesion is a fracture of the posterior glenoid rim (Figure 12.6*A*).
- The humeral head is held in fixed internal rotation with glenohumeral joint-space widening (Figure 12.5*A*).
- Associated lesser tuberosity fracture may be seen with posterior dislocation.

## Proximal Subluxation-Pseudosubluxation
Refer to Figure 12.7.

- Decreased acromiohumeral distance (<7 mm) is associated with a massive rotator cuff tear. This is typically associated with muscular atrophy.
- Bony remodeling (acetabularization) of the undersurface of the acromion may be present.

## Inferior Subluxation-Pseudosubluxation

- Inferior subluxation of the humeral head from the glenoid—associated with a large posttraumatic hemarthrosis or lipohemarthrosis

## Treatment Options

- Acute anterior dislocation is treated with prompt closed reduction and immobilization followed by physical therapy.
- Surgical treatment for anterior dislocations depends on complications and includes but is not limited to glenoid augmentation with more than 20% of glenoid bone loss and various treatments of large and/or engaging

Hill-Sachs lesions that involve more than 25% of the humeral head.

- Acute inferior dislocation is treated with prompt closed reduction and immobilization. Surgical treatment may be subsequently performed for capsulolabral and rotator cuff repair.
- Acute posterior dislocation is treated with prompt closed reduction and immobilization in external rotation for 4-6 weeks.

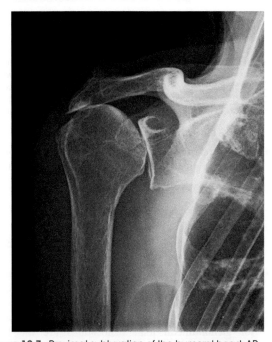

**Figure 12.7.** Proximal subluxation of the humeral head. AP radiograph of the right shoulder demonstrates proximal subluxation of the humeral head from the glenoid fossa with marked narrowing and near obliteration of the subacromial space and bony remodeling (acetabularization) of the undersurface of the acromion consistent with a massive chronic full-thickness rotator cuff tear.

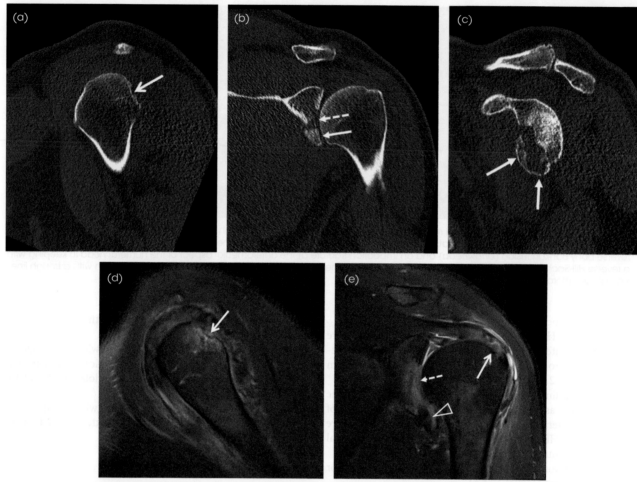

**Figure 12.8.** Hill-Sachs and bony Bankart lesions on the CT and MR images after closed reduction of the recurrent anterior glenohumeral joint dislocation in a middle-aged patient. (*A*) Sagittal reformatted CT image of the left shoulder shows a moderate-size Hill-Sachs lesion at the posterosuperolateral aspect of the humeral head (*arrow*). Coronal (*B*) and sagittal (*C*) reformatted CT images of the same shoulder show a large displaced bony Bankart lesion (*solid tip arrows*) with approximately 40% glenoid bone loss seen in (*C*). In (*B*) note a large bone defect in glenoid articular surface (*dashed arrow*). (*D*) T2W FS sagittal MR image of the same shoulder redemonstrates a moderate-sized Hill-Sachs lesion (*arrow*) with subjacent bone marrow edema. Note associated soft tissue edema. (*E*) Coronal T2W FS MR image demonstrates a large displaced bony Bankart lesion (*arrowhead*) with an associated large defect in the glenoid articular surface (*dashed arrow*). Note a high-grade partial-thickness undersurface supraspinatus tendon tear (*arrow*), periarticular soft tissue edema, tearing of the superior labrum, and mild thickening of the subacromial-subdeltoid bursa.

- Surgical treatment for posterior dislocations may be indicated in patients with recurrent posterior instability.

### Key Points

- The shoulder is one of the most frequently dislocated joints in the body.
- Anterior glenohumeral joint dislocations are much more common than other types, comprising approximately 95% of all shoulder dislocations.
- Common bone injuries associated with anterior glenohumeral joint dislocations are the bony Bankart (fracture of the anterior inferior glenoid rim) and Hill-Sachs lesions (impaction fracture at the posterosuperolateral aspect of the humeral head) and possible greater tuberosity fracture.

- Bone injuries associated with posterior glenohumeral joint dislocations are the reverse bony Bankart (fracture of the posterior glenoid rim) and reverse Hill-Sachs lesions (impaction fracture at the anteromedial aspect of the humeral head) and possible lesser tuberosity fracture.
- Diagnosis of glenohumeral joint dislocations is made on radiographs. Post closed reduction images must be obtained to assure adequate reduction.
- CT examination is useful in evaluation of associated bone lesions and glenoid bone loss.
- MRA is the study of choice in the evaluation of associated glenolabral and rotator cuff injuries.
- Treatment for acute glenohumeral joint dislocations is prompt closed reduction with immobilization and subsequent physical therapy. Surgical treatment is indicated for complicated dislocations with instability.

## Recommended Reading

Demehri S, Hafezi-Nejad N, Fishman EK. Advanced imaging of glenohumeral instability: the role of MRI and MDCT in providing what clinicians need to know. *Emerg Radiol.* 2017 Feb;24(1):95–103. doi:10.1007/s10140-016-1429-7.

Sheehan SE, Gaviola G, Gordon R, Sacks A, Shi LL, Smith SE. Traumatic shoulder injuries: a force mechanism analysis-glenohumeral dislocation and instability. *AJR Am J Roentgenol.* 2013 Aug;201(2):378–93. doi:10.2214/AJR.12.9986.

## References

1. Bencardino JT, Gyftopoulos S, Palmer WE. Imaging in anterior glenohumeral instability. *Radiology.* 2013 Nov;269(2):323–37. doi:10.1148/radiol.13121926.

2. Griffith JF, Antonio GE, Yung PS, et al. Prevalence, pattern, and spectrum of glenoid bone loss in anterior shoulder dislocation: CT analysis of 218 patients. *AJR Am J Roentgenol.* 2008;190(5):1247–54.

3. Gyftopoulos S, Albert M, Recht MP. Osseous injuries associated with anterior shoulder instability: what the radiologist should know. *AJR Am J Roentgenol.* 2014 Jun;202(6):W541–50. doi:10.2214/AJR.13.11824.

4. Gyftopoulos S, Yemin A, Beltran L, Babb J, Bencardino J. Engaging Hill-Sachs lesion: is there an association between this lesion and findings on MRI? *AJR Am J Roentgenol.* 2013 Oct;201(4):W633–38. doi:10.2214/AJR.12.10206.

5. Rouleau DM, Hebert-Davies J, Robinson CM. Acute traumatic posterior shoulder dislocation. *J Am Acad Orthop Surg.* 2014 Mar;22(3):145–52. doi:10.5435/JAAOS-22-03-145. [Erratum: *J Am Acad Orthop Surg.* 2014 Jun;22(6):401.]

# CHAPTER 13

# Humerus Trauma

Michael O'Keeffe, Kiran Khursid, Peter L. Munk, and Mihra S. Taljanovic

## Basic Anatomy and Mechanism of Injury

### Basic Anatomy

The humerus is the long bone of the arm connecting the shoulder to the elbow. It is roughly divided into 3 sections:

1. The *upper/proximal* section consists of the head, neck, and 2 tuberosities, greater and lesser. The constriction below the tuberosities is called the *surgical neck of the humerus*, a commonly fractured part of the bone. The anatomic neck connects the humeral head (epiphysis) with the proximal humeral metaphysis and is uncommonly injured.
2. The *mid/diaphysis* section is cylindrical at the proximal aspect and flattens to become prismatic distally.
3. The *lower/distal* section consists of 2 epicondyles (medial and lateral); 2 processes, the trochlea and capitellum (capitulum); and 3 fossae, the radial, coronoid, and olecranon.

At the shoulder, the head of humerus articulates with the glenoid fossa of the scapula, forming the glenohumeral joint. Distally, the capitellum and trochlea of the humerus articulate with the head of the radius and trochlear notch of the ulna, respectively, forming the elbow joint.

### Mechanism of Injury

Fractures of the humerus are common presentations to emergency departments and a number of fracture patterns are frequently encountered.

Fractures of the surgical neck of the humerus are extremely common. In the elderly, these fractures are often caused by a fall on an outstretched hand (FOOSH) with the force being transmitted to the neck of the humerus or direct fall onto the shoulder. In younger patients, a high-energy trauma with direct impact, such as motor vehicle collision, is the most likely etiology. These fractures can cause significant morbidity because of pain and restricted range of motion.

Proximal humerus fractures are often classified with the *Neer classification*, which is based on the number of fracture parts and degree of displacement (Figure 13.1). The Neer classification system divides the proximal humerus into 4 parts (greater tuberosity, lesser tuberosity, articular surface, and shaft) and considers not the fracture line, but the displacement as being significant to classification. A fracture part is considered displaced if the fragment is displaced by more than 1 cm or if there is larger than a 45-degree angulation (Figures 13.2 and 13.3).

- One-part fractures (70-80% of the proximal humerus fractures) may involve 1-4 parts, however, without significant displacement or angulation (Figure 13.1A).
- Two-part fractures (approximately 20% of proximal humerus fractures) may involve 2-4 parts; one of the parts is displaced more than 1 cm or angulated more than 45 degrees. The most commonly involved is the surgical neck followed by the greater tuberosity (Figure 13.1B). These fractures may be seen in association with anterior glenohumeral joint dislocation.
- Three-part fractures (approximately 5% of proximal humerus fractures) involve 3-4 parts; 2 of the parts are displaced more than 1 cm or angulated more than 45 degrees. The most common pattern includes the greater tuberosity and humeral shaft, which are displaced with respect to the lesser tuberosity and articular surface. Alternatively, the lesser tuberosity and humeral shaft are displaced with respect to the greater tuberosity and articular surface (Figure 13.1C).
- Four-part fractures (<1% of proximal humerus fractures) involve more than 4 parts; 3 parts are displaced more than 1 cm or angulated more than 45 degrees (Figure 13.1D). With this type of injury, the articular surface is no longer attached to any parts of the humerus that are attached to soft tissues. ON of the humeral head is a common complication.

*Fractures of the mid shaft (diaphysis) of the humerus* often occur secondary to direct trauma such as injury secondary to falls (Figure 13.4). Radial nerve injury may be seen with mid humeral shaft fracture where the nerve travels within the spiral groove located in the posterior aspect of the shaft, resulting in wrist drop, muscular weakness, and sensory loss along the distribution of the nerve.

Descriptive classification of the humeral shaft fractures is frequently used in everyday practice based on

- Fracture location (eg, proximal, middle, or distal third)
- Fracture pattern (eg, spiral, transverse, comminuted)

*Pathological fractures* may occur in any bone, but the long bones such as the humerus are quite susceptible. A history of fracture with minimal or no history of trauma should raise suspicion of a pathological fracture.

| **(a) One-Part Fracture** | |
|---|---|
| No or minimal displacement and no or minimal angulation of any or all of the four anatomic segments(Anatomic neck/articular surface, Shaft/Surgical Neck, Greater Tuberosity, Lesser Tuberosity) | 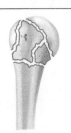 |

| **(b) Two-Part (one segment displaced)** | |
|---|---|
| Articular Segment (Anatomic Neck) | 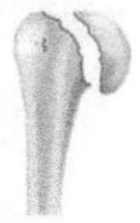 |
| Shaft Segment (Surgical Neck), displaced segment may be impacted or unimpacted, without or with comminution | 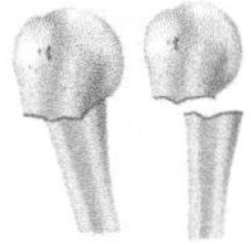 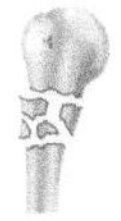 |
| Greater Tuberosity segment | 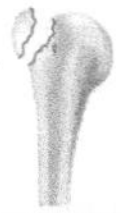 |
| Lesser Tuberosity Segment | 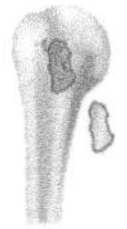 |

| **(c) Three-Part (two segments displaced; one tuberosity remains in continuity with humeral head)** | |
|---|---|
| Surgical Neck and Greater Tuberosity Segments | 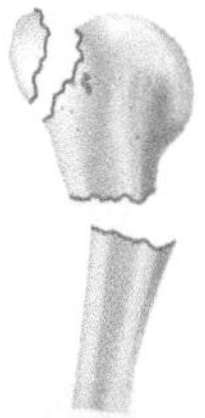 |
| Surgical Neck and Lesser Tuberosity Segments | 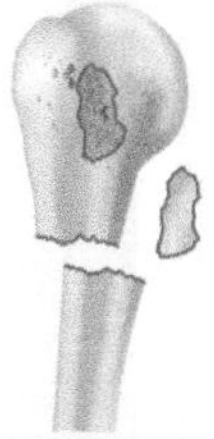 |

| **(d) Four-Part (three segments displaced)** | |
|---|---|
| Surgical neck, Greater and Lesser Tuberosity Segments | 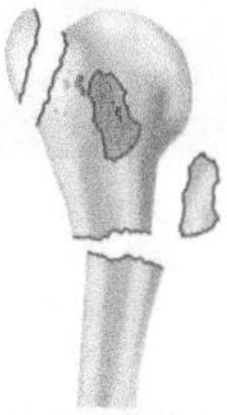 |

**Figure 13.1.** Neer 4-segment (greater tuberosity, lesser tuberosity, articular surface and shaft) classification of the proximal humerus fractures: (A) 1-part, (B) 2-part, (C) 3-part, and (D) 4-part fractures. A fracture part is considered displaced if the fragment is displaced by more than 1 cm or if there is greater than 45-degree angulation.

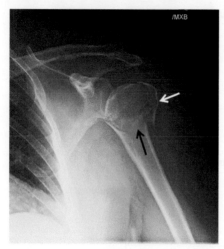

**Figure 13.2.** Two-part Neer fracture. Humeral surgical neck fracture in a 62-year-old woman after a fall. AP view of the left shoulder shows a nondisplaced fracture of the surgical neck of the humerus (*black arrow*) and a mildly displaced greater tuberosity fracture. Note minimal inferior pseudosubluxation of the humeral head secondary to hemarthrosis. This fracture healed with conservative treatment.

*Fractures of the distal humerus* frequently occur in the supracondylar region (Figure 13.5), especially in children. Displaced supracondylar fractures may be complicated by intraarticular extension into the elbow joint, radial nerve injury, or brachial artery injury. Fractures of the medial epicondyle of the humerus can also be associated with ulnar nerve injury.

Distal humerus fractures are often classified based on *AO/OTA classification.* Owing to the frequent involvement of the growth plate in children, these are associated with development of serious complications, such as Volkmann ischemic contracture.

- Extraarticular (A)—extraarticular (supracondylar), 80% extension type (Figure 13.5)
- Partial articular (B)—single column (isolated condylar, coronal shear, epicondyle)

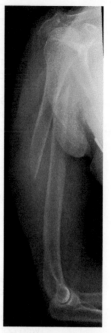

**Figure 13.4.** Displaced mid humeral diaphyseal fracture in a 74-year-old woman after a ground-level fall. AP radiograph of the right humerus shows a displaced and rotated oblique fracture of the mid humeral diaphysis/shaft. This fracture was treated operatively with plate and screw fixation. The patient also had associated radial nerve contusion with transient palsy, which completely resolved in a few months.

- Complete articular (C)—intraarticular, both columns fractured with no portion of the joint contiguous with the shaft (complete articular)

## Imaging Strategy
- Dedicated radiographs of the shoulder, humerus, and elbow are used.
- CT examination is frequently used in preoperative planning.
- MRI is rarely indicated.

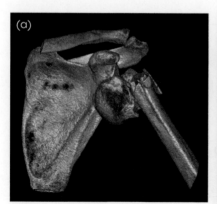
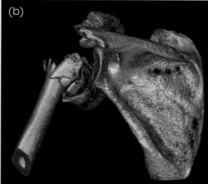
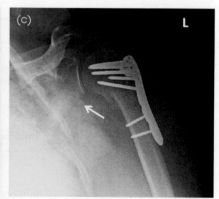

**Figure 13.3.** Three-part Neer fracture. Subcoracoid anterior glenohumeral joint dislocation in a 57-year-old man after a fall 15 feet from a ladder. 3D reformatted CT images of the left shoulder show a comminuted displaced 3-part fracture of the proximal humerus viewed from the anterior aspect in (*A*) and from the posterior aspect in (*B*). Note involvement of the surgical neck and greater tuberosity and anterior dislocation of the glenohumeral joint. (*C*) Grashey AP radiograph of the left shoulder. The fracture was treated with ORIF with a periarticular locking plate and multiple screws. Note anatomically reduced glenohumeral joint and a small displaced fracture fragment off the anterior inferior glenoid rim consistent with bony Bankart lesion (*arrow*).

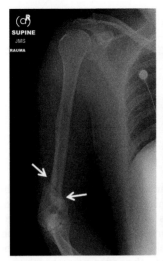
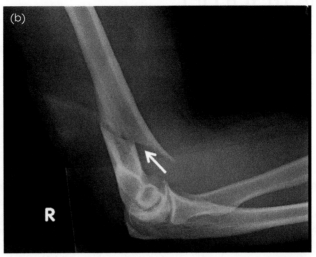

**Figure 13.5.** Humeral supracondylar fracture in a 45-year-old man after a car fell on his arm while he was working underneath it. (*A*) AP radiograph of the right humerus and (*B*) lateral radiograph of the right elbow show a moderately displaced oblique supracondylar fracture of the distal humerus (*arrows*), which was treated operatively with a lateral periarticular locking plate and multiple screws.

■ US examination is useful in suspected radial nerve injuries.

## Imaging Findings
■ Radiographs are used to describe the anatomic location, open versus closed fracture, number of fracture fragments, impaction, displacement, rotation and angulation of the fracture fragments, and presence of articular extension or subluxation/dislocation.
■ Pseudosubluxation of the glenohumeral joint–Inferior subluxation of the humeral head is associated with proximal humerus fractures seen in the presence of hemarthrosis or lipohemarthrosis.
■ CT examination with coronal, sagittal, and 3D reformatted images (Figures 13.3*A* and 13.3*B*) provides more detailed evaluation of the fracture patterns.
■ MRI is rarely needed for acute injuries. It may be used to evaluate for concomitant rotator cuff tears associated with proximal humerus fractures.

## Treatment Options
■ Proximal humerus fractures–Most proximal humerus fractures are minimally displaced and can be treated nonoperatively. Displaced comminuted fractures are treated operatively (Figure 13.3*C*). Extensive physiotherapy is required postoperatively.
■ Most humeral shaft fractures may be treated nonoperatively. Absolute indications for operative treatment are open fractures, neurovascular injuries, ipsilateral forearm fracture with floating elbow, and compartment syndrome.
■ Most distal humerus fractures are treated operatively.

## Key Points
■ Fractures of the humerus are commonly associated with trauma and may involve the proximal humerus (most commonly the surgical neck), the humeral diaphysis or the distal humerus (most commonly the supracondylar region).
■ Multidetector computed tomography (MDCT) is particularly useful for assessment of proximal humerus fractures and for preoperative planning.
■ Fractures of the humeral diaphysis may be associated with radial nerve injury, whereas supracondylar fractures are sometimes associated with brachial artery injuries.
■ Fractures of the medial epicondyle of the humerus can also be associated with ulnar nerve injury.

## References
1. Brorson S, Bagger J, Sylvest A, et al. Diagnosing displaced four-part fractures of the proximal humerus: a review of observer studies. *Int Orthop*. 2009;33(2):323–27.
2. Murray IR, Amin AK, White TO, Robinson CM. Proximal humeral fractures: current concepts in classification, treatment and outcomes. *J Bone Joint Surg Br*. 2011;93(1):1–11.
3. Sandstrom CK, Kennedy SA, Gross JA. Acute shoulder trauma: what the surgeon wants to know. *Radiographics*. 2015;35:475–92.
4. Sheehan SE, Dyer GS, Sidockson AD, Patel KI, Khurana B. Traumatic elbow injuries: what the orthopedic surgeon wants to know. *Radiographics*. 2013;33:869–88.

# CHAPTER 14

# Elbow Trauma

Michael O'Keeffe, Kiran Khursid, Peter L. Munk, and Mihra S. Taljanovic

## Basic Anatomy and Mechanism of Injury

### Basic Anatomy

The elbow is a synovial hinge joint consisting of 3 articulating bones, including the humerus, ulna, and radius. It is surrounded by a common capsule. The joints forming the elbow are the

- Humeroulnar (humerotrochlear, ulnohumeral) joint
- Humeroradial (radiocapitellar) joint
- Proximal radioulnar joint

Additional stability to the elbow joint is provided by the joint capsule, which is thickened peripherally to form collateral ligaments (ie, the radial and ulnar collateral ligamentous complexes). The humeral epicondyles are located outside the joint capsule. The anterior and posterior fat pads are extrasynovial and located under the fibrous joint capsule, which explains their displacement with the presence of elbow joint effusion.

- The *ulnar collateral ligament complex* originates from the medial humeral epicondyle and attaches to the coronoid process and adjacent proximal ulna and olecranon.
- The *radial collateral ligament complex* extends from the lateral humeral epicondyle and attaches to the annular ligament, which encircles the radial head, and onto the supinator crest of the ulna.

The collateral ligaments of the elbow are described in detail in Chapter 105, "Internal Derangements of the Elbow."

Bursae serve to limit the friction between adjacent structures. The subcutaneous olecranon bursa is frequently distended with traumatic conditions of the elbow.

The range of movement at the elbow varies from 0 degrees of elbow extension to 150 degrees of elbow flexion. Pronation and supination occur at the nearby radioulnar joint, but not at the elbow joint itself.

### Mechanism of Injury

The elbow joint may be injured secondary to direct trauma or with transmitted forces from an injury such as a fall on an outstretched hand.

Fractures of the olecranon process of the ulna are common injuries, often sustained following a direct fall onto the elbow. These can vary from nondisplaced fractures to more complex, displaced injuries that demonstrate intraarticular extension into the elbow joint (Figure 14.1). Because of the disruption of the articular surface of the elbow joint in this type of injury, operative management with ORIF is the treatment of choice.

Fractures of the neck and head of the radius are also common injuries, particularly in the adult population. These often occur following direct trauma to the elbow joint (Figure 14.2). Clinically, they often present with pain and decreased range of motion, particularly with pronation and supination.

Nondisplaced radial head fractures can be subtle on radiographs. These should always be suspected in cases of direct trauma to the elbow with a joint effusion and decreased range of motion. Short interval follow-up radiographs in 7-10 days or MRI is recommended for further evaluation.

The elbow joint is the second most commonly dislocated large joint of the body (after the glenohumeral joint). The most common direction of dislocation is posterior (Figure 14.3). This occurs most often secondary to a fall on an arm with the elbow flexed.

Elbow dislocation may occur in isolation (simple) or in association with fractures (complex) such as the coronoid or olecranon process of the ulna and/or the radial head. Associated injury to the ulnar nerve is not uncommon in elbow dislocation as it passes near the medial epicondyle of the distal humerus.

Soft tissue injury to the elbow can involve any of the supporting structures of the elbow and is further described in Chapter 105, "Internal Derangements of the Elbow."

## Imaging Strategy

- Dedicated AP, oblique, and lateral radiographs are the mainstay of initial assessment and follow-up of elbow fractures and dislocations. These can provide useful pre- and postreduction assessment.
- More complex elbow fractures and fracture/dislocation injuries, which involve comminuted bone fragments and intraarticular extension, frequently require CT examination for preoperative planning (Figure 14.4).
- MRI is the imaging modality of choice in the diagnosis of occult elbow fractures and is performed in some institutions in the setting of acute trauma with suspected occult radial head fractures that cannot be seen on radiographs.

## Imaging Findings

- With olecranon fractures, look for the degree of comminution, articular extension, and displacement and distraction of fracture fragments.

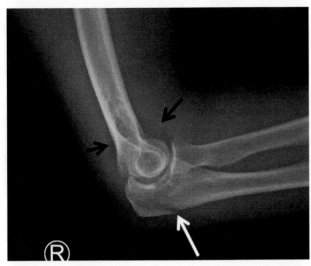

**Figure 14.1.** Olecranon fracture. Minimally displaced transverse intraarticular olecranon fracture in a 48-year-old man. Lateral radiograph of the elbow shows a minimally displaced fracture line (*white arrow*) and elevation of the anterior and posterior fat pads (*black arrows*) consistent with a joint effusion. The fracture was treated with ORIF.

- AO/OTA classification is the simplest of several existing classifications and divides the olecranon fractures into extraarticular, intraarticular, and intraarticular fractures with associated radial head fracture.
- With radial head and neck fractures, look for the degree of comminution, displacement, and articular surface depression. Mason classification of radial head fractures is shown in Table 14.1.

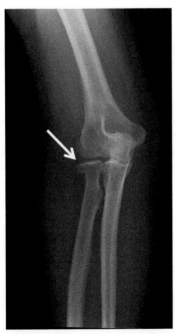

**Figure 14.2.** Radial head fracture. Mildly displaced (Mason type I) radial head fracture in a 48-year-old male patient after a fall. AP radiograph of the elbow shows a mildly displaced intraarticular fracture of the radial head (*arrow*), which was treated conservatively.

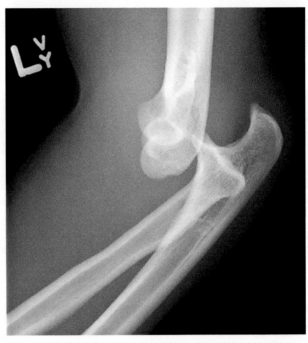

**Figure 14.3.** Posterior dislocation of the elbow joint. Lateral radiograph of the elbow shows posterior dislocation of the proximal radius and ulna with respect to the distal humerus with substantial overlying soft tissue swelling.

- With elbow dislocations, look for the direction in which the distal fragments are displaced and for the presence of associated fractures (ulnar coronoid, olecranon process, radial head).
- On post closed reduction radiographs, look for congruency of the elbow joint.
- CT examination can better delineate the degree of comminution, orientation of the fracture fragments, and intraarticular bone fragments.
- Bone contusion on MRI will show high signal intensity on fluid-sensitive sequences, whereas the fracture line, if present, will often show linear low signal intensity.

## Treatment Options
- Nondisplaced olecranon fractures and displaced fractures in low-demand elderly patients are treated conservatively. Transverse olecranon fractures without comminution and comminuted and displaced olecranon fractures require surgical treatment most of the time.
- Nondisplaced and minimally displaced (type I) radial head fractures are treated conservatively. Displaced fractures (type II-IV) require surgical treatment, which varies from ORIF to radial head excision or replacement depending on injury and fracture severity.
- All elbow dislocations are initially close reduced and splinted. Simple dislocations without associated fractures may be treated conservatively, whereas complex dislocations with associated fractures require surgical treatment.

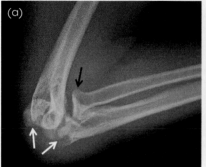 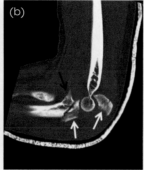 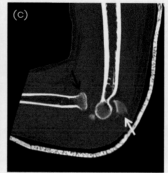 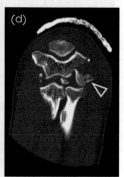

**Figure 14.4.** Anterior dislocation of the elbow. Dislocation associated with a comminuted displaced and distracted olecranon fracture and a comminuted displaced capitellar fracture in a 30-year-old man who fell from the border fence. (*A*) Lateral radiograph of the elbow shows anterior dislocation of the radial head with respect to the distal humerus (*black arrow*) and a distracted transverse fracture of the olecranon (*white arrows*). (*B*) and (*C*) sagittal and (*D*) coronal reformatted CT images of the same elbow obtained for preoperative planning show anterior dislocation of the elbow (*black arrows*) with a displaced, distracted, transverse olecranon fracture (*white arrows*) and a displaced comminuted capitellar fracture (*arrowhead*).

## Table 14.1. Mason Classification of the Radial Head Fractures

| Type I | Minimally displaced fracture, no mechanical block to rotation, intraarticular displacement <2 mm |
|---|---|
| Type II | Displaced fracture >2 mm or angulated, possible mechanical block to forearm rotation |
| Type III | Comminuted and displaced fracture, mechanical block to motion |
| Type IV (Hotchkiss modification) | Radial head fracture with elbow dislocation |

### Key Points

- Fractures of the bones about the elbow joint can result from either direct trauma or transmitted forces such as from a fall on an outstretched hand.
- The olecranon and radial head/neck are the most commonly fractured bones involved in the elbow joint in the adult population. This is in contrast to the pediatric population, in which supracondylar fractures of the distal humerus are more common.
- The elbow joint is the second most commonly dislocated joint in the body after the glenohumeral joint. It is most commonly dislocated posteriorly, often after a fall onto a flexed elbow.
- Treatment options for olecranon and radial head fractures vary from conservative to surgical management depending on complexity of injury.

- All elbow dislocations are initially close reduced and splinted. Further conservative versus operative treatment depends on complexity of injury.

### References

1. Goldflam K. Evaluation and treatment of the elbow and forearm injuries in the emergency department. *Emerg Med Clin North Am.* 2015;33(2):409–21.
2. Kuhn MA, Ross G. Acute elbow dislocations. *Orthop Clin North Am.* 2008;39(2):155–61.
3. Rosas HG, Lee KS. Imaging acute trauma of the elbow. *Semin Musculoskelet Radiol.* 2010;14(4):394–411.
4. Sheehan SE, Dyer GS, Sidockson AD, Patel KI, Khurana B. Traumatic elbow injuries: what the orthopedic surgeon wants to know. *Radiographics.* 2013;33:869–88.

# CHAPTER 15

# Radius and Ulna Trauma

Michael O'Keeffe, Kiran Khursid, Peter L. Munk, and Mihra S. Taljanovic

## Basic Anatomy and Mechanism of Injury

### Basic Anatomy
The 2 bones of the forearm include the radius and ulna, which connect the elbow and the wrist joints.

### Principle Articulations
- The *proximal and distal radioulnar joints* are formed by articulation between the upper and lower ends of the radius and ulna, respectively. The shafts of the radius and ulna are connected by an intraosseous membrane.
- Superiorly, the head of radius and trochlear notch of the ulna articulate with the distal humerus to form the *elbow joint*.
- Inferiorly, the distal radius articulates with the carpal bones (scaphoid and lunate) forming the radiocarpal or *wrist joint*.
- At the ulnar side of the wrist, the triangular fibrocartilage separates the distal ulna from the triquetrum.

### Mechanism of Injury
Fractures of the forearm are most often caused by direct trauma. Fractures are often displaced because of the degree of force required to fracture either the radius or ulna. Redistribution of these forces can also result in dislocation of some of the previously mentioned articulations.

### Nightstick Fractures
Nightstick fractures are isolated ulnar fractures, typically at the mid diaphysis, which usually result from a direct blow.

### Monteggia Fracture-Dislocation
The Monteggia fracture-dislocation injury consists of a displaced fracture of the proximal ulnar diaphysis (in type IV, there is an additional fracture of the proximal radial diaphysis) with an associated dislocation of the radial head. The most common mechanism is a fall on an outstretched hand.

The Bado classification describes Monteggia fracture-dislocations according to the direction of dislocation of the radial head:

- Type I: Anterior dislocation of the radial head (most common) (Figure 15.1)
- Type II: Posterior dislocation of the radial head (Figure 15.2)
- Type III: Lateral dislocation of the radial head
- Type IV: Anterior dislocation of the radial head with proximal radial and ulnar fractures

### Galeazzi Fracture-Dislocation
This injury involves a fracture of the distal radial diaphysis or metadiaphysis with associated disruption of the distal radioulnar joint (DRUJ) (Figure 15.3). These are most commonly caused by a fall on an outstretched hand, however, they are more common in the pediatric population.

### Essex-Lopresti Fracture-Dislocation
The injury is named after Peter Essex-Lopresti who first described it in 1951. Essex- Lopresti fracture-dislocation is a rare injury that encompasses the triad of a comminuted radial head fracture, DRUJ dislocation, and interosseous membrane disruption, all resulting in DRUJ instability (Figure 15.4). This injury usually occurs from a fall from a height with high-impact trauma to the forearm.

The triad of injury is difficult to diagnose because initial attention is usually given to the radial head injury. This often results in overlooking the DRUJ injury, which can cause later complications, including proximal migration of radius.

Major complications of forearm fractures include

- Neurovascular injury, particularly to the median, radial, and ulnar nerves with resultant paresthesia in the distribution of these nerves is a serious complication.
- Nonunion or malunion, although a serious complication, is relatively uncommon, particularly with modern surgical techniques including ORIF.
- Compartment syndrome is associated with increased pressure in one or more of the anatomical compartments of the forearm with resultant insufficient blood supply. This can occur secondary to the initial trauma or following attempted surgical repair and can lead to permanent neurovascular deficit.

## Imaging Strategy
- Radiographs are the mainstay in initial evaluation and treatment follow-up of forearm fractures.
- In addition to forearm radiographs, dedicated radiographs of the elbow and wrist joint are needed.
- CT examination may help in further characterization of radial head, ulnar coronoid, and olecranon fractures.

### Imaging Findings
- Radius and ulnar diaphyseal fractures—Describe the location, amount of comminution, displacement, degree of angulation and rotation at the fracture site according to the position of the distal fragment. Angulation at the

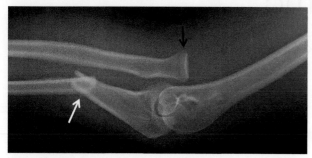

**Figure 15.1.** Type I Monteggia fracture-dislocation in a 22-year-old woman after a motor vehicle collision. Lateral radiograph of the left elbow shows a displaced, angulated, transverse fracture of the proximal ulnar diaphysis (*white arrow*) associated with anterior dislocation of the radial head (*black arrow*). The patient was treated with plate and screw fixation of the ulnar fracture and closed reduction of the radial head dislocation.

fracture site may also be described according to orientation of the angle apex.

- Monteggia fracture-dislocation (Figures 15.1 and 15.2)—Look for the complexity of the proximal ulnar fracture, possible proximal radius fracture and direction of the radial head dislocation. Look for additional fractures.

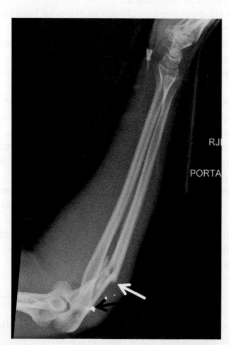

**Figure 15.2.** Type II Monteggia fracture-dislocation in a 22-year-old man after a gunshot wound. Lateral radiograph of the left forearm shows a mildly posteriorly displaced, mildly comminuted, transverse fracture of the proximal ulnar diaphysis (*white arrow*) with multiple metallic bullet fragments in the adjacent soft tissues associated with posterior dislocation of the radial head (*black arrow*). The patient was treated with plate and screw fixation of the ulnar fracture and closed reduction of the radial head dislocation.

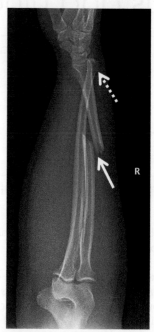

**Figure 15.3.** Galeazzi fracture-dislocation in a 38-year-old man after an all-terrain vehicle accident. An AP radiograph of the right forearm shows a displaced oblique fracture of the mid radial diaphysis (*white arrow*) associated with dislocation of the DRUJ (*dashed arrow*). The patient was treated with plate and screw fixation of the radial fracture and closed reduction of the DRUJ.

- Galeazzi fracture-dislocation (Figure 15.3)—Look for the complexity of the radial diaphyseal fracture. Look for DRUJ dislocation or subluxation, which may not be readily evident on the initial radiographs.
- Essex-Lopresti fracture-dislocation (Figure 15.4)—Look for the complexity of the radial head fracture and dislocation and/or subluxation of the DRUJ, which may not be readily evident on initial radiographs.

## Treatment Options

- Radius and ulna diaphyseal fractures—Depending on the amount of displacement (50%) and angulation (<10 degrees), isolated nightstick fractures of the ulnar diaphysis may be treated nonoperatively. Significantly displaced and angulated ulnar diaphyseal and both bone (radius and ulna) diaphyseal fractures are typically treated operatively.
- Monteggia fracture/dislocation—Most of these fractures in adults are treated operatively. In children, stable fractures are treated with casting following successful closed reduction.
- Galeazzi fracture-dislocation is treated with ORIF of the radial diaphyseal or metadiaphyseal fractures and closed reduction of the DRUJ.
- Essex-Lopresti fracture-dislocation is treated with radial head excision or replacement with complex fractures and closed reduction of the DRUJ.

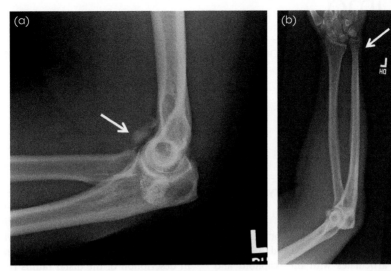

**Figure 15.4.** Essex-Lopresti fracture-dislocation in a 61-year-old man who fell from a ladder. (*A*) Lateral radiograph of the left elbow shows a displaced comminuted radial head fracture (*arrow*). (*B*) Lateral radiograph of the left forearm shows disruption/dislocation of the DRUJ (*arrow*). The patient was treated with radial head replacement and closed reduction of the DRUJ.

## Key Points

- Depending on their complexity, isolated fractures of the ulnar diaphysis may be treated nonoperatively or operatively, whereas both bone (radius and ulna) diaphyseal fractures are typically treated operatively.
- Fractures of the radius or ulna are usually caused by direct trauma and are often displaced.
- Forearm fractures can be associated with dislocation of the DRUJ (Galeazzi and Essex-Lopresti fracture-dislocations) or dislocation of the radial head (Monteggia fracture-dislocation).

## References

1. Konrad GG, Kundel K, Kreuz PC, et al. Monteggia fractures in adults: long-term results and prognostic factors. *J Bone Joint Surg Br.* 2007;89(3):354–60.
2. Reckling FW. Unstable fracture-dislocations of the forearm (Monteggia and Galeazzi lesions). *J Bone Joint Surg Am.* 1982;64(6):857–63.
3. Sheehan SE, Dyer GS, Sodickson AD, Patel KI, Khurana B. Traumatic elbow injuries: what the orthopedic surgeon wants to know. *Radiographics.* 2013;33(3):869–88. doi:10.1148/rg.333125176.

# CHAPTER 16

# Wrist Trauma

Michael O'Keeffe, Kiran Khursid, Peter L. Munk, and Mihra S. Taljanovic

## Basic Anatomy and Mechanism of Injury

### Basic Anatomy

The wrist is a complex joint consisting of 3 compartments including the radiocarpal, distal radioulnar and midcarpal joints. The distal radius articulates with the scaphoid and lunate bones at the scaphoid and lunate fossae. The triangular fibrocartilage (TFC) separates the distal ulna from the triquetrum. Ulnar variance compares the length of the distal radius and ulna, measured at the distal aspect of the distal radioulnar joint (DRUJ). The difference between ulnar and radial length of less than 1mm is considered neutral ulnar variance. A distal ulnar length of greater than 1mm more than that of the distal radius implies positive ulnar variance, and a distal radial length of more than 1mm greater than that of the distal ulna suggests negative ulnar variance. The negative ulnar variance is associated with lunatomalacia (Kienböck disease) and ulnar impingement syndrome (bony remodeling with subsequent degenerative changes of the DRUJ). The positive ulnar variance is associated with ulnar impaction/abutment syndrome with development of BME and subchondral cystlike changes in the proximal ulnar corner of the lunate, proximal radial aspect of the triquetrum, and the distal ulnar head with central degeneration and subsequent tearing of the TFC. Normal alignment and measurements of the wrist are shown in Figure 16.1.

The carpus is made of 8 small bones arranged in 2 rows. The proximal row contains the scaphoid, lunate, triquetrum, and pisiform bones, and the distal row contains the trapezium, trapezoid, capitate, and hamate bones arranged from radial to ulnar sides (Figure 16.2). The midcarpal joint communicates normally with the common carpometacarpal joint (second through fifth). The trapezium articulates with the first metacarpal base at the first carpometacarpal joint, which does not communicate with the midcarpal or common carpometacarpal joints. Movements at the wrist include flexion, extension, adduction, abduction, and circumduction.

### Distal Radius and Ulna Fractures

Fractures of the distal radius are extremely common. They occur in all age groups, often because of a fall on an outstretched hand (FOOSH). This mechanism usually results in dorsiflexion and ulnar deviation of the hand, in combination with supination of the carpus against the fixed pronated forearm. The elderly are particularly susceptible to distal radius fractures because of increased rates of osteoporosis. Distal radius fractures in older patients typically result from low-energy trauma (eg, falls), whereas in younger patients, these fractures result from high-energy trauma (eg, motor vehicle collisions). Associated injuries of the DRUJ, radial and ulnar styloid process, and soft tissue/ligaments are common. There are several classifications of distal radius fractures including the Frykman classification, which is based on joint involvement (Table 16.1). There are also several eponyms used in description of the distal radius fractures that are listed in Table 16.2.

The most common eponymous fracture of the distal radius is the *Colles* fracture, which involves a distal radial metaphysis with dorsal displacement and angulation of the distal fracture fragment (Figure 16.3).

Approximately 1 in 6 of all fractures presenting to the emergency department are of the distal radius. Some of the intraarticular distal radius fractures are complex and involve both the radiocarpal joint and DRUJ (Figure 16.4). Die-punch fractures are intraarticular fractures characterized by a depression of the lunate fossa at the distal radial articular surface (Figure 16.5).

Distal radius fractures are commonly associated with fractures of the ulnar styloid process. This is often a *stable* injury that usually heals with conservative management. More substantial fractures through the base of the ulnar styloid can lead to significant ligamentous injury of the triangular fibrocartilage complex (TFCC), which can lead to long-term wrist instability.

### Carpal Bone Fractures

Carpal bone fractures may occur in isolation or in predictable combinations as a result of a FOOSH. These fractures can also result from crashing injuries. Most carpal bone fractures occur at the *zone of vulnerability*, which follows the direction of the major volar extrinsic wrist ligaments, which are described in Chapter 106, "Internal Derangements of the Wrist and Hand." The starting point is the radial styloid process. It includes the waist and proximal pole of the scaphoid and the scapholunate joint, extending distally through the body of the capitate and the capitolunate joint. It then turns ulnarly to include the base of the hamate, the lunotriquetral joint, and finally the ulnar styloid process (Figure 16.6).

Carpal bone subluxations result from ligamentous disruption involving the lunate, scaphoid, and capitate. They may or may not be associated with carpal fractures or dislocations. The alignment of the long axis of the capitate, lunate, and scaphoid on the lateral view is assessed for carpal instability. The scapholunate angle normally ranges between 30 and 60 degrees, and the normal capitolunate angle is less than 30 degrees (Figure 16.7). In a true lateral projection, the distal radius, lunate, capitate, and third metacarpal base should be aligned, which is termed the *link joint*. With the normal

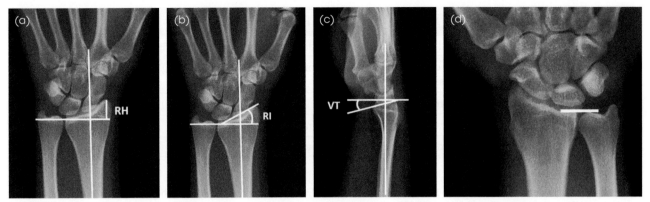

**Figure 16.1.** Normal measurements on PA and lateral wrist radiographs. (*A*) Normal radial height (RH) on the PA wrist radiograph measures 11 mm. (*B*) Normal radial inclination (RI) on the PA wrist radiograph measures approximately 22 degrees. (*C*) Normal volar tilt (VT) of the distal radial articular surface on the lateral wrist radiograph measures approximately 11 degrees. (*D*) PA radiograph of the wrist shows neutral ulnar variance with the equal length of the radius and ulna (*white line*).

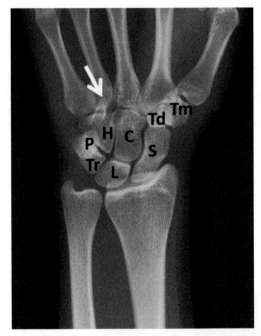

**Figure 16.2.** Normal carpal bones. PA radiograph of the wrist shows normal carpal bones, 4 in the proximal and 4 in the distal row. Note hook of the hamate (*arrow*). H = hamate; L = lunate; P = pisiform; S = scaphoid; Td = trapezoid; Tm = trapezium; Tr = triquetrum.

alignment of the carpal bones, in the PA projection of the wrist, the 3 carpal arcs (*Gilula arcs*) should not be disrupted (Figure 16.8). The first smooth arc outlines the proximal convexity of the proximal carpal row, and the second arc traces the distal concave surfaces of this row. The third arc follows the main proximal curvatures of the capitate and hamate bones.

*Dorsal intercalated segmental instability* (DISI) is a deformity with dorsal tilting of the lunate with the scapholunate angle measuring more than 80 degrees. This abnormality is associated with intrinsic scapholunate and extrinsic dorsal intercarpal ligament injuries.

*Volar intercalated segmental instability* (VISI) is a deformity with volar tilting of the lunate and decreased scapholunate angle. This abnormality is associated with intrinsic lunotriquetral and extrinsic dorsal radiocarpal ligament injuries.

### Scaphoid Fractures

The scaphoid is the most commonly fractured carpal bone (75% of cases). Scaphoid fractures tend to occur in younger adults with normal bone density. Similar mechanisms of injury tend to result in distal radius fractures in the elderly.

Scaphoid fractures most commonly affect the waist of the bone (70-80%) (Figure 16.9) with the proximal pole (15-20%) and distal pole and tubercle (5-10%) less commonly fractured. Fracture lines may have horizontal oblique, transverse, or vertical oblique orientations. Because of retrograde blood supply through the distal pole, the proximal scaphoid pole is susceptible to ON (Figure 16.10).

| Table 16.1. Frykman Classification of Distal Radius Fractures | |
| --- | --- |
| **Type I**<br>Transverse metaphyseal fracture (Smith/Colles) | **Type II**<br>Type I + ulnar styloid fracture |
| **Type III**<br>Fractures of the radiocarpal joint (Barton/reverse Barton/chauffeur) | **Type IV**<br>Type III + ulnar styloid fracture |
| **Type V**<br>Transverse fracture involving the DRUJ | **Type VI**<br>Type V + ulnar styloid fracture |
| **Type VII**<br>Comminuted fracture involving both the radiocarpal and radioulnar joints | **Type VIII**<br>Type VII + ulnar styloid fracture |

| Table 16.2. Eponyms (Names) Frequently Used in Description of Distal Radius Fractures | |
| --- | --- |
| Die-punch | Depressed fracture of the lunate fossa of the articular surface of the distal radius |
| Barton | Fracture-dislocation of radiocarpal joint with intraarticular fracture involving the volar or dorsal lip (volar Barton or dorsal Barton fracture) |
| Chauffer | Radial styloid fracture |
| Colles | Low-energy, dorsally displaced, extraarticular fracture |
| Smith | Low-energy, volarly displaced, extraarticular fracture |

Scapholunate dissociation (Figure 16.11) is caused by scapholunate ligament injury/disruption and is often associated with sports injuries. Without treatment, subsequent wrist instability can lead to debilitating degenerative changes. The most common pattern of progressive instability causing advanced OA of the radiocarpal and midcarpal joints is scapholunate advanced collapse, termed *SLAC wrist* (Figure 16.12).

Scaphoid nonunion advanced collapse (SNAC) wrist is another complication associated with scaphoid fracture nonunion, which is characterized by advanced collapse and progressive OA of the wrist (Figure 16.13).

**Other Carpal Bone Fractures**

The triquetrum is the second most common carpal bone fracture comprising 7-20% of all carpal bone fractures. Chip fractures of the dorsal surface of the triquetrum are the most common type (Figure 16.14). They may be associated with dorsal avulsion of the dorsal radiocarpal ligament. This fracture is best seen on lateral radiographs and frequently has associated soft tissue edema. Triquetral body fractures (transverse or vertical) are less common and occur in conjunction with perilunate fracture-dislocations as a part of greater arc injuries. Pisiform fractures are rare and may be associated with ulnar nerve injury.

Lunate fractures are rare. Chip fractures from the dorsal or volar surface of the lunate may occur either as isolated injuries or in combination with fracture-dislocations about the lunate bone. Transverse fractures of the lunate that involve the entire width of the distal radial joint surface and other fractures of the lunate body occur occasionally.

Trapezium fractures are most comon at its radial margin and may be associated with subluxation or dislocation of the first carpometacarpal joint. Avulsion of the volar ridge of the trapezium, at the attachment of the transverse carpal ligament, is less common.

The trapezoid is keystone-shaped and is the least commonly injured carpal bone. It is hypothesized that the mechanism of isolated trapezoid injury is because of axial loading or bending through the index finger metacarpal, which results in a coronally oriented fracture.

Capitate fractures are uncommon in isolation and may occur in association with scaphoid fractures, perilunate dislocations, and rarely with fractures of other carpal bones. Transverse fractures of the capitate waist or head are most common. Capitate head fractures, with or without displacement, associated with scaphoid waist fractures in the absence of perilunate dislocation are called *scaphocapitate*

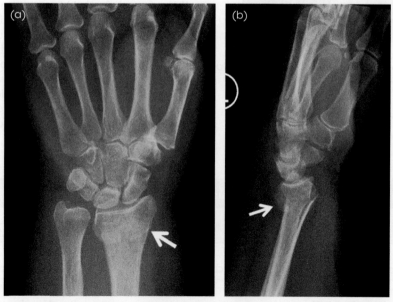

**Figure 16.3.** Colles distal radius fracture in a 65-year-old man after a fall. (*A*) PA radiograph of the wrist shows a mildly impacted transverse extraarticular fracture of the distal radial metaphysis (*arrow*). (*B*) Lateral radiograph of the same wrist shows mild dorsal displacement and mild dorsal angulation (*arrow*) of the principal distal fragment.

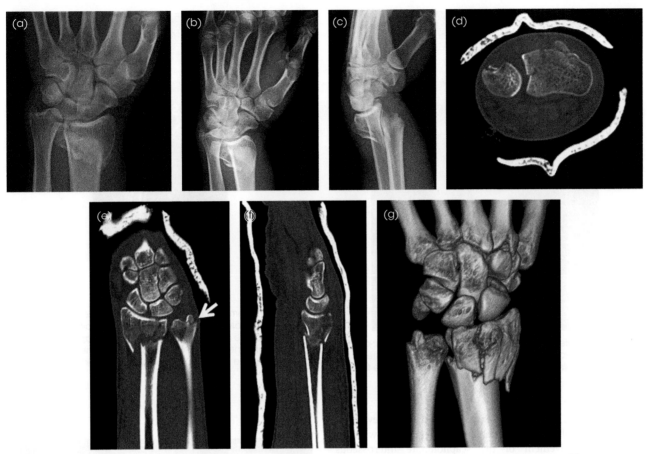

**Figure 16.4.** Displaced comminuted intraarticular distal radius and mildly displaced ulnar styloid process fractures in a 30-year-old man after a fall from a border fence. (*A*) PA, (*B*) oblique, and (*C*) lateral radiographs of the wrist show a comminuted dorsally displaced and dorsally angulated intraarticular fracture of the distal radial metaphysis and epiphysis with disruption of the DRUJ. There is a mildly displaced ulnar styloid process fracture. (*D*) Axial, (*E*) coronal, (*F*) sagittal, and (*G*) 3D reformatted images of the same wrist after closed reduction and splinting show improved alignment of the radial fracture with residual mild dorsal displacement of the principal distal fragment. In (*E*), note a mildly displaced ulnar styloid process fracture (*arrow*). The patient was treated with volar plate and screw fixation of the distal radius fracture and temporary Kirschner wire pinning of the DRUJ.

*syndrome* and are most likely the result of transient perilunate dislocation.

Hamate fractures may involve the hook (Figure 16.15) or the body. Fractures of the body may occur in isolation or in combination with perilunate dislocations. Fractures of the dorsal surface of the hamate body (often in coronal plane) occur in association with subluxations and dislocations of the fourth and fifth metacarpal bases at the mobile fourth and fifth carpometacarpal joints (Figure 16.16).

**Carpal and Fracture-Dislocations**

Carpal instability represents subluxation of the carpal bones, which occurs because of ligamentous disruption and involves the lunate, scaphoid, and capitate. It may or may not be associated with carpal fractures or dislocations, particularly involving the scaphoid. The key in recognizing carpal instability is noting the abnormal alignment of the link joint on the lateral view. The major volar extrinsic wrist ligaments follow the *greater arc* of the carpus, which is the zone of fracture-dislocations. The lesser carpal arc outlines

the radial, distal, and ulnar sides of the lunate, which is the zone of dislocations. The volar aspect of the capitolunate joint is termed the *space of Poirier*, which is not protected by ligaments (Figure 16.17). Carpal dislocations are divided into lunate and perilunate.

*Perilunate dislocations* are devastating injuries, which may or may not be associated with fractures. Without fractures, they are associated with injuries of the lesser arc with disrupted ligaments about the lunate. The lunate stays in place while the carpus dislocates (Figure 16.18).

Perilunate dislocations with fractures result in greater arc injury and are twice as common as perilunate dislocations without associated fractures. There are several types of perilunate fractures-dislocations, including transradial styloid, transscaphoid, transcapitate, transtriquetral, and transulnar styloid (Figure 16.19).

*Lunate dislocations* are the most severe form of carpal instability. The lunate dislocates volarly and the capitate stays aligned with the distal radius and third metacarpal (Figure 16.20). Lunate dislocations may be associated with median nerve injury. The mechanism of injury involves high-impact

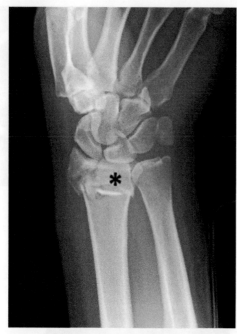

**Figure 16.5.** Die-punch distal radius fracture in a 68-year-old man. Oblique radiograph of the wrist shows a comminuted intraarticular distal radius fracture with depressed lunate fossa at the articular surface of the distal radius (*asterisk*).

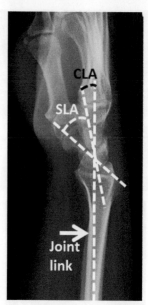

**Figure 16.7.** Normal scapholunate (SLA) and capitolunate (CLA) angles. Lateral radiograph of the wrist shows normal alignment of the distal radius with the lunate, capitate, and third metacarpal bones (joint link). The normal SLA measures 30-60 degrees and the normal CLA measures less than 30 degrees.

trauma to the wrist during extension and ulnar deviation. The pattern of injury progresses through 4 stages with sequential involvement of the scapholunate interosseous ligament, capitolunate joint, lunotriquetral interosseous ligament, and the dorsal radiocarpal ligament. The lunate rotates and dislocates, usually into the carpal tunnel. The Mayfield

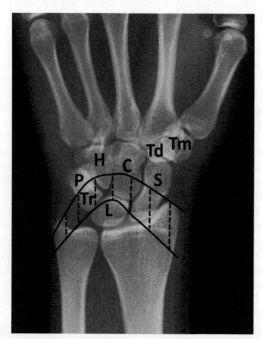

**Figure 16.6.** Zone of vulnerability shown on PA wrist radiograph. Most carpal bone fractures occur in the zone of vulnerability (*between the 2 black lines*), which follows the direction of the major volar extrinsic wrist ligaments.

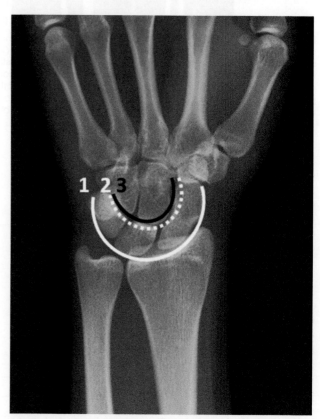

**Figure 16.8.** Arcs of Gilula. The first smooth arc (1) outlines the proximal convexity of the proximal carpal row, whereas the second arc (2) traces the distal concave surfaces of this row. The third arc (3) follows the main proximal curvatures of the capitate and hamate bones.

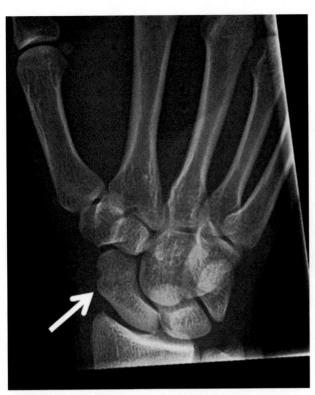

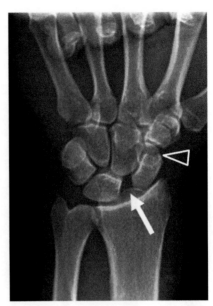

**Figure 16.11.** Scapholunate dissociation. Clenched-fist radiograph of the wrist shows widening of the scapholunate interval consistent with scapholunate ligament tear (*arrow*). The rotation of the scaphoid may produce the signet ring sign (*arrowhead*).

**Figure 16.9.** Nondisplaced scaphoid waist fracture in a 19-year-old man after a fall from a roof. PA radiograph of the wrist with ulnar deviation shows a nondisplaced scaphoid waist fracture (*arrow*). This fracture was healed with conservative treatment.

classification of lunate and perilunate dislocations is shown in Table 16.3.

## Imaging Strategy

- Radiographs (PA, oblique 45-degree pronation and lateral) are the mainstay in the initial evaluation and treatment follow-up of wrist fractures/injuries. Normal radiographic measurements of the distal radius and ulna articular surfaces and acceptable ranges are shown in Figure 16.1.
- The PA view with ulnar deviation radiograph (*scaphoid view*) is of value in the evaluation of scaphoid fractures (Figure 16.9).
- The supination oblique view with extension provides good visualization of the pisiform, triquetrum, pisotriquetral joint, and hook of the hamate.
- The carpal tunnel view is useful in the evaluation of the hook of the hamate, volar ridge of the trapezium, and pisiform fractures.
- A PA radiograph of the wrist with a clenched fist is often useful for assessment of scapholunate interval injuries (Figure 16.11).
- CT examination with coronal, sagittal, and 3D reformats is frequently performed in preoperative planning for further evaluation of articular involvement and complexity of distal radius (Figure 16.4*D*–*G*) and carpal bone fractures. Sagittal oblique reformatted images along the long axis of the scaphoid bone are useful for evaluation of scaphoid fractures.
- MRI is the imaging modality of choice in evaluation of radiographically occult fractures and associated soft tissue injuries.
- With suspected scapholunate dissociation with scapholunate ligament injury, MRA or MRI may be

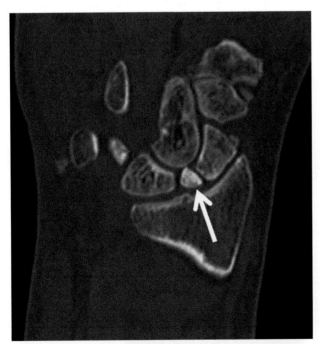

**Figure 16.10.** Scaphoid fracture nonunion with proximal pole ON. Coronal reformatted CT image of the wrist shows a nonunited fracture of the proximal scaphoid pole. Note a diminutive sclerotic proximal pole consistent with ON (*arrow*).

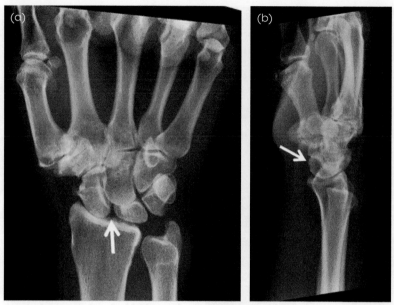

**Figure 16.12.** SLAC wrist in a 52-year-old man. (*A*) PA radiograph of the wrist shows widening of the scapholunate interval (*arrow*) consistent with scapholunate ligament disruption. Note proximal migration of the capitate with narrowing of the capitolunate joint. (*B*) Lateral radiograph of the wrist shows dorsal tilt of the lunate (*arrow*) consistent with DISI deformity.

performed. Likewise, both of these imaging modalities are frequently performed in the evaluation of other wrist ligament injuries and the TFCC.

### Imaging Findings

- Distal radius and ulna fractures—Describe anatomic location, articular involvement, open versus closed, and the amount of comminution, displacement, and angulation at the fracture site with respect to the orientation of the distal fragment. Angulation may also be described according to the orientation of the apex.

- Scapholunate dissociation—More than 4 mm of scapholunate interval widening (Terry Thomas sign) indicates potential scapholunate ligament injury. This condition may also be known as *rotary subluxation of the scaphoid* (Figure 16.11).
- Scapholunate ligament widening is more pronounced on clenched-fist view and PA view with ulnar deviation (scaphoid view). The scaphoid rotates to a more transverse position, which frequently increases the scapholunate angle to greater than 60 degrees. The rotation of the scaphoid may produce an appearance termed

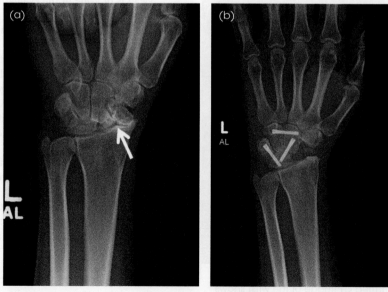

**Figure 16.13.** SNAC wrist in a 46-year-old man 4 years after trauma and untreated scaphoid fracture. (*A*) PA radiograph of the wrist shows a scaphoid fracture nonunion (*arrow*) with associated carpal collapse and panscaphoid OA. (*B*) PA radiograph of the wrist. The patient was treated with scaphoid excision and partial carpal, 4-corner fusion (lunate, triquetrum, capitate, and hamate).

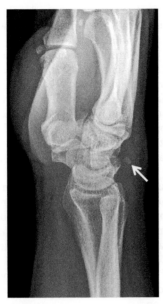

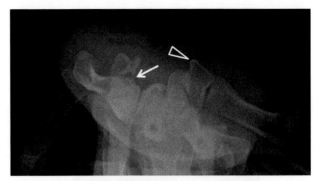

**Figure 16.15.** Hook of the hamate fracture. Carpal tunnel radiograph of the wrist shows a mildly displaced fracture at hook of the hamate base (*arrow*). Note the trapezial ridge (*arrowhead*).

**Figure 16.14.** Triquetral fracture. Lateral radiograph of the wrist shows a mildly displaced small chip fracture of the dorsal surface of the triquetrum (*arrow*) with associated soft tissue edema.

the *signet ring sign* (flexed proximal scaphoid pole seen end on) (Figure 16.11).

- Anterior bowing of the pronator quadratus muscle fat pad indicates the presence of wrist injury.
- SLAC wrist is characterized by widening of the scapholunate interval, scaphoid flexion and lunate extension, and proximal migration of the capitate with DISI deformity. The disease progresses from OA between the scaphoid and radial styloid to the entire radioscaphoid joint and later on capitolunate joint (Figure 16.12).

- SNAC wrist is associated with nonunited scaphoid fracture. The disease progresses from OA localized to the radial side of the scaphoid and radial styloid to panscaphoid OA (Figure 16.13).
- Perilunate dislocations—Most commonly, the carpus dislocates dorsally and the lunate stays aligned with the distal radius. Dorsal perilunate dislocations (Figs. 16.18 and 16.19) are more common than volar, and fractures-dislocations are more common than pure dislocations.
- Lunate dislocations—The lunate dislocates volarly, and the carpus stays aligned with the distal radius and third metacarpal (Figure 16.20).

## Treatment Options
- Most distal radius fractures respond well to conservative management with closed reduction and casting.

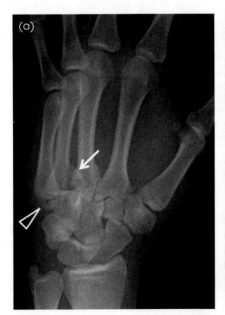

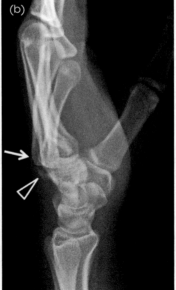

**Figure 16.16.** Hamate body fracture with dorsal subluxation of the fourth and fifth carpometacarpal joints. (*A*) Oblique and (*B*) lateral radiographs of the wrist show an intraarticular fracture of the dorsal distal hamate body (*arrowhead*) with misalignment of the fourth and fifth carpometacarpal joints. In (*A*), note an associated intraarticular fracture of the fourth metacarpal base (*arrow*). In (*B*), the *arrow* points to dorsal subluxation of the fourth and fifth metacarpal bases.

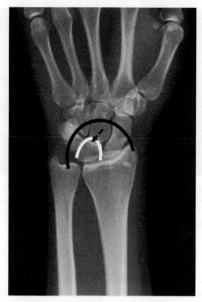

**Figure 16.17.** Greater and lesser carpal arcs. On the PA radiograph of the wrist note greater (*black line*) and lesser (*white line*) carpal arcs. *Arrow* points to the space of Poirier.

- Scaphoid fractures-Acute proximal pole fractures are treated with ORIF; acute nondisplaced waist fractures may be treated with cast immobilization or ORIF; and displaced waist fractures should be treated with ORIF. Acute distal pole and tubercle fractures are treated with short-term immobilization.
- Other than scaphoid carpal bone fractures—most nondisplaced or minimally displaced fractures may be treated conservatively with 4-6 weeks of splint or cast immobilization.
- The displaced lunate body and trapezoid fractures may be treated surgically.
- Intraarticular trapezium fractures with 2 mm or more of displacement or subluxation of the first carpometacarpal joint, displaced capitate fractures, and dorsal fractures of the hamate body in association with fourth and fifth carpometacarpal joint dislocation are treated with closed reduction and percutaneous pinning.
- Displaced hook of hamate fractures can be treated with ORIF or excision, and nonunited fractures are treated with excision.
- Perilunate and lunate dislocations require prompt closed reduction followed by open reduction, ligament repair, and fixation with or without carpal tunnel release.

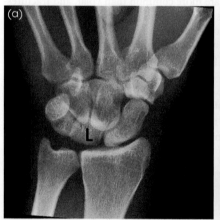
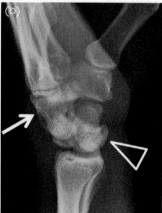
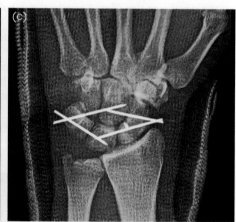

**Figure 16.18.** Dorsal perilunate dislocation in a 34-year-old man after an ATV accident. (A) PA radiograph of the wrist shows abnormal alignment of the lunate (L) and capitate with disruption of the Gilula arcs. (B) Lateral radiograph of the wrist shows dorsal dislocation of the capitate/carpus (*arrow*) in relation to lunate (*arrowhead*), which remains in anatomic alignment with the distal radius. (C) PA radiograph of the wrist. This injury was treated with closed reduction, scapholunate ligament repair, and percutaneous pinning of the carpal joints.

- Relative indications for surgical treatment of distal radius fractures that are prone to further displacement or impaired healing with long-term disability include
  - Comminution of the dorsal or volar cortex
  - Inability to complete a closed reduction of the fracture
  - Substantial loss of normal volar angulation of the distal radius (dorsal angulation >5 degrees or >20 degrees of the contralateral distal radius), although larger degrees of angulation may be acceptable for conservative treatment depending on clinical indications
  - More than 5 mm of radial shortening
  - Intraarticular extension with loss of congruity of the articular surface of the radiocarpal joint greater than 2 mm

| Table 16.3. Mayfield Classification of Carpal Dislocations and Lunate and Perilunate Dislocations | |
| --- | --- |
| Stage I | Scapholunate dissociation |
| Stage II | Stage I: + lunocapitate disruption |
| Stage III | Stage II: + lunotriquetral disruption, "perilunate" |
| Stage IV | Lunate dislocated from lunate fossa (usually volar), associated with median nerve compression |

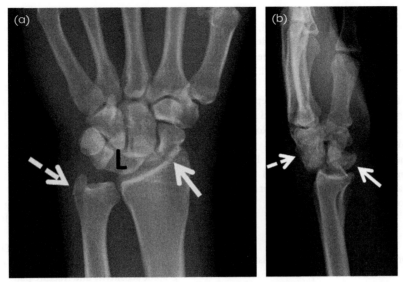

**Figure 16.19.** Transscaphoid, transulnar styloid perilunate fracture-dislocation in a 38-year-old man. (*A*) PA radiograph of the wrist shows disruption of the Gilula arcs, a displaced scaphoid waist fracture (*arrow*), and a minimally displaced ulnar styloid process fracture (*dashed arrow*). (*B*) Lateral radiograph of the wrist shows dorsal dislocation of the capitate/carpus (*dashed arrow*) in relation to lunate (*arrow*), which remains in anatomic alignment with the distal radius. L = lunate.

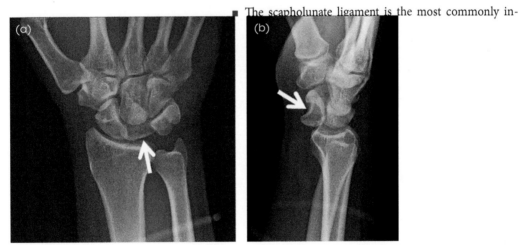

**Figure 16.20.** Lunate dislocation in a 53-year-old man after a fall. (*A*) PA radiograph of the wrist shows a pie-shaped lunate (*arrow*) with disruption of the proximal and mid carpal arcs. (*B*) Lateral radiograph of the wrist shows volar dislocation of the lunate (*arrow*) in relation to the capitate/carpus, distal radius, and third metacarpal.

## Key Points

- The distal radius is the most commonly fractured bone about the wrist. Many fractures respond well to conservative management with immobilization and pain relief. However, complex and unstable fractures require surgical repair.
- Radiographs are the mainstay in initial evaluation and treatment follow-up of wrist fractures, although CT examination is often performed and helpful in preoperative planning of complex fractures. MRI is the study of choice in evaluation of radiographically occult fractures.
- The scaphoid is the most commonly fractured carpal bone and, because of its retrograde blood supply, ON of the proximal pole can occur.
- The scapholunate ligament is the most commonly injured wrist ligament.
- If left untreated, scapholunate ligamentous injury or ON of the scaphoid can lead to chronic degenerative changes and instability of the wrist which can be seen with SLAC and SNAC wrist.
- Carpal dislocations require prompt closed reduction followed by open reduction, ligament repair, and fixation with or without carpal tunnel release.
- Dorsal fractures of the hamate body in association with fourth and fifth carpometacarpal joint dislocations are treated with closed reduction and percutaneous pinning.

## Recommended Reading

Porrino JA Jr, Maloney E, Scherer K, Mulcahy H, Ha AS, Allan C. Fracture of the distal radius: epidemiology and premanagement radiographic characterization. *AJR Am J Roentgenol*. 2014;203(3):551–59. doi:10.2214/AJR.13.12140.

Scalcione LR, Gimber LH, Ho AM, Johnston SS, Sheppard JE, Taljanovic MS. Spectrum of carpal dislocations and fracture-dislocations: imaging and management. *AJR Am J Roentgenol*. 2014;203(3):541–50. doi:10.2214/AJR.13.11680.

Taljanovic MS, Karantanas A, Griffith JF, DeSilva GL, Rieke JD, Sheppard JE. Imaging and treatment of scaphoid fractures and their complications. *Semin Musculoskelet Radiol*. 2012;16(2):159–73. doi:10.1055/s-0032-1311767.

## References

1. Foster RJ. Stabilization of ulnar carpometacarpal dislocations or fracture dislocations. *Clin Orthop Relat Res*. 1996 Jun;(327):94–97.

2. Hey HW, Chong AK, Murphy D. Prevalence of carpal fracture in Singapore [Erratum in *J Hand Surg Am*. 2011;36(9):1567]. *J Hand Surg Am*. 2011;36(2):278–83. doi:10.1016/j.jhsa.2010.11.009.

3. Komura S, Yokoi T, Nonomura H, Tanahashi H, Satake T, Watanabe N. Incidence and characteristics of carpal fractures occurring concurrently with distal radius fractures. *J Hand Surg Am*. 2012;37(3):469–76. doi:10.1016/j.jhsa.2011.11.011.

4. Lichtman DM, Bindra RR, Boyer MI, et al. Treatment of distal radius fractures. *J Am Acad Orthop Surg*. 2010;18(3):180–89.

5. Lögters T, Windolf J. Fractures of carpal bones [in German]. *Chirurg*. 2016;87(10):893–906. doi:10.1007/s00104-016-0274-2.

6. Murthy NS, Ringler MD. MR imaging of carpal fractures. *Magn Reson Imaging Clin N Am*. 2015;23(3):405–16. doi:10.1016/j.mric.2015.04.006.

7. Welling RD, Jacobson JA, Jamadar DA, Chong S, Caoili EM, Jebson PJ. MDCT and radiography of wrist fractures: radiographic sensitivity and fracture patterns. *AJR Am J Roentgenol*. 2008;190(1):10–16.

# CHAPTER 17

# Hand Trauma

Michael O'Keeffe, Kiran Khursid, Peter L. Munk, and Mihra S. Taljanovic

## Basic Anatomy and Mechanism of Injury

### Basic Anatomy

Each of the 5 digits of the hand have a metacarpal articulating with the distal carpal row at the carpometacarpal (CMC) joints, which has a zig-zag appearance on PA hand and wrist radiographs. All digits have proximal phalanges that articulate with metacarpals at the metacarpophalangeal (MCP) joints. The thumb has a distal phalanx that articulates with the proximal phalanx at the interphalangeal (IP) joint. The index, middle, ring, and small (little) fingers have middle and distal phalanges that articulate at the proximal interphalangeal (PIP) and distal interphalangeal (DIP) joints. These multiple synovial joints allow tremendous mobility of the hand, varying from strong grip to delicate fingertip movements.

Fractures of the metacarpals and phalanges (Figure 17.1) are common and account for approximately 10% of all fractures. These injuries may be related to sports or work trauma or result from a fall. Osseous injuries are frequently associated with ligamentous or tendon injury.

Metacarpal fractures may result from a direct blow to the hand or rotational injury from an axial load. High-energy injuries may result in multiple fractures. Closed injuries with multiple fractures or dislocations and crush injuries may be complicated by compartment syndrome, a serious condition that threatens tissue viability and requires prompt surgical treatment.

Metacarpal fractures may involve the base, diaphysis/shaft, neck, and head. The "boxer" fracture (Figure 17.2) involves the distal aspect of the fifth metacarpal and is so named because of its association with punching injuries. Base of the thumb (first metacarpal) fractures may be intraarticular or extraarticular. Intraarticular fractures may be simple (Bennett) (Figure 17.3) or comminuted (Rolando) (Figure 17.4), which is less common than the Bennett fracture. Subluxations and dislocations of the first carpometacarpal joint may occur with or without associated first metacarpal base fractures.

Volar plate injury/fracture results from hyperextension of the PIP joint, resulting in an avulsion type injury from the middle phalangeal volar plate, also known as a *jammed finger*. Severe injuries may be associated with dorsal dislocation of the PIP joint. Patients present with swelling, deformity, pain (worse with movement), and/or inability to move the joint. Volar plate middle phalangeal base fractures are common, and if they involve less than 30% of the articular surface, they are consider stable (Figure 17.5). Volar plate fractures with more than 50% articular surface involvement represent unstable injuries, and those with 30-50% involvement are considered tenuous.

Dorsal dislocations of the PIP joints (Figure 17.6) are more common than volar ones. Volar dislocations of the PIP joints lead to disruption of the central extensor tendon slip, collateral ligament injury, and formation of the boutonniere deformity with flexion of the PIP and extension of the DIP joints (Figure 17.7).

Mallet finger injuries consist of tendinous or bony avulsion (Figure 17.8) of the extensor tendon from the distal phalangeal base. This injury occurs when the DIP joint is forcefully flexed such as when hit by a basketball. The patients present with inability to actively extend the distal phalanx, while still being able to passively extend it. A complication of mallet finger injury is the swan neck deformity with hyperextension of the PIP joint and flexion at the DIP joint.

Dorsal dislocations of the DIP joints may be associated with fractures. Distal phalangeal tuft crush injuries are frequent (Figure 17.9). The mechanism of injury is direct trauma to the distal phalanx. The patients present with pain and visible nail bed involvement.

Ulnar collateral ligament (UCL) injuries of the thumb (skier or gamekeeper thumb) occur with a forceful abduction of the thumb, such as during a fall while skiing. Patients present with swelling and pain around the thumb MCP joint and weak pinch. The ligament is usually avulsed from the proximal phalangeal base attachment site. The diagnosis can often be made on radiographs by seeing an avulsion fracture on the ulnar side of the base of proximal phalanx of the thumb (Figure 17.10). The first MCP joint may appear asymmetrically widened at the ulnar aspect and/or radially subluxated. *Stener lesions* consist of displacement of the UCL superficial to the adductor aponeurosis. This lesion may be clinically palpable, but radiological diagnosis can be made on US or MRI. MR images of gamekeeper thumb and Stener lesions are shown in Chapter 106, "Internal Derangement of the Wrist and Hand."

## Imaging Strategy

- Dedicated hand radiographs including PA, oblique, and lateral views are performed for initial evaluation and treatment follow-up of metacarpal and phalangeal fractures and fracture-dislocations.
- In finger fractures, dedicated PA, oblique and lateral radiographs of the affected digit may be needed.
- Post closed reduction radiographs should be obtained.
- Cross-sectional imaging is rarely needed in acute hand trauma.

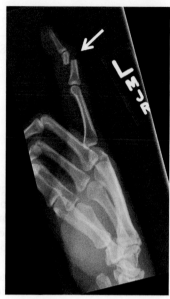

**Figure 17.1.** Near amputation of the index finger in a 30-year-old woman who was using a meat cleaver to cut chicken and accidentally cut her finger. Lateral radiograph of the index finger shows a volarly displaced transverse fracture of the middle phalangeal shaft (*arrow*). This injury required operative treatment with ORIF of the middle phalangeal fracture and repair of the flexor and extensor tendon lacerations.

- With suspected ligamentous injuries, US or MRI examinations are performed on a nonemergent basis if clinically indicated.

**Imaging Findings**
- Metacarpal fractures—Look for the location of the fracture (base, shaft, neck, and head), comminution, amount of displacement, degree of angulation, articular

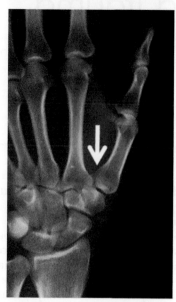

**Figure 17.3.** Bennett fracture in a 30-year-old man with trauma to the hand following a bicycle accident. Cropped oblique radiograph of the hand shows a minimally displaced intraarticular fracture of the left first metacarpal base (*arrow*) with associated mild soft-tissue edema. This fracture healed with nonoperative treatment.

extension, associated dislocation, and whether the fracture is open or closed (Figure 17.2).
- Bennett fracture—Intraarticular fracture of the first metacarpal base with the bone fragment attached to the volar oblique ligament. The bone fragment articulates with the trapezium (Figure 17.3).
- Rolando fracture—Comminuted intraarticular fracture of the first metacarpal base (Figure 17.4).

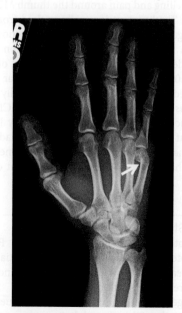

**Figure 17.2.** Boxer fracture in a 22-year-old man with hand trauma after punching a wall. Oblique radiograph of the hand shows a transverse, mildly volarly displaced fracture of the fifth metacarpal neck with moderate volar angulation of the principal distal fragment (*arrow*). This fracture was treated with closed reduction and splinting.

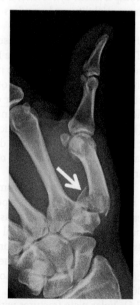

**Figure 17.4.** Rolando fracture of the first metacarpal base in a 35-year old man. Oblique radiograph of the thumb shows a mildly displaced comminuted intraarticular fracture of the first metacarpal base (*arrow*) with involvement of the CMC joint. The fracture was treated with ORIF with 2 K-wires.

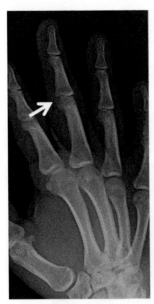

**Figure 17.5.** Volar plate fracture in a 23-year-old man with finger hyperextension injury. Oblique radiograph of the fingers shows a small mildly displaced fracture fragment (*arrow*) at the volar aspect of the middle phalangeal base, which was treated nonoperatively.

- Volar plate injury—Look for a small avulsed bone fragment at the volar aspect of the middle phalangeal base (Figure 17.5). Look for associated subluxation or dislocation of the PIP joint (Figure 17.6).

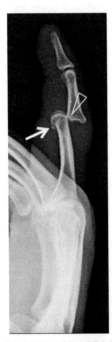

**Figure 17.6.** Dorsal dislocation of the PIP joint and volar plate fracture in a 56-year-old man. Lateral radiograph of the index finger shows dorsal dislocation of the middle phalanx at the PIP joint with an associated displaced small volar plate fracture (*arrow*). *Arrowhead* points to the donor site. After 2 unsuccessful closed reduction attempts, the patient was treated operatively with radial and UCL release, PIP joint reduction, and temporary pinning.

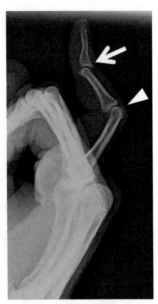

**Figure 17.7.** Boutonniere deformity of the little finger in a 32-year-old man with a basketball-related injury. Lateral radiograph of the little finger shows fixed flexion of the PIP joint (*arrowhead*) in keeping with central slip extensor tendon rupture. Note hyperextension of the DIP joint with mild dorsal subluxation of the distal phalanx (*arrow*).

- Mallet finger injury—Look for fixed flexion of the DIP joint and an avulsed bone fragment off the dorsal aspect of the distal phalangeal base (Figure 17.8).
- Boutonniere deformity—Look for hyperextension of the DIP joint and flexion of the PIP joint (Figure 17.7).

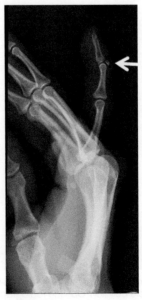

**Figure 17.8.** Mallet finger injury in a 39-year-old woman after a fall. Lateral radiograph of the hand shows a mildly dorsally displaced small avulsed bone fragment off the dorsal aspect of the little finger distal phalangeal base (*arrow*) with associated mild flexion deformity of the DIP joint and mild soft-tissue edema. This fracture was treated nonoperatively.

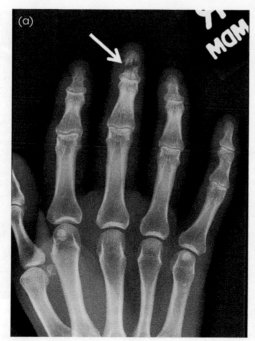
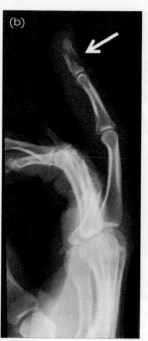

**Figure 17.9.** Crush injury of the middle finger distal phalanx in a 41-year-old woman. (*A*) PA and (*B*) lateral radiographs of the fingers show a moderately dorsally displaced, mildly comminuted, extraarticular fracture of the right middle finger distal phalangeal tuft extending to the nail bed (*arrows*), which required operative treatment.

- Ulnar collateral ligament injury of the thumb MCP joint— Look for a small avulsed bone fragment off the ulnar aspect of the proximal phalangeal base (Figure 17.10), asymmetric joint space widening and/or radial subluxation.
- US and MRI are helpful in evaluation of ligamentous or tendon injuries.

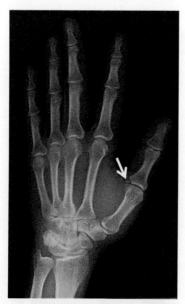

**Figure 17.10.** Gamekeeper thumb injury in a 36-year-old man after a motor vehicle collision. Oblique radiograph of the hand shows a small avulsed bone fragment off the ulnar aspect of the thumb proximal phalangeal base (*arrow*) consistent with UCL bony avulsion injury. This injury was treated nonoperatively.

## Treatment Options

- Metacarpal fractures—Nondisplaced or mildly displaced metacarpal fractures may respond to conservative management with closed reduction and immobilization. However, displaced and open fractures or those with intraarticular extension and displacement of the articular surface and/or dislocation may require operative management, ranging from Kirschner (K)-wire fixation to ORIF.
- Phalangeal fractures—Extraarticular fractures with less than 10 degrees angulation or less than 2 mm shortening and no rotational deformity are treated conservatively with closed reduction and buddy taping or splinting. Irreducible or unstable fractures require surgical fixation.
- PIP and DIP joint dislocations and fracture-dislocations—Anatomic reduction must be achieved. Stable injuries are treated with closed reduction and splinting. Irreducible fractures and fracture-dislocations and those with involvement of more than 40% articular surface require surgical treatment.
- Volar plate injury/fracture—Fractures that involve less than 40% of the articular surface or with less than 30 degrees of flexion are reducible and can be managed conservatively with splinting. Other fractures often require operative management.
- Mallet finger injury—In the acute setting, most of these injuries may be treated conservatively with extension splinting of the affected DIP joint for 6-8 weeks. Surgical treatment is indicated with volar subluxation of the distal phalanx and may be indicated with greater than 50% articular surface involvement or more than 2 mm articular gap. Chronic injuries (>12 weeks) usually require surgical treatment.

- Gamekeeper thumb and Stener lesion—If the joint is unstable and with the presence of Stener lesion, surgical repair is required, otherwise conservative management with a thumb spica cast is indicated.
- Crush injuries of the distal phalangeal tuft with involvement of the nail bed—Open fractures often require reduction. Nail bed removal or repair may be required.

---

### Key Points

- The hand is composed of a complex anatomical arrangement of bone and soft tissue.

  The network of synovial joints and overlying tendons allows for extensive mobility in the hand.
- Metacarpal and phalangeal fractures are common, as are dislocations of the IP and MCP joints.
- Most hand fractures are stable and can be treated with closed reduction and immobilization. Significantly displaced fractures and those with substantial intraarticular extension often require operative repair including K-wire stabilization or ORIF. In general, the treatment option that achieves the desired reduction and degree of fixation, allows early motion, and minimizes soft-tissue injury should be preferred.

### Recommended Reading

Leggit JC, Meko CJ. Acute finger injuries: part II. Fractures, dislocations, and thumb injuries. *Am Fam Physician.* 2006;73(5):827–34.

Jones NF, Jupiter JB, Lalonde DH. Common fractures and dislocations of the hand. *Plast Reconstr Surg.* 2012;130(5):722e–36e. doi:10.1097/PRS.0b013e318267d67a.

### References

1. Cheah AE, Yao J. Hand fractures: indications, the tried and true and new innovations. *J Hand Surg Am.* 2016;41(6):712–22. doi:10.1016/j.jhsa.2016.03.007.
2. Cotterell IH, Richard MJ. Metacarpal and phalangeal fractures in athletes. *Clin Sports Med.* 2015;34(1):69–98. doi:10.1016/j.csm.2014.09.009.
3. Giddins GE. The non-operative management of hand fractures. *J Hand Surg Eur Vol.* 2015;40(1):33–41. doi:10.1177/1753193414548170.
4. Kadow TR, Fowler JR. Thumb injuries in athletes. *Hand Clin.* 2017;33(1):161–73. doi:10.1016/j.hcl.2016.08.008.
5. Shaftel ND, Capo JT. Fractures of the digits and metacarpals: when to splint and when to repair? *Sports Med Arthrosc.* 2014;22(1):2–11. doi:10.1097/JSA.0000000000000004.

# 3

# Pelvis and Lower Extremity

Edited by Mihra S. Taljanovic and Tyson S. Chadaz

# CHAPTER 18

# Pelvic Bone Trauma

Winnie A. Mar and Tyson S. Chadaz

## Mechanism of Injury

The pelvis is an inherently stable structure composed of the sacrum and the paired innominate bones, each of which consists of an ilium, pubis, and ischium. Strong pelvic ligaments hold the pelvis together, including the anterior and posterior SI joint ligaments, and the sacrospinous and sacrotuberous ligaments. The anterior arch consists of the pubic rami and the pubic symphysis. The stronger posterior arch consists of the ilium posterior to the acetabulum, sacrum, and SI joint.

Two-thirds of all pelvic fractures are stable. The most common of these is an inferior pubic ramus fracture (Figure 18.1). This is usually seen in osteoporotic patients from a fall. An isolated sacral fracture usually occurs from a fall and is typically transverse and below the level of the SI joint. A Duverney fracture is an isolated iliac wing fracture (Figure 18.2), which usually occurs from high-energy trauma.

Pelvic avulsion fractures are also stable and typically affect adolescents in whom the apophysis is weaker than the attaching muscle and tendons. An acute pelvic avulsion fracture occurs with a forceful, unbalanced muscle contraction and usually results in severe pain. Chronic avulsion fractures are a result of microtrauma. Ischial tuberosity avulsion injuries from the hamstring tendons are the most common avulsion injuries and are usually seen in sprinters, cheerleaders, and dancers. An avulsion injury from the anterior superior iliac spine at the origin of the sartorius muscle is the next most common. Avulsion injuries can also occur at the anterior inferior iliac spine from the rectus femoris tendon.

Unstable pelvic fractures disrupt the posterior pelvic arch and are usually high-energy fractures. They can be associated with hemorrhage, bladder or urethral injury. Lateral compression fractures are the most common of the unstable fractures and can result from a pedestrian or motor vehicle passenger being struck on the side. An internal rotation force is involved, generally narrowing the pelvis. Anteroposterior (AP) compression fractures are the next most common pelvic ring fracture, typically resulting from high-energy blunt trauma, and can occur after being struck from the front or back in a motor vehicle crash, as a pedestrian, as a crush injury or from a motorcycle crash. Vertical shear fractures involve a craniocaudal force on the pelvis, typically from a fall from a height onto an extended leg, and are rotationally and vertically unstable.

Acetabular fractures occur when the femoral head or neck impacts on the acetabulum. They usually result from a high-energy motor vehicle accident or a fall onto the greater trochanter and are also associated with 20% of pelvic ring fractures. Significant pelvic hemorrhage or bladder injury can accompany these high-energy fractures. Acetabular fractures in the osteoporotic elderly are less common but increasing.

Pelvic insufficiency fractures are common, but often unsuspected fractures are most commonly seen in osteoporotic elderly patients. Patients can present with low back pain, groin, or gluteal pain. Common locations include the sacrum, pubic bones within the parasymphyseal region, medial iliac bone, iliac wing, pubic rami, and the supracetabular region.

## Imaging Strategy

Evaluation begins with radiographs. In the setting of acute trauma, an AP pelvic radiograph is first performed. Inlet and outlet views help detect sacral fractures and involve angling the x-ray tube without moving the patient. Inlet views better depict AP and rotational displacement. Outlet views help detect SI joint widening and vertical displacement. Judet views are helpful for surgical management planning in acetabular fractures. CT is routinely performed for better delineation of pelvic and acetabular fractures. 3D reformatted images are helpful for classifying acetabular fractures. CT angiography may be performed when significant hemorrhage and active bleeding is suspected. Unstable patients should have angiography, embolization for treatment of active bleeding, or urgent fixation and possible pelvic packing. CT cystography should be performed for patients with hematuria and a pelvic fracture, and if negative for leak, retrograde urethrogram should be performed.

In the nonemergent setting, if radiographs are negative but there is high clinical suspicion for fracture, CT or MRI should be performed. With avulsion fractures, the AP pelvic radiograph usually suffices for diagnosis. Comparison to the contralateral side can be performed to detect subtle abnormalities. Pelvic insufficiency fractures are best evaluated with MRI or bone scintigraphy as they can be occult on radiographs particularly in osteoporotic patients.

## Imaging Findings and Classifications

### Avulsion Fractures

- Acute avulsion fractures appear as curvilinear bone fragments with sharp margins adjacent to the site of origin (Figure 18.3).
- Subacute healing avulsion fractures can appear aggressive on radiographs with irregular margins, osteolysis, and bone destruction.
- Chronic avulsion injuries show a bony protuberance with smooth margins.

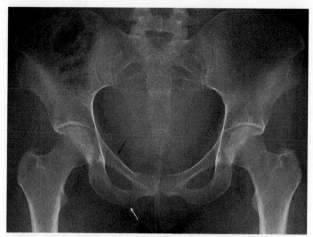

Figure 18.1. Nondisplaced right superior and inferior pubic rami fractures. AP radiograph of the pelvis shows nondisplaced superior (*black arrow*) and inferior (*white arrow*) pubic rami fractures.

### Pelvic Ring Fractures

- The Young and Burgess classification of pelvic ring fractures incorporates the mechanism of injury and helps determine treatment (Figure 18.4).
- Lateral compression fractures are categorized type I through III.
  - Type I involves a horizontal pubic ramus or medial acetabular fracture along with a crush fracture of the sacrum (Figure 18.5).
  - Type II involves internal rotation of the ilium with ipsilateral SI joint diastasis or a vertical posterior ilium fracture. A crescent of bone may be attached to the posterior ilium signifying that the posterior SI ligament remains intact.

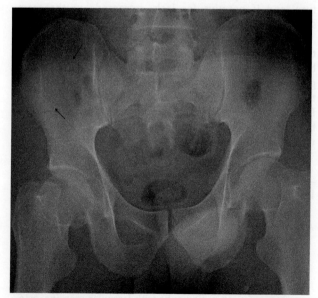

Figure 18.2. Duverney fracture. AP radiograph of the pelvis shows a mildly comminuted, nondisplaced right iliac wing fracture (*arrows*) consistent with a Duverney fracture. There is no SI joint or pubic symphysis widening.

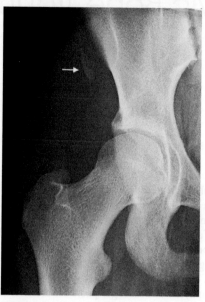

Figure 18.3. Anterior superior iliac spine avulsion fracture. AP radiograph of the right hip shows an avulsion fracture of the anterior superior iliac spine (*arrow*).

- Type III involves additional external rotation of the contralateral hemipelvis resulting in bilateral SI joint widening, also referred to as a *windswept pelvis*.
- Anteroposterior compression fractures are described as follows:
  - The iliac wings appear broader because of the external rotation.
  - Type I injury is rare and involves only anterior ring disruption with vertical fractures of the pubic rami or pubic symphysis widening less than 2.5 cm.
  - Type II injury, also referred to as an *open book* fracture, is an AP compression injury with widening of the pubic symphysis and SI joints. There is usually greater than 2.5 cm of pubic symphysis widening with disruption of the sacrotuberous, sacrospinous, and anterior SI joint ligaments.
  - Type III injury involves additional posterior SI joint ligament disruption with increased widening of the joint space (Figure 18.6). Posterior displacement of the ilium is best seen on CT examination.
- Vertical shear injury involves the following:
  - There is cephalad displacement of the iliac crest and vertical displacement of the SI joint seen at the inferior margin related to posterior SI ligament tear (Figure 18.7).
  - There is either pubic symphysis widening or vertical pubic rami fractures.
  - Vertical shear mimics AP compression type III because of a disarticulated pelvis. Evaluation for cephalad displacement of the iliac crest is the key to making this diagnosis.
  - Severe SI joint widening with less than 2.5 cm pubic symphysis diastasis suggests a vertical shear fracture.
- Judet and Letournel classification divides acetabular fractures into elemental fractures and associated fractures (Figure 18.8)

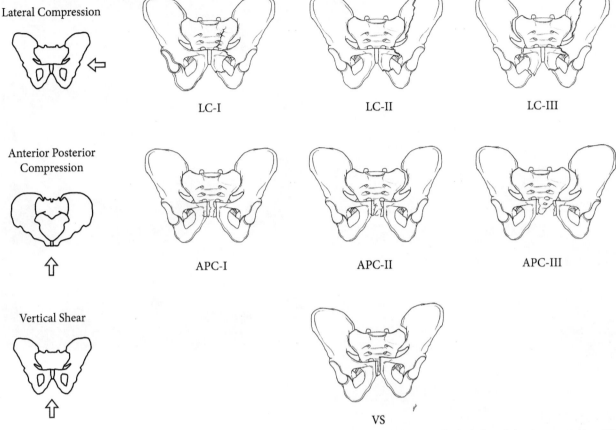

**Figure 18.4.** Artist drawing showing different type of pelvic fractures with mechanism of injury. Illustrated are lateral compression (LC) fractures types I-III, AP compression (APC) fractures types I-III, and vertical shear (VS) fracture. © 2016 Lauren Kalinoski.

- Elemental acetabular fractures consist of wall, column, and transverse fractures, with posterior wall and transverse fractures being most common.
  - Wall fractures involve the non-weight-bearing acetabular rim and can be seen with hip dislocation.
  - Column fractures separate the weight-bearing acetabulum from the remainder of the pelvis, extending through the obturator foramen into the pubic ramus.
  - A transverse fracture separates the superior pelvis from the inferior pelvis and is the only elemental fracture that involves both columns.
  - When evaluating the acetabulum on radiographs, the iliopectineal line corresponds to the anterior column, and the ilioischial line corresponds to the posterior column.
  - A column fracture line is in the coronal plane, and the transverse fracture line is in the sagittal plane.
  - Posterior column fractures extend from the greater sciatic notch through the posterior acetabulum, obturator foramen, and into the ischiopubic ramus.
  - Anterior column fractures extend from the iliac wing, through the anterior acetabulum into the obturator foramen and ischiopubic ramus (Figure 18.9).
- Associated acetabular fractures most commonly involve both columns, and are transverse and posterior wall, T-shaped, anterior wall or column with posterior hemitransverse and posterior column with posterior wall.
- It is important to evaluate for any intraarticular bony fragments, which are best seen on CT studies.

**Pelvic Insufficiency Fractures**
- They can be radiographically occult and are better evaluated on MRI and bone scintigraphy.
- Nondisplaced fracture lines can be seen with surrounding BME on MRI and radiotracer uptake on bone scintigraphy.
- Sacral insufficiency fractures most commonly involve vertical fractures of the sacral alae resembling the so-called H sign.

## Treatment Options

**Stable Pelvic Fractures**
- Conservative treatment

**Unstable Pelvic Ring Fractures**
- Surgical fixation is performed.
- SI joint diastasis or distracted sacral fractures are treated with transverse lag screws.

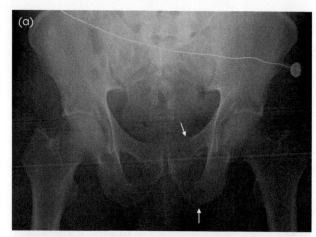

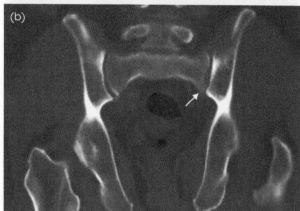

**Figure 18.5.** Lateral compression type I pelvic fracture. AP radiograph of the pelvis (*A*) shows left inferior and superior pubic rami fractures (*arrows*). There is no SI joint widening. Coronal CT reformatted image of the pelvis (*B*) of the same patient better shows a zone I left sacral ala crush fracture (*arrow*) without SI joint widening.

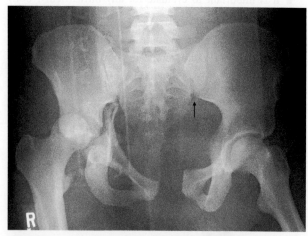

**Figure 18.6.** AP compression type III pelvic fracture. AP radiograph of the pelvis shows an AP compression fracture type III with widening of the pubic symphysis, left SI joint (*arrow*), and apparent broadening of the left iliac wing. There is also a transverse right acetabular fracture. Despite the malalignment of the pubic symphysis related to the right acetabular fracture, there is no cephalad displacement of the left iliac wing to suggest vertical shear injury, which can appear similar.

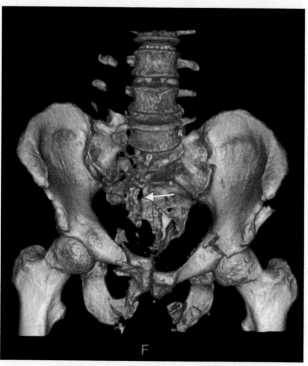

**Figure 18.7.** Vertical shear pelvic fracture. A vertical shear fracture with cephalad displacement of the right ilium, bilateral inferior and superior pubic rami fractures, a vertical right sacral fracture (*arrow*), and right L3-L5 transverse process fractures is shown in a 3D reformatted CT image.

- Acetabular fractures are frequently treated with reconstruction plates and screws.
- Active bleeding is treated with embolization.

**Acetabular Fractures**
- Displaced or unstable fractures are treated with surgical fixation, typically with reconstruction plates and screws.
- Conservative management is used for stable nondisplaced fractures or minimally displaced fractures.

**Pelvic Avulsion Fractures**
- Conservative management is used for the vast majority of pelvic avulsion fractures.
- If the avulsed fragment is distracted more than 2 cm, it is likely to heal with fibrous union, which results in prolonged recovery.

**Pelvic Insufficiency Fractures**
- Conservative management
- Surgical fixation if more than 1 cm of displacement, persistent pain, or evidence of neurologic injury

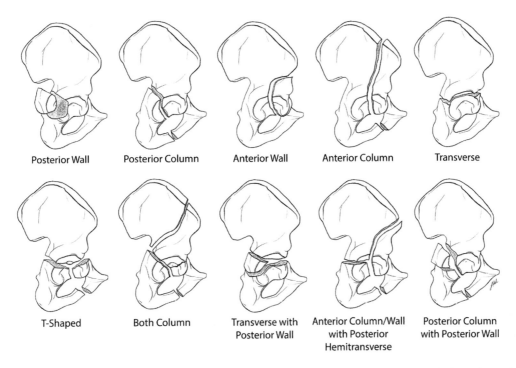

**Figure 18.8.** Artist drawing showing the Judet and Letournel classification of acetabular fractures. Illustrated are elemental (posterior wall, posterior column, anterior wall, anterior column, transverse) and associated (T-shaped, both column, transverse with posterior wall, anterior column/wall with posterior hemitransverse, and posterior column with posterior wall) fractures. © 2016 Lauren Kalinoski

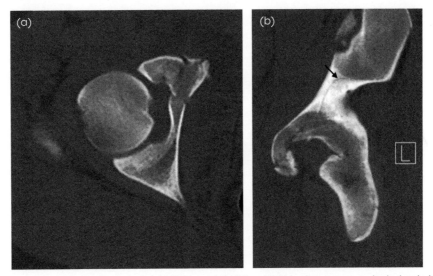

**Figure 18.9.** Anterior column acetabular fracture. Axial CT image (*A*) of the right hip shows a comminuted anterior column fracture. Sagittal reformatted CT image (*B*) of the same hip shows extension of the acetabular fracture superiorly into the iliac wing (*arrow*). Patient also had the right inferior pubic ramus fracture (*not shown*).

### Key Points
- Most pelvic fractures are stable.
- Unstable pelvic fractures disrupt the posterior pelvic arch/ring.
- Pelvic fractures may be associated with significant hemorrhage or bladder or urethral injury.
- In acetabular fractures, the iliopectineal line corresponds to the anterior column and the ilioischial line corresponds to the posterior column.

- It is important to recognize pelvic avulsion fractures as they may simulate tumor or osteomyelitis during the healing phase.

### Recommended Reading
Khurana B, Sheehan SE, Sodickson AD, Weaver MJ. Pelvic ring fractures: what the orthopedic surgeon wants to know. *Radiographics*. 2014;34:1317–33.

### References

1. Durkee NJ, Jacobson J, Jamadar D, Karunakar MA, Morag Y, Hayes C. Classification of common acetabular fractures: radiographic and CT appearances. *AJR Am J Roentgenol.* 2006;187:915–25.
2. Lawrence DA, Menn K, Baumgaertner M, Haims AH. Acetabular fractures: anatomic and clinical considerations. *AJR Am J Roentgenol.* 2013;201:W425–36.
3. Stevens MA, El-Khoury GY, Kathol MH, Brandser EA, Chow S. Imaging features of avulsion injuries. *Radiographics.* 1999;19:655–72.
4. Young JW, Burgess AR, Brumback RJ, Poka A. Pelvic fractures: value of plain radiography in early assessment and management. *Radiology.* 1986;160:445–51.
5. Taljanovic MS, Jones MD, Ruth JT, Benjamin JB, Sheppard JE, Hunter TB. Fracture fixation. *Radiographics.* 2003;23:1569–90.

# CHAPTER 19

# Hip Trauma

Winnie A. Mar and Tyson S. Chadaz

## Mechanism of Injury

Femoral neck and intertrochanteric fractures are the most common types of hip fractures. They are often associated with osteopenia and result from low-energy falls. Patients present with an externally rotated, flexed leg. Femoral neck fractures are intracapsular and have a slower healing time than extracapsular fractures. Because of the tenuous femoral head blood supply, femoral neck fractures carry an increased risk of ON.

An intertrochanteric fracture usually results from a fall laterally onto the greater trochanter. Intertrochanteric fractures are extracapsular and are not predisposed to ON.

An isolated greater trochanter fracture usually occurs in osteoporotic women, after a fall on the hip or, less commonly, as an avulsion fracture by the gluteal muscles. However, most greater trochanter fractures have intertrochanteric extension. An isolated lesser trochanter fracture is suspicious for an underlying metastatic lesion in an adult without significant trauma.

Hip dislocations usually result from high-energy trauma, such as a motor vehicle collision where the knee hits the dashboard or a fall onto an abducted hip. Approximately 90% of hip dislocations are posterior. Patients with posterior hip dislocations present with the leg in adduction and internal rotation. Hip dislocations increase the risk of ON; thus prompt diagnosis and relocation is crucial. A minority of posterior hip dislocations are associated with sciatic nerve injury.

### Other Types of Hip Dislocation

Anterior hip dislocations are less common than posterior ones, representing approximately 10% of all hip dislocations. They are usually inferior and less commonly superior. Anterior-inferior dislocations occur when the hip is forced into abduction and external rotation and are uncommonly associated with acetabular fractures. However, impaction fractures of the femoral head are commonly present.

Central hip dislocations are associated with fractures of the acetabulum with protrusion of the femoral head into the pelvis. Femoral shaft fractures may also occur in association with hip dislocations.

Asymmetric bilateral hip dislocations are rare, with a small number of cases reported in literature, and comprise posterior dislocation of one of the hips and anterior of the other.

## Imaging Strategy

Imaging should begin with AP and either true lateral or frog-leg lateral radiographs. If radiographs are negative and there is high clinical suspicion for fracture, as in a patient who cannot bear weight, MRI is the study of choice. Bone scans are much less sensitive and may require up to 72 hours in order to show uptake in osteopenic patients.

Patients with hip dislocations should have a CT scan to evaluate for any intraarticular fragments. CT examination should be performed after closed reduction to decrease the likelihood of subsequent ON. Other fractures in the pelvis, including pubic rami or sacral fractures or soft tissue injuries, can be found on CT or MRI.

## Imaging Findings and Classifications

Femoral neck fractures are most commonly subcapital, but can also be transcervical or basicervical.

- Basicervical fractures are most commonly stress fractures but can occur in young people during high-impact trauma.
- The degree of displacement is important to assess, because the risk of ON increases with the degree of displacement.
- The Garden classification (Figure 19.1) is commonly used and is as follows:
  - Type I—nondisplaced incomplete, including valgus-impacted fractures (Figure 19.2); can be easily missed
  - Type II—complete nondisplaced fractures
  - Type III—partially displaced complete fractures, varus angulated
  - Type IV—fully displaced complete fractures (Figure 19.3)
- A lateral sclerotic triangle at the fracture site may be seen on radiographs or CT study with valgus-impacted fractures.
- A medial sclerotic triangle may be seen in nondisplaced varus-impacted fractures.
- Radiographically occult fractures will appear as BME on fluid-sensitive MRI sequences with a linear hypointense fracture line seen on all sequences (Figure 19.4).
- Intertrochanteric fractures appear as a diagonal fracture line extending from the greater trochanter laterally to the lesser trochanter medially (Figure 19.5).
  - Classification is based on the number of fracture fragments, ranging from a 2-part fracture to a 4-part fracture.
- Isolated greater trochanter fractures are rare, and MRI is useful to verify that an occult intertrochanteric fracture is not present.

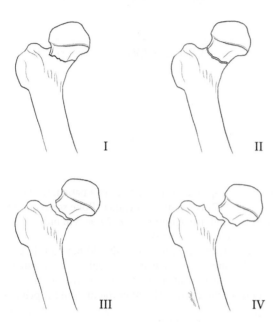

**Figure 19.1.** Illustration showing the Garden classification of femoral neck fractures. © 2016 Lauren Kalinoski.

- When an avulsion fracture of the lesser trochanter is seen in an adult, there should be a high index of suspicion for underlying metastasis (Figure 19.6).
- With hip dislocations, it is important to evaluate for intraarticular bone fragments, which may prevent adequate relocation of the hip and can result in accelerated OA (Figure 19.7). On radiographs, this may appear as hip joint space widening or incongruence.
- With posterior hip dislocations, on radiographs, the hip is usually posteriorly and superiorly dislocated and

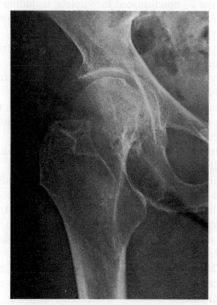

**Figure 19.2.** Valgus-impacted subcapital femoral neck fracture on radiograph. A frontal radiograph of the hip shows an impacted subcapital femoral neck fracture with associated valgus angulation, Garden I classification.

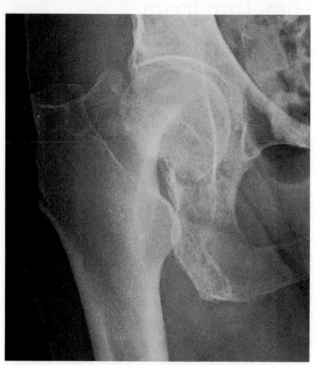

**Figure 19.3.** Displaced femoral neck fracture on radiograph. A frontal radiograph of the hip shows a displaced subcapital femoral neck fracture, Garden IV classification.

internally rotated, placing the greater trochanter in profile.
- There may be an associated posterior acetabular wall or column fracture or femoral head fracture or impaction similar to a Hill-Sachs lesion. An intraarticular fracture fragment can also occur from the insertion site of the ligamentum teres.
- Anterior hip dislocations are usually inferior (Figure 19.8) and less commonly superior. Impaction fractures of the femoral head are commonly present.
- Central hip dislocations involve a fracture of the acetabulum with protrusion of the femoral head into the pelvis (Figure 19.9).

---

## Treatment Options

### Femoral Neck Fractures
- Garden I or II—internal fixation with 3 percutaneously placed cannulated lag screws
- Displaced Garden III or IV—hip arthroplasty
- Nonsurgical treatment for poor surgical candidates or nonambulatory patients

### Intertrochanteric Fractures
- Intramedullary nail fixation
- Dynamic hip screw (for stable fractures), consisting of a lateral femoral diaphyseal cortical plate and hip screw, which allows settling and increased apposition of the fracture, improving the chances of healing

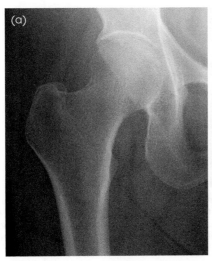
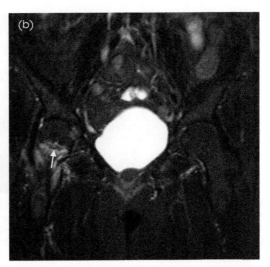

**Figure 19.4.** Radiographically occult femoral neck fracture seen on MRI. A frontal radiograph of the hip (*A*) shows no abnormality. A coronal STIR MR image of the pelvis (*B*) shows high signal intensity BME and a low signal intensity transverse fracture line (*arrow*) in the femoral neck related to a nondisplaced, radiographically occult fracture.

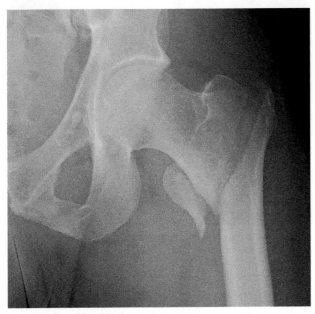

**Figure 19.5.** Intertrochanteric femur fracture on radiograph. A frontal radiograph of the hip shows an intertrochanteric fracture with detachment of the lesser trochanter (3-part fracture) with associated varus angulation.

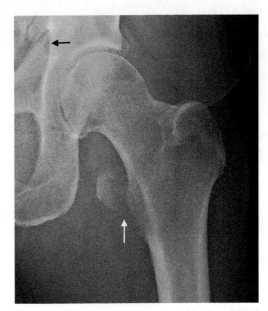

**Figure 19.6.** Pathologic avulsion fracture of the lesser trochanter associated with metastatic disease. A frontal radiograph of the hip shows a lesser trochanter avulsion fracture secondary to an osteolytic metastasis (*white arrow*). Additional medial acetabular metastasis is present (*black arrow*).

## Hip Dislocation

- Prompt relocation to prevent ON
- Surgery if removal of intraarticular fragment or fixation of acetabular wall fracture is needed

## Key Points

- The greater degree of femoral neck fracture displacement, the greater the likelihood of ON.
- For intertrochanteric fractures, the number of fracture parts is important to assess.

- It is important to assess for an intraarticular fragment after hip dislocation, best seen on CT.
- There is a high association of underlying metastasis with lesser trochanter fractures in adults.
- MRI is the study of choice in the evaluation of occult hip fractures.

## Recommended Reading

Sheehan SE, Shyu JY, Weaver MJ, Sodickson AD, Khurana B. Proximal femoral fractures: what the orthopedic surgeon wants to know. *Radiographics*. 2015;35:1563–84.

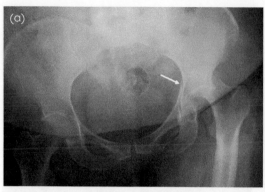
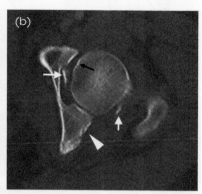

**Figure 19.7.** Posterior hip dislocation associated with intraarticular fracture fragments. A frontal radiograph of the pelvis (*A*) shows a posterior dislocation of the left femoral head with associated acetabular fracture (*arrow*). Axial CT image post closed reduction (*B*) shows relocated left hip with intraarticular bone fragments (*white arrows*). Note irregularity of the fractured posterior acetabular wall consistent with a fracture (*arrowhead*). There is a minimal impaction of the femoral head anterior to the fovea capitis (*black arrow*).

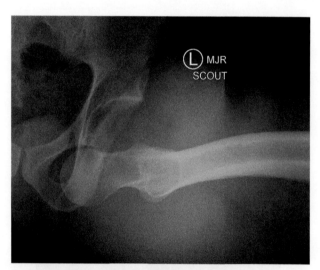

**Figure 19.8.** Anterior hip dislocation. A frontal radiograph of the left hip shows anterior-inferior dislocation of the femoral head projecting over the obturator ring.

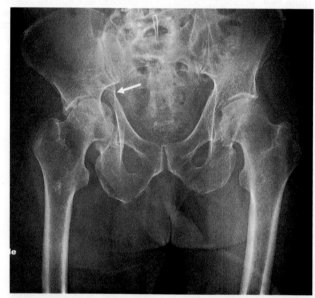

**Figure 19.9.** Central hip dislocation. A frontal radiograph of the pelvis shows central dislocation of the right femoral head with a displaced acetabular fracture (*arrow*).

## References

1. Damany DS, Parker MJ. Varus impacted intracapsular hip fractures. *Injury.* 2005;36:627–9.
2. Feldman F, Staron RB. MRI of seemingly isolated greater trochanteric fractures. *AJR Am J Roentgenol.* 2004;183:323–9.
3. Harris J Jr. Hips and proximal femurs. In: Pope T, Harris JJr, ed. *Harris and Harris Radiology of Emergency Medicine.* 5th ed. Philadelphia, PA: Lippincott Williams & Wilkins; 2013:831–60.
4. Kirby MW, Spritzer C. Radiographic detection of hip and pelvic fractures in the emergency department. *AJR Am J Roentgenol.* 2010;194:1054–60.
5. Mitchell MJ, Ho C, Resnick D, Sartoris DJ. Diagnostic imaging of lower extremity trauma. *Radiol Clin North Am.* 1989;27:909–28.
6. Phillips CD, Pope TL Jr, Jones JE, Keats TE, MacMillan RH 3rd. Nontraumatic avulsion of the lesser trochanter: a pathognomonic sign of metastatic disease? *Skeletal Radiol.* 1988;17:106–10.
7. Sanders S, Tejwani N, Egol KA. Traumatic hip dislocation—a review. *Bull NYU Hosp Jt Dis.* 2010;68:91–96.
8. Zoga A. Osseous pathology: hip and proximal femur. In: Sonin A, ed. *Diagnostic Imaging Musculoskeletal: Trauma.* Altona, Manitoba: Amirsys; 2010:5.8–5.36.

# CHAPTER 20

# Femur Trauma

Winnie A Mar and Tyson S. Chadaz

## Mechanism of Injury

The femur is the longest and strongest bone in the body often requiring high-energy trauma for fracture. Subtrochanteric fractures are usually high-energy fractures, but are also seen in osteoporotic patients after low-energy trauma and those on bisphosphonate treatment. When a low-energy subtrochanteric fracture is seen, a pathologic etiology must be considered, including metastasis or bisphosphonate treatment. Bisphosphonate-related fractures can also be seen within the femoral shaft.

The femoral shaft is the strongest part of the femur and femoral shaft fractures usually occur in young patients after high-energy trauma. These fractures may be associated with significant life-threatening trauma elsewhere.

Distal femoral fractures are relatively uncommon and may be supracondylar or intercondylar. The mechanism is an axial loading injury with valgus or varus stress. They occur in low-energy trauma usually in elderly osteoporotic women and high-energy trauma, typically in younger men. They may be associated with popliteal artery injuries.

## Imaging Strategy

Evaluation of femoral fractures begins with AP and lateral radiographs of the femur. Radiographic coverage should include the hip and knee joints to evaluate for associated fractures. Distal femoral fractures are often subsequently evaluated with CT for intraarticular extension or osseous fragments that may be difficult to visualize on radiographs, particularly in osteoporotic patients.

## Imaging Findings and Classifications

### Subtrochanteric Fractures

- Located 5 cm or less distal to the lesser trochanter and are usually spiral or comminuted (Figure 20.1).
- The distal femoral fragment is typically medially angulated because of the pull of the adductor muscles.
- The proximal fragment is abducted, externally rotated, and flexed because of the abductor musculature.
- It is important to note if there is involvement of the lesser trochanter or the piriformis fossa, which is the entry site

for the intramedullary nail located just medial to the greater trochanter (Figure 20.2).

### Bisphosphonate-Associated Fractures

- These fractures may occur anywhere from the subtrochanteric femur to the distal femoral shaft with involvement of the lateral cortex.
- A lateral beak of periosteal thickening is often seen, and typically these fractures are transverse with no or minimal comminution (Figure 20.3).
- In the setting of a bisphosphonate-associated fracture, it is important to evaluate the contralateral femur as these fractures frequently occur bilaterally.

### Femoral Shaft Fractures

- These fractures are classified by the Orthopedic Trauma Association as simple, wedge, and complex fractures (Figure 20.4).
- Simple fractures may be transverse, oblique, or spiral.
- Wedge fractures have a butterfly fragment.
- Complex fractures are comminuted or segmental fractures. These fractures commonly have varus angulation because of the pull of thigh musculature.
- Distal femoral shaft or supracondylar fractures typically have posterior displacement and angulation of the principal distal fragment because of the pull of the gastrocnemius muscle.

### Distal Femoral Fractures

- These fractures may be extraarticular supracondylar, partial articular condylar, or intraarticular intercondylar fractures.
- Supracondylar fractures tend to be comminuted. Condylar fractures may be oriented sagittally or coronally (Figure 20.5). A coronal (Hoffa) fracture is important to note as it will require a condylar buttress plate.

## Treatment Options

### Subtrochanteric Fractures

- Antegrade intramedullary nail

### Femoral Shaft Fractures

- Antegrade intramedullary nail
- Retrograde intramedullary nail

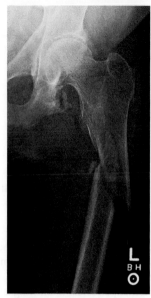

**Figure 20.1.** Subtrochanteric femur fracture. A frontal radiograph of the proximal femur shows a spiral, mildly comminuted subtrochanteric fracture with medial angulation of the principal distal fragment. The fracture does not involve the lesser trochanter or the piriformis fossa. Incidentally noted is irregularity of the ischium related to remote trauma.

### Distal Femoral Fractures

- Intraarticular distal femoral fractures are treated with ORIF (plate and screw fixation) or total knee arthroplasty.
- Extraarticular distal femoral fractures may be treated with intramedullary nail.

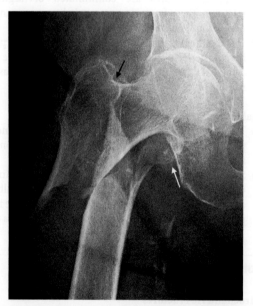

**Figure 20.2.** Subtrochanteric femur fracture with involvement of the lesser trochanter a.k.a. reverse obliquity intertrochanteric fracture. A frontal radiograph of the proximal femur shows a spiral subtrochanteric fracture with medial displacement of the principal distal fragment. The fracture involves the lesser trochanter (*white arrow*) but does not involve the piriformis fossa (*black arrow*). This fracture pattern may also be described as reverse obliquity intertrochanteric fracture.

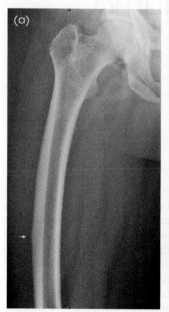
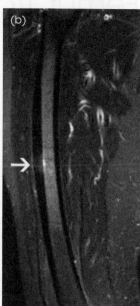

**Figure 20.3.** Bisphosphonate-related incomplete femoral shaft fracture. Frontal radiograph of the femur (*A*) shows bowing, lateral cortical thickening and periosteal reaction with an incomplete transverse lucency (*arrow*) in this patient on long-term bisphosphonate therapy consistent with an incomplete atypical femoral fracture. Coronal T2W FS MR image of the femur (*B*) shows corresponding BME and a hypointense incomplete transverse fracture line (*arrow*) in the same region.

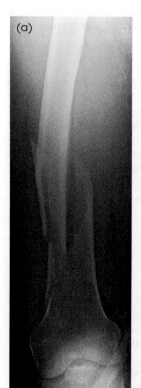
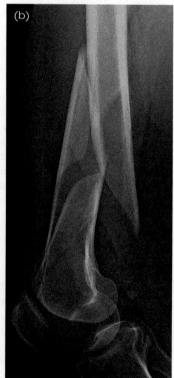

**Figure 20.4.** Displaced comminuted spiral wedge fracture of the distal femoral shaft. Frontal (*A*) and lateral (*B*) radiographs of the femur show a comminuted, spiral wedge fracture of the distal femoral shaft with anterior displacement of the principal distal fragment and butterfly fragments.

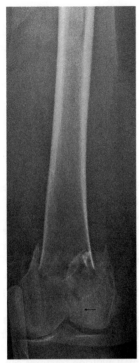

**Figure 20.5.** Comminuted intraarticular distal femur fracture. A frontal radiograph of the femur shows a comminuted supracondylar femoral fracture with intraarticular extension into the intercondylar notch (*arrow*) (T-shaped fracture).

## Key Points

- Subtrochanteric fractures are usually high-energy fractures, but are also seen in osteoporotic patients after low-energy trauma and those on bisphosphonate treatment.
- It is important to evaluate for secondary signs suggesting bisphosphonate-related fractures, particularly in low-energy trauma.

- Femoral shaft fractures may be associated with life-threatening trauma elsewhere.
- Intraarticular extension of distal femoral fractures is important to note as this will affect management.

### Recommended Reading

Mitchell MJ, Ho C, Resnick D, Sartoris DJ. Diagnostic imaging of lower extremity trauma. *Radiol Clin North Am.* 1989;27:909–28.

### References

1. Ehlinger M, Ducrot G, Adam P, Bonnomet F. Distal femur fractures. Surgical techniques and a review of the literature. *Orthop Traumatol Surg Res.* 2013;99(3):353–60.
2. Hak DJ, Mauffrey C, Hake M, Hammerberg EM, Stahel PF. Ipsilateral femoral neck and shaft fractures: current diagnostic and treatment strategies. *Orthopedics.* 2015;38:247–51.
3. Marsh JL, Slongo TF, Agel J, et al. Fracture and dislocation classification compendium—2007: Orthopaedic Trauma Association classification, database and outcomes committee. *J Orthop Trauma.* 2007;21(10 suppl):S1–133.
4. Sheehan SE, Shyu JY, Weaver MJ, Sodickson AD, Khurana B. Proximal femoral fractures: what the orthopedic surgeon wants to know. *Radiographics.* 2015;35:1563–84.
5. Shane E, Burr D, Abrahamsen B, et al. Atypical subtrochanteric and diaphyseal femoral fractures: second report of a task force of the American Society for Bone and Mineral Research. *J Bone Miner Res.* 2014;29:1–23.
6. Zoga A. Osseous pathology: hip and proximal femur. In: Sonin A, ed. *Diagnostic Imaging Musculoskeletal: Trauma.* Altona, Manitoba: Amirsys; 2010:5.8–5.36.

# CHAPTER 21

# Knee Trauma

Winnie A. Mar and Tyson S. Chadaz

## Mechanism of Injury

Most tibial plateau fractures occur with valgus and axial loading during high-energy trauma, such as a pedestrian struck by a car bumper, and low-energy trauma, such as a fall from standing height. Fractures with compression (Schatzker type II and III) typically occur in patients who are middle-aged or older with associated osteopenia. Schatzker type IV medial tibial plateau fractures occur with varus stress and axial loading and are usually high-energy injuries in younger patients. They represent 10% of all tibial plateau fractures and carry the worst prognosis. There may be associated popliteal artery or peroneal nerve injury. Schatzker type V and VI are also high-energy injuries with a complex mechanism of injury involving valgus and varus stresses with axial loading.

Knee dislocations are uncommon and are seen in high-energy trauma with hyperextension or dashboard injury. Patients can present with knee deformity, but the dislocation frequently has already been reduced in the field. Severe ligamentous and vascular injuries may be associated.

Patellar fractures usually result from sudden tension on the extensor mechanism resulting in a transverse fracture, or less commonly, a direct fall on the knee anteriorly.

Avulsion fractures of the knee are important to identify as these often portend more significant ligamentous injuries. A Segond fracture is an avulsion fracture of the lateral tibia from the mid third lateral capsular ligament and may involve the anterolateral ligament (ALL). It has a high association with anterior cruciate ligament (ACL) tears. This injury occurs during forceful internal rotation of the knee with varus stress. An avulsion fracture of the proximal fibular tip at the attachment of the arcuate ligament, conjoined tendon and popliteofibular and fabellofibular ligaments is termed an *arcuate fracture* or *arcuate sign* and has a high association with posterolateral corner injuries. An ACL bony avulsion fracture from the tibial eminence is frequently associated with ligamentous and meniscal injuries in adults typically from a hyperextension injury in a high-energy trauma. In children, a tibial spine avulsion fracture results from tibial internal rotation in a flexed knee and is usually isolated.

## Imaging Strategy

Radiographs are performed first when evaluating for trauma about the knee. Standard views include AP and lateral or cross-table lateral projections. Oblique views should be performed if there is suspicion for a tibial plateau fracture. An axial patellofemoral view should be performed if there is suspicion for a patellar fracture.

In tibial plateau fractures, CT or MRI is often performed to accurately depict the degree of depression, as this may modify the surgical plan. Conventional angiography or CT angiography should be performed to evaluate for popliteal artery injury in a patient with diminished pulses after a knee dislocation or high-energy tibial plateau fracture.

When certain avulsion fractures are seen about the knee, including the arcuate fracture/sign, Segond fracture, or tibial eminence avulsion, MRI should be performed, as these seemingly innocuous small avulsion fractures can indicate significant ligamentous or meniscal injury.

## Imaging Findings and Classifications

- Patients with tibial plateau fractures always have a joint effusion on radiographs.
- If nondepressed, the fracture may be difficult to detect.
- A lipohemarthrosis indicates an intraarticular fracture (Figure 21.1).

The Schatzker classification for tibial plateau fractures is widely used (Figure 21.2).

- Most fractures involve the lateral plateau.
- Type I is a nondepressed vertical fracture of the lateral tibial plateau (Figure 21.3).
- Type II is a depressed vertical/split fracture of the lateral tibial plateau (Figure 21.4).
- Type III is a depressed compression fracture of the lateral tibial plateau (Figure 21.5).
- Type IV is a medial tibial plateau fracture (Figure 21.6).
- Type V is a bicondylar fracture (Figure 21.7).
- Type VI is any fracture with a transverse metaphyseal component (Figure 21.8).

Tibial plateau fractures are often associated with other injuries.

- Schatzker type I fractures are associated with medial collateral ligament (MCL) and ACL tears.
- Schatzker type II fractures are associated with MCL and medial meniscal tears.
- Schatzker type IV fractures are associated with lateral collateral ligament (LCL) and posterolateral corner injuries.

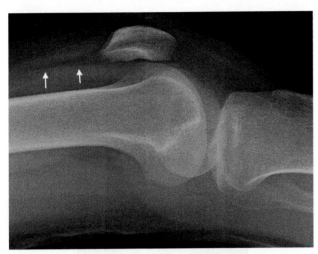

**Figure 21.1.** Lipohemarthrosis. A cross-table lateral radiograph of the knee shows a lipohemarthrosis (*arrows*), indicating an intraarticular fracture in this patient with a Schatzker type I lateral tibial plateau fracture.

### Femorotibial Joint Dislocations

- Knee dislocations are described with the direction of the tibia with respect to the femur.
- Anterior, posterior, medial, lateral, and rotary femorotibial dislocations may occur.
- Anterior dislocations are more common than posterior dislocations (Figure 21.9).

- Rotary femorotibial dislocations are further subdivided into anteromedial, posteromedial, anterolateral, and posterolateral directions.

### Proximal Tibiofibular Joint Dislocations

- Proximal tibiofibular joint dislocations are the least common type of knee dislocations.
- There are 3 types including anterolateral, posteromedial, and superior dislocations, which are based on the position of the fibular head relative to the tibia.

### Patellar Fractures

- Patellar fractures may be horizontal, vertical, or stellate (Figure 21.10).
- It is important to differentiate this from a normal variant bipartite or multipartite patella, which usually occurs in the superolateral quadrant of the patella.

### Patellar Dislocations

- Acute patellofemoral joint dislocations are most common in young, athletic individuals and are most commonly lateral.
- These injuries result from a twisting motion with a flexed knee and less commonly from medial impact to the knee. Other types of patellar dislocations are rare.
- The patella dislocates laterally, with resultant injury of the medial soft tissue patellofemoral supporting structures.
- Lateral patellofemoral dislocations are most commonly transient.

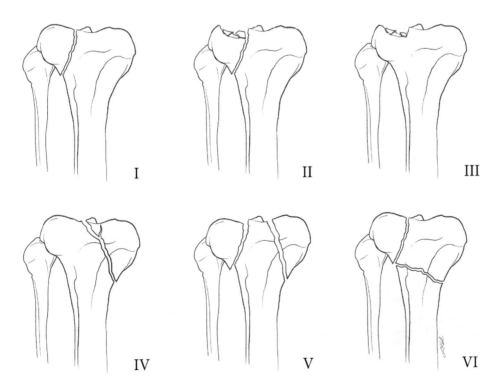

**Figure 21.2.** Illustration shows the Schatzker classification for tibial plateau fractures. © 2016 Lauren Kalinoski.

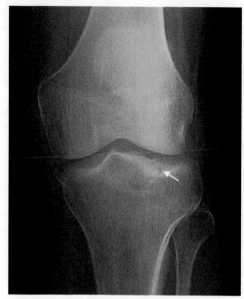

**Figure 21.3.** Schatzker type I vertical fracture of the lateral tibial plateau is seen on AP radiograph (*arrow*).

- With spontaneous reduction, the medial facet of the patella impacts the anterior aspect of the lateral femoral condyle, which may result in bone contusion and/or osteochondral fracture of the medial patellar facet and impaction injury at the peripheral aspect of the lateral femoral condyle (Figure 21.11).
- Predisposing factors include: patella alta, shallow trochlear groove, and increased tibial tubercle-trochlear groove (TT-TG) distance with more lateral position of the tibial tuberosity (>2 cm).

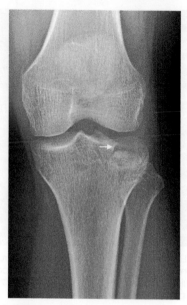

**Figure 21.5.** Schatzker type III tibial plateau fracture. AP radiograph of the knee shows a Schatzker type III depressed lateral tibial plateau fracture (*arrow*).

**Avulsion Fractures**
- A Segond fracture (Figure 21.12*A*) has a very high association with ACL (Figure 21.12*B*) and meniscal tears, which are well depicted by MRI.
- In a reverse Segond fracture, a small avulsed fragment of the medial tibia by the deep capsular MCL will be seen and is associated with posterior cruciate ligament (PCL) and medial meniscal tears.

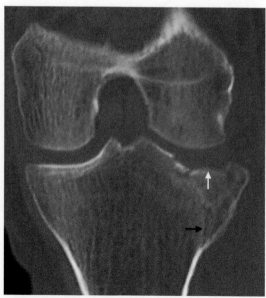

**Figure 21.4.** Schatzker type II lateral tibial plateau fracture. Coronal reformatted CT image shows a Schatzker type II split depressed lateral tibial plateau fracture (*white arrow*) with a vertical cleavage fracture line (*black arrow*).

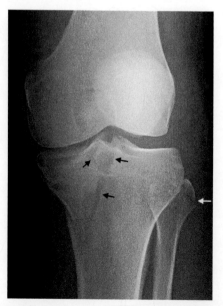

**Figure 21.6.** Schatzker type IV medial tibial plateau fracture. AP radiograph of the knee shows a Schatzker type IV medial tibial plateau fracture extending into the tibial eminence (*black arrows*) with narrowing of the medial compartment and widening of the lateral compartment. There is also a proximal fibular avulsion fracture (*white arrow*) related to the lateral compartment distraction injury.

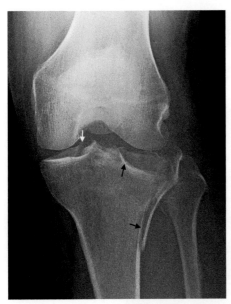

**Figure 21.7.** Schatzker type V bicondylar tibial plateau fracture. AP internal oblique radiograph of the knee shows a lateral tibial plateau depressed fracture (*black arrows*) in addition to a medial tibial plateau fracture (*white arrow*) consistent with Schatzker type V classification.

- The arcuate fracture/sign is highly associated with posterolateral corner injuries including cruciate and collateral ligaments, posterolateral capsule, and meniscal tears. It will appear as an elliptical, horizontally oriented avulsion fracture of the proximal fibula.
- Unrecognized posterolateral corner injuries can result in ACL reconstruction failure and chronic instability with premature OA.

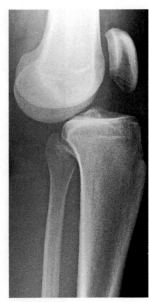

**Figure 21.9.** Anterior knee dislocation. Lateral radiograph of the knee shows an anterior tibiofemoral joint dislocation.

- A larger, irregular fibular avulsion fragment is seen with biceps femoris avulsion, which is associated with LCL and popliteus tendon tears and Segond fractures.
- ACL or less commonly PCL avulsion injuries will present as small to large avulsed bone fragments of the tibial eminence.

**Deep Femoral Notch Sign with Anterior Cruciate Ligament Tear**

- An indentation at the lateral femoral condyle joint surface that measures more than 1.5-2 mm in depth (Figure

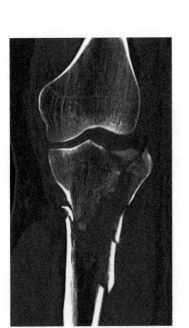

**Figure 21.8.** Schatzker type VI tibial plateau fracture. Coronal reformatted CT image of the knee shows a lateral tibial plateau comminuted fracture with oblique proximal tibial metadiaphyseal extension (Schatzker type VI).

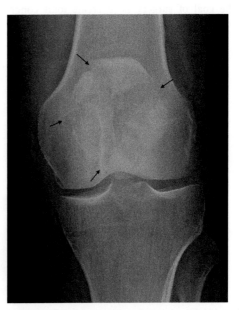

**Figure 21.10.** Patellar fracture. AP radiograph of the knee shows a stellate comminuted patellar fracture (*arrows*) with distraction of the fracture fragments.

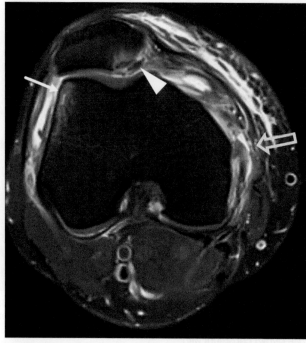

**Figure 21.11.** Transient lateral patellar dislocation. Axial proton density weighted (PDW) FS MR image of the knee demonstrates BME in the anterior lateral femoral condyle (*arrow*), osteochondral fracture fragment of the medial patellar facet (*arrowhead*) with subjacent BME and femoral disruption of the medial patellofemoral ligament (*open arrow*) consistent with transient lateral dislocation of the patella.

21.13) consistent with impaction injury secondary to pivot shift mechanism
- High correlation with ACL tears

## Treatment Options

### Tibial Plateau Fractures
- The goal of surgery is to create joint congruence to prevent OA.

- Vertical split fractures are typically treated with transverse cancellous screws.
- Degree of depression for surgery is controversial, but typically patients with greater than 3 mm of depression or distraction should have surgery.
- Significantly depressed fractures can be reduced arthroscopically with cartilage repair.
- Schatzker type IV and VI fractures need surgical fixation with buttress plates and cancellous screws.
- Schatzker type V fractures may be treated surgically as described or with external fixation or splinting because of the high risk of infection and wound dehiscence.

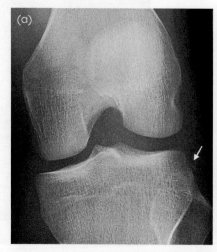
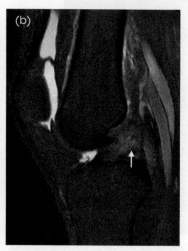

**Figure 21.12.** Segond fracture in association with ACL tear. AP radiograph of the knee (*A*) shows an avulsion fracture from the peripheral lateral tibial epiphysis (*arrow*) consistent with a Segond fracture. Sagittal PDW FS MR image (*B*) shows an associated ACL tear (*arrow*).

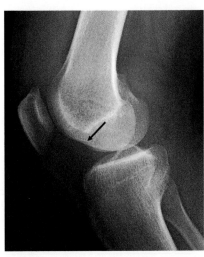

**Figure 21.13.** Deep femoral notch sign. Lateral knee radiograph demonstrates a deep lateral femoral condyle notch measuring more than 1.5-2 mm in depth (*arrow*).

## Knee Dislocations
- Prompt relocation, bypass graft for vascular injury, ligament reconstruction

## Patellar Fractures
- Conservative management if less than 2 mm articular step-off
- Surgical management with tension band and wires or cannulated or lag screw fixation

## Avulsion Fractures
- Repair of ligamentous and meniscal injuries
- Internal fixation for a large separated tibial eminence avulsion (optional)

## Key Points
- Oblique radiographs are helpful for detecting tibial plateau fractures.
- CT is useful in quantifying the degree of depression in tibial plateau fractures, which affects management.

- The Schatzker classification is useful in assessment of tibial plateau fractures.
- Tibial plateau fractures most commonly involve the lateral tibial plateau.
- Certain avulsion fractures/signs about the knee, such as the Segond fracture, arcuate fracture/sign, and deep femoral notch sign, are often associated with significant ligamentous injury and should be evaluated with MRI.
- Neurovascular injuries may be associated with knee dislocations.
- Patellar dislocations are most commonly lateral and transient.

### Recommended Reading
Markhardt BK, Gross JM, Monu JU. Schatzker classification of tibial plateau fractures: use of CT and MR imaging improves assessment. *Radiographics.* 2009;29:585–97.

### References
1. Gimber LH, Scalcione LR, Rowan A, Hoardy JC, Melville DM, Taljanovic MS. Multiligamentous injuries and knee dislocations. *Skeletal Radiol.* 2015:44:1559–72.
2. Gottsegen CJ, Eyer BA, White EA, Learch TJ, Forrester D. Avulsion fractures of the knee: imaging findings and clinical significance. *Radiographics.* 2008;28:1755–70.
3. Ha AS, Porrino JA, Chew FS. Radiographic pitfalls in lower extremity trauma. *AJR Am J Roentgenol.* 2014;203:492–500.
4. Juhng SK, Lee JK, Choi SS, Yoon KH, Roh BS, Won JJ. MR evaluation of the "arcuate" sign of posterolateral knee instability. *AJR Am J Roentgenol.* 2002;178:583–88.
5. Kakazu R, Archdeacon MT. Surgical management of patellar fractures. *Orthop Clin North Am.* 2016;47:77–83.
6. Markhardt BK, Gross JM, Monu JU. Schatzker classification of tibial plateau fractures: use of CT and MR imaging improves assessment. *Radiographics.* 2009;29:585–97.
7. Robertson A, Nutton RW, Keating JF. Dislocation of the knee. *J Bone Joint Surg Br.* 2006;88:706–11.
8. Stevens MA, El-Khoury GY, Kathol MH, Brandser EA, Chow S. Imaging features of avulsion injuries. *Radiographics.* 1999;19:655–72.

# CHAPTER 22

# Tibia and Fibula Trauma

Winnie A. Mar and Tyson S. Chadaz

## Mechanism of Injury

Tibial shaft fractures are relatively common. The clinical presentation is pain, swelling, and inability to bear weight. These usually result from a high-energy trauma, such as motor vehicle accident, pedestrian struck, or motorcycle crash. Spiral fractures result from indirect forces, such as low-energy twisting injury or fall, and direct forces result in transverse or comminuted fractures. Fractures tend to be open because the bone is very close to the skin anteriorly; thus, infection is a common complication. Tibial fractures may heal slowly and can take up to 2 years. Higher-energy injuries may also result in concomitant fracture of the fibula. Compartment syndrome may develop because of edema and hemorrhage and occurs more commonly with tibial shaft fractures and in younger patients.

A fibular fracture may result from a direct blow, or varus or valgus injury of the knee. Isolated fibular head or neck fractures are uncommon and may be associated with ligamentous injuries of the knee. Proximal fibular fractures may be associated with external rotation injury of the ankle, often called *Maisonneuve fractures*. Proximal fibular fractures can be associated with peroneal nerve injury.

## Imaging Strategy

Imaging should begin with AP and lateral radiographs of the entire tibia and fibula. Additional radiographs of the pelvis, femur, knee, and ankle may be obtained as additional fractures may be present.

## Imaging Findings

- Tibial shaft fractures can be transverse, oblique, spiral, or segmental.
- Segmental fracture affects 2 or more levels, creating a separate fracture fragment.
- The mid and distal thirds of the tibia are commonly involved.
- The degree of comminution, displacement, angulation, and rotation should be noted.
- An open fracture occurs where bone is exposed and should be noted (Figure 22.1).
- An associated fibular fracture is common and may or may not be at the same level of the tibial fracture.
- If an isolated fibular fracture is seen, radiographs of the ankle should be performed to evaluate for medial or posterior malleolar fractures or medial ankle mortise

widening, termed *Maisonneuve injury with associated syndesmotic injury* (see Figure 23.5 in Chapter 23, "Ankle Trauma").

## Treatment Options

- Intramedullary nail, plate, or external fixation
- Casting for low-energy fractures without significant displacement

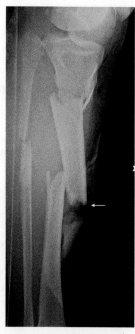

**Figure 22.1.** Open segmental tibial shaft fracture and segmental fibular shaft fracture. A lateral view of the tibia and fibula shows a comminuted, overriding segmental fracture of the proximal to mid tibial shaft which is open with exposed bone (*arrow*). A segmental proximal fibular shaft fracture is also seen.

## Key Points

- Tibial shaft fractures are common with potential complications of infection, compartment syndrome, and delayed union.
- The ankle should be closely evaluated when an isolated fibular fracture is found.

**Recommended Reading**

Mitchell MJ, Ho C, Resnick D, Sartoris DJ. Diagnostic imaging of lower extremity trauma. *Radiol Clin North Am.* 1989;27:909–28.

**References**

1. McMahon SE, Little ZE, Smith TO, Trompeter A, Hing CB. The management of segmental tibial shaft fractures: a systematic review. *Injury.* 2015;47(3):568–73.

2. Mitchell MJ, Ho C, Resnick D, Sartoris DJ. Diagnostic imaging of lower extremity trauma. *Radiol Clin North Am.* 1989;27:909–28.

3. Park S, Ahn J, Gee AO, Kuntz AF, Esterhai JL. Compartment syndrome in tibial fractures. *J Orthop Trauma.* 2009;23:514–18.

4. Resnick D. Physical injury: extraspinal sites. In: Resnick D, ed. *Diagnosis of Bone and Joint Disorders.* 3rd ed. Philadelphia, PA: Saunders; 2005:831–78.

# CHAPTER 23

# Ankle Trauma

Pavan Parasu and Winnie A. Mar

## Mechanism of Injury

Most ankle injuries occur because of a low-energy twisting trauma, usually an inversion injury, with a planted foot and angulation or rotation of the leg. The most common type of ankle sprain results from inversion-type twisting of the foot with injury of the LCL complex, whereas the less common eversion sprain occurs when the ankle rolls too far outward resulting in deltoid ligament injury.

Clinically, the ankle is painful and swollen, and the patient cannot bear weight and has focal bone tenderness. The most common mechanism of injury is *supination external rotation* (SER), in which the lateral structures are injured first, accounting for 40-75% of all ankle fractures. *Supination adduction* (SAD) trauma is primarily caused by a compression force on the medial malleolus with traction of the lateral aspect of the ankle. In the *pronation external rotation* (PER) mechanism, the primary stressor is on the deltoid ligament. With the *pronation-abduction* (PAB) mechanism, abduction of the talus causes traction of the medial ankle and compression of the lateral ankle structures.

A distal tibial plafond (Pilon) fracture is caused by an axial load on the tibial plafond with associated valgus or varus stress. This may occur from a fall from height or a motor vehicle accident and can be associated with additional fractures of the pelvis, spine, or contralateral limb.

The Maisonneuve fracture is seen when an abduction force is transferred superiorly along the tibiofibular interosseous membrane to the proximal fibula while the foot is pronated. This fracture is associated with a fall from a height or motor vehicle collision.

Ankle sprains as well as crush injuries can cause osteochondral lesions of the talus, which are osteochondral impaction injuries. They are also referred to as *osteochondral fractures* or *defects*.

## Imaging Strategy

Ankle injuries are first evaluated with radiographs. AP and lateral views should always be obtained. The lateral view helps to delineate posterior malleolus and lateral malleolar fractures. The mortise view is taken as an AP view with 15-25 degree internal rotation of the foot. The fifth metatarsal base should always be included on the lateral image, as its fracture may clinically simulate an ankle injury. In the setting of an isolated medial malleolus or posterior malleolus fracture with ankle mortise widening, radiographs of the entire tibia and fibula should be obtained to evaluate for a proximal fibular fracture (Maisonneuve fracture). CT examination can be useful for preoperative planning in Pilon fractures or other complex cases with marked comminution or severe displacement, as well as to detect fractures that are not well seen on radiographs. An MRI may be useful in determining associated ligamentous injury. CT examination or preferably MRI can be used to assess for osteochondral lesions, as one-third of these may be radiographically occult.

### Optional Stress Views

Manual external rotation stress testing can evaluate syndesmotic and deep deltoid ligament injuries and is performed in the supine position. On the AP view, the difference in the width of the superior clear space between the medial and lateral sides of the tibiotalar joint should be less than 2 mm. The gravity stress view is as effective as the manual stress test in detection of medial clear space widening. This test is performed with the patient in the lateral decubitus position on the side of the affected ankle with the distal leg, ankle, and foot allowed to hang dependent off the end of the examination table whereas a mortise view is obtained.

## Imaging Findings and Classifications

The Lauge-Hansen and Weber classifications for ankle fractures are widely used (Table 23.1).

### Lauge-Hansen Classification

- Injuries are classified by the mechanism of injury, referring to the position of the foot and the direction of trauma.
- Injuries occur in a predictable manner depending on the degree of force applied.
- The findings of the previous stages are always seen, for example, an SER stage III injury will have the findings of an SER I–II injury as well. In SER and SAD injuries, the lateral structures are injured first, whereas the medial structures are injured first in PER and PAB injuries.

### Weber Classification

- Ankle injuries are categorized by the level of the fibular fracture, with Weber A being distal to ankle mortise, Weber B at and above the level of the ankle joint, and Weber C above the level of the ankle joint.
- Weber A corresponds to the SAD mechanism; Weber B is equivalent to SER; and Weber C corresponds to the PER mechanism.

**Table 23.1. Lauge-Hansen and Weber Classifications for Ankle Fractures**

| LAUGE-HANSEN (MECHANISM) | WEBER CLASSIFICATION | IMAGING FINDINGS |
|---|---|---|
| Supination adduction (SAD) | A | SAD I: Distal lateral malleolar fracture or lateral mortise widening<br>SADII: Vertical medial malleolar fracture |
| Supination external rotation (SER) | B | SER I: Lateral clear space widening<br>SERII: Spiral fibular fracture at mortise<br>SER III: Posterior malleolar fracture<br>SER IV: Transverse medial malleolar fracture |
| Pronation external rotation (PER) | C | PER I: Medial mortise widening or fracture<br>PER II: Tibiofibular widening<br>PER III: Spiral fibular fracture typically 6 cm above mortise<br>PER IV: Posterior malleolar fracture |
| Pronation-abduction (PAB) | | PAB I: Medial mortise widening or medial maleollar fracture<br>PAB II: Posterior malleolar fracture<br>PAB III: Oblique lateral malleolar fracture above mortise |

### Supination External Rotation (Weber B) Injuries

- In the most common mechanism, SER (Weber B) injuries, the lateral structures of the ankle joint are the first to be compromised.
- As the force continues, eventually the medial structures are damaged.
- Stage I is a stable injury involving anterior inferior tibiofibular ligament sprain, which may be radiographically occult, or seen as widening of the lateral clear space greater than 6 mm.
- In stage II, a spiral fracture of the lateral malleolus becomes evident (Figure 23.1); the isolated spiral fracture of the fibula is the most common ankle fracture.
- In stage III, the posterior malleolus is fractured.
- In stage IV, a fracture of the medial malleolus or medial joint space widening is seen (Figure 23.2).

### Supination Adduction (Weber A) Injuries

- Stage I SAD (Weber A) injury results in a transverse distal lateral malleolus fracture or widening of the lateral clear space (Figure 23.3).
- Stage II injuries involve a vertical fracture through the medial malleolus.

### Pronation External Rotation (Weber C) Injuries

- With a stage I PER injury (Weber C), the deltoid ligament is ruptured, which results in widening of the medial clear space or a transverse avulsion fracture of the medial malleolus.
- Further stress causes progression to a stage II injury with rupture of the anterior talofibular ligament and interosseous membrane and widening of the tibiofibular joint space.

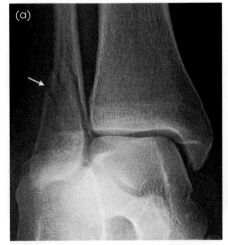 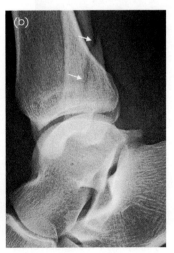

**Figure 23.1.** Weber B (SER II) injury. Oblique (*A*) and lateral (*B*) radiographs of the ankle show a Weber B, SER stage II injury with a spiral intraarticular distal fibular fracture (*arrow*). There is no medial ankle mortise widening. In the oblique projection, the fracture line (*arrows*) starts high laterally and in the lateral projection, high posteriorly extending anteromedial and superior to anterior respectively.

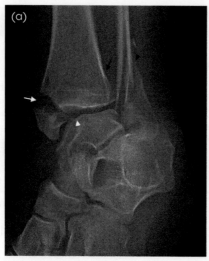
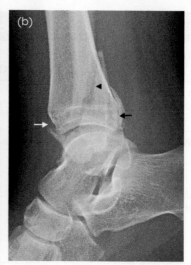

**Figure 23.2.** Weber B (SER IV) injury. Oblique (*A*) and lateral (*B*) radiographs of the ankle show a Weber B, SER stage IV injury, trimalleolar ankle fracture with an osteochondral lesion of the medial talar dome (*arrowhead*). The trimalleolar fracture comprises a transverse medial malleolar fracture (*white arrow*), spiral lateral malleolar fracture (*black arrowhead*) and posterior malleolar fracture (*black arrow*).

- A stage III injury involves a spiral fracture of the fibula, approximately 6 cm above the tibiotalar joint (Figure 23.4).
- A stage IV injury has an additional posterior malleolar fracture.

**Pronation-Abduction Injury**
- Stage I PAB injury presents as a transverse fracture of the medial malleolus or rupture of the deltoid ligament, which may be radiographically occult and is difficult to differentiate from a stage I PER injury.
- Further abduction of the talus progresses to a stage II injury, where a posterior malleolus injury is also seen.
- The lateral ankle components are the next to be involved in stage III injuries, with an oblique fracture of the fibula

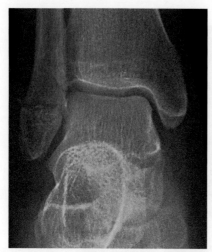

**Figure 23.3.** Weber A (SAD) injury. An AP radiograph of the ankle shows a Weber A, SAD injury with a distal fibular fracture below the level of the ankle mortise.

extending from medial to lateral, in addition to the injuries seen in stages I and II.

**Maisonneuve Fracture**
- Combination of a spiral fracture of the proximal fibula and an injury to the distal tibiofibular syndesmosis/interosseous membrane (Figure 23.5).
- It may occur with fractures of the medial or posterior malleolus as well as rupture of the deltoid ligament.
- The normal tibiofibular overlap on the AP views of the ankle should be more than 6 mm with decrease in overlap indicating syndesmotic injury.

**Pilon Fracture**
- The extent of distal tibial plafond (Pilon) fractures is often underestimated on radiographs.
- A longitudinally oriented fracture of the distal tibia that extends to the articular surface is typically seen (Figure 23.6).
- This fracture is usually comminuted, and there may be a degree of tibial depression.
- CT examination is valuable in determining the location of major fragments for surgical planning and often better delineates injuries to the tibiofibular syndesmosis.

**AO/OTA Foundation Classification of Distal Tibial Plafond (Pilon) Fractures**
- Type A is an extraarticular injury (divided into A1, A2, and A3 depending on severity of comminution).
- Type B is a partial articular injury (divided into B1, B2, and B3 depending on severity of comminution); with these injuries, a portion of the distal tibial metadiaphysis is in continuity with the distal tibial articular surface.
- Type C is a complete articular injury (divided into C1, C2, and C3 depending on severity of comminution).

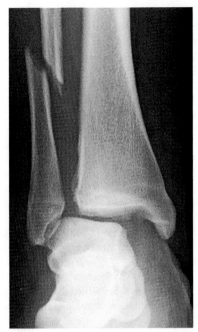

**Figure 23.4.** Weber C (PER III) injury. An AP radiograph of the ankle shows a Weber C fracture, PER injury, with a displaced high distal fibular shaft fracture 7 cm above the ankle joint and marked widening of the medial ankle mortise related to deltoid ligament tear. Note syndesmotic space widening consistent with disruption.

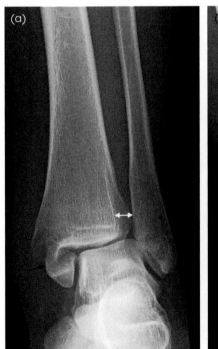
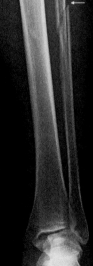

**Figure 23.5.** Maisonneuve injury. Oblique radiograph of the ankle (*A*) shows widening of the lateral tibiofibular clear space (*double arrows*) consistent with syndesmotic injury and a displaced, transverse medial malleolus fracture (*black arrow*). No fibular fracture is seen. An AP radiograph of the tibia and fibula (*B*) shows an oblique proximal fibular shaft fracture (*arrow*).

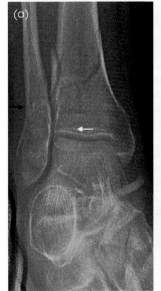
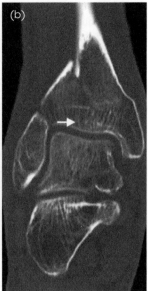

**Figure 23.6.** Distal tibial Pilon fracture. AP (*A*) radiograph of the ankle shows a comminuted distal tibial fracture with intraarticular extension (*white arrow*) and a distal fibular fracture (*black arrow*). A coronal reformatted CT image (*B*) of the ankle confirms the distal tibial intraarticular fracture (*arrow*).

## Osteochondral Lesions of the Talar Dome
- These lesions tend to be smaller and thinner laterally, larger and more depressed medially, and can be classified as follows:
  - Stage I—subchondral bone compression
  - Stage II—partially detached osteochondral fragment
  - Stage III—completely detached but nondisplaced osteochondral fragment (with fluid deep to the fragment)
  - Stage IV—displaced osteochondral fragment
  - Stage V—subchondral cyst formation

## Tibiotalar Joint Dislocations
- These dislocations can be associated with malleolar fractures, termed a *fracture-dislocation*. Often times, the talar dome is displaced anteriorly.

---

## Treatment Options

### Malleolar Fractures
- For stable fractures: closed reduction
- For unstable fractures: ORIF

### Tibial Pilon Fractures
- External or internal fixation

### Osteochondral Lesions of the Talar Dome
- Lower stage lesions may be managed conservatively.
- Operative management is required for stage III lesions and higher.

## Key Points

- The Lauge-Hansen classification of ankle fractures is based on the mechanism of injury; the most common mechanism is SER.
- The Weber classification of ankle fractures is based on the fibular fracture location relative to the ankle mortise.
- Evaluation of the entire fibula is needed for a Maisonneuve fracture, in which there is an isolated medial or posterior malleolus fracture or medial ankle mortise widening.
- CT examination is helpful in preoperative planning for distal tibial Pilon fractures, which are generally underestimated radiographically.
- An osteochondral lesion of the talar dome with fluid deep to the fragment is an unstable injury and requires surgical treatment.

## Recommended Reading

Okanobo H, Khurana B, Sheehan S, Duran-Mendicuti A, Arianjam A, Ledbetter S. Simplified diagnostic algorithm for Lauge-Hansen classification of ankle injuries. *Radiographics.* 2012;32(2):E71–E84.

## References

1. Arimoto HK, Forrester DM. Classification of ankle fractures: an algorithm. *AJR Am J Roentgenol* 1980;135(5):1057–63.
2. Clare MP. A rational approach to ankle fractures. *Foot Ankle Clin.* 2008;13(4):593–610.
3. Crist BD, Khazzam M, Murtha YM, Della Rocca GJ. Pilon fractures: advances in surgical management. *J Am Acad Orthop Surg.* 2011;19:612–22.
4. Kosuge D, Mahadevan D, Chandrasenan J, Pugh H. Managing type II & IV LH SER ankle fractures: current orthopaedic practice. *Ann R Coll Surg Engl.* 2010;92(8):689–92.
5. Melenevsky Y, Mackey RA, Abrahams RB, Thomson NB 3rd. Talar fractures and dislocations: a radiologist's guide to timely diagnosis and classification. *Radiographics.* 2015;35:765–79.
6. Mitchell MJ, Ho C, Resnick D, Sartoris DJ. Diagnostic imaging of lower extremity trauma. *Radiol Clin North Am.* 1989;27:909–28.
7. Okanobo H, Khurana S, Sheehan B, Duran-Mendicuti A, Arianjam A, Ledbetter S. Simplified diagnostic algorithm for Lauge-Hansen classification of ankle injuries. *Radiographics.* 2012:32(2):E71–E84.
8. Pope T, Bloem HL, Beltran J, Morrison WB, Wilson DJ. *Musculoskeletal Imaging.* 2nd ed. Philadelphia, PA: Elsevier Health Sciences; 2014.

# CHAPTER 24

# Foot Trauma

Winnie A. Mar and Tyson S. Chadaz

## Mechanism of Injury

Foot fractures are common. The calcaneus is the largest bone in the foot and supports the axial load of the body. It is the most frequently fractured tarsal bone. Calcaneal fractures typically occur from axial loading in high-energy traumas, such as a motor vehicle accident (MVA) or fall from a height, with 10% occurring bilaterally. Other axial loading injuries can be associated, including burst fractures of the thoracolumbar spine. Because of the thin skin surrounding the calcaneus, open fractures with subsequent infection and skin necrosis are potential complications.

Talar neck and body fractures and talar or subtalar joint dislocations are generally high-energy fractures associated with MVA or fall from a height. Patients present with dorsal midfoot swelling and painful midfoot range of motion. A lateral talar process fracture is commonly seen in snowboarders and occurs with axial loading of the dorsiflexed, everted, or externally rotated foot. A dorsal avulsion fracture of the talus at the location of the anterior ankle joint capsule insertion is relatively common and occurs with extreme plantar flexion and axial loading.

Most navicular body fractures are secondary to high-energy trauma, and avulsion fractures are caused by ankle inversion or eversion injuries.

The subtalar joint is an articulation between the talus and calcaneus at 3 facets, the posterior, middle, and anterior. The posterior facet is located in the posterior subtalar joint, and the middle and anterior facets are located in the anterior subtalar joint, which is in continuity with the talonavicular joint. At the lateral aspect between the posterior and anterior subtalar joints, there is a laterally based, fan-shaped space termed the *sinus tarsi* with associated interosseous and cervical neck ligaments. Subtalar dislocations result from a high-energy mechanism, most frequently in the medial direction. Approximately 25% of subtalar dislocations are open. The Chopart joint is the articulation between the hindfoot and midfoot in particular between the talar head, navicular, anterior process of the calcaneus, and cuboid. Dislocations of the Chopart joint are uncommon.

The Lisfranc joint comprises the articulation of the tarsal and metatarsal bones, which are connected with numerous tarsometatarsal and intermetatarsal ligaments. The Lisfranc ligament complex extends from the medial cuneiform to the second and third metatarsal bases and is an important stabilizer of the midfoot (Figure 24.1). A Lisfranc fracture-dislocation may occur from high-energy trauma or low-energy fall, by axial loading of the plantar flexed foot or abduction of the forefoot. Fractures/dislocations commonly affect the first and second metatarsal bases followed by medial or lateral dislocation depending on the direction of the force.

Metatarsal fractures are common and can occur from direct trauma with an object falling on the foot or an indirect twisting injury of the hindfoot while the forefoot remains planted. The fifth metatarsal is the most commonly injured, followed by the third metatarsal. Fifth metatarsal base avulsion fractures are common and occur with ankle inversion injury. They are a result of a bony avulsion fracture at the attachment of the peroneus brevis tendon or the lateral cord of the plantar fascia. A Jones fracture is located at the junction of the proximal fifth metatarsal metaphysis and diaphysis, approximately 2.5 cm (1 in.) distal to the base. In contrast, fifth metatarsal proximal diaphyseal fractures are usually stress fractures.

Phalangeal fractures usually result from direct trauma, such as from a stubbed toe or an object falling onto the toe.

## Imaging Strategy

Radiographs should be performed first in the evaluation of foot trauma. Standard views of the foot are AP, lateral, and oblique. For phalangeal fracture assessment, a lateral view with coned-down views of the toes and displacement of the nonaffected toes is helpful. An axial Harris view of the calcaneus should be performed if there is suspicion of a calcaneal fracture. CT with multiplanar reformats is commonly used for preoperative assessment of calcaneal fractures and can show tendon entrapment (Figure 24.2).

In assessment of the talus, radiographs of the ankle using AP, lateral, and mortise views, as well as foot radiographs are performed. CT examination can be performed to evaluate for potentially radiographically occult fractures, including lateral talar process fractures, dorsal avulsion fractures, or osteochondral lesions. CT examination is also frequently performed for talar head, neck, and body fractures for presurgical planning to assess the degree of displacement, joint reduction, comminution, and intraarticular involvement.

Weight-bearing radiographs should be performed if there is clinical suspicion for Lisfranc or Chopart joint injury. Approximately 50% of Lisfranc injuries are not visible on non-weight-bearing radiographs.

## Imaging Findings and Classifications

- The Böhler angle can help detect an occult calcaneal fracture and show the degree of depression.

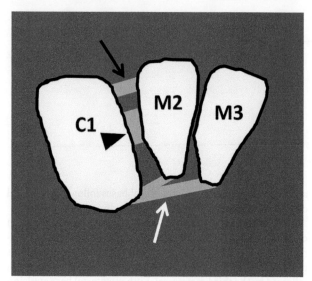

**Figure 24.1.** Lisfranc ligament. Drawing shows 3 components of the Lisfranc ligament with the dorsal band (*black arrow*) between the dorsal aspects of the medial cuneiform (C1) and second metatarsal base (M2), interosseous band (*arrowhead*) between the central aspects of C1 and M2, and a bifid plantar band (*white arrow*) between the plantar aspects of C1 and M2 and C1 and third metatarsal base (M3).

- One line is drawn from the anterior process of the calcaneus to the superior aspect of the posterior facet.
- Another line is drawn from the superior aspect of the posterior facet to the superior aspect of the posterior calcaneal tuberosity (Figure 24.3).
- A normal Böhler angle measures between 20 and 40 degrees.

**Calcaneal Fractures**
- Calcaneal fractures can be divided into intraarticular and extraarticular.

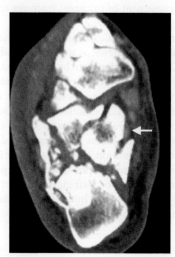

**Figure 24.2.** Severely comminuted calcaneal fracture. Axial CT image shows a severely comminuted and moderately displaced calcaneal fracture with entrapment of the flexor hallucis longus tendon between the fracture fragments (*arrow*).

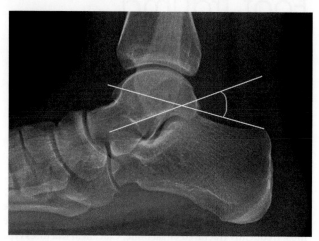

**Figure 24.3.** Normal Böhler angle. A lateral radiograph of a normal foot shows a normal Böhler angle with lines drawn from the anterior process of the calcaneus to the superior aspect of the posterior facet and the posterior facet superiorly to the superior margin of the posterior calcaneal tuberosity. A normal Böhler angle measures between 20 and 40 degrees.

- The degree of comminution laterally and medially is important to note, as this can affect surgical fixation.
- Intraarticular calcaneal fractures are most common and involve the posterior subtalar joint (Figure 24.4).
- It is important to note the degree of displacement and number and location of fracture lines involving the posterior subtalar joint.
- Sanders classification is based on the number of articular fragments seen on the coronal CT image at the widest point of the posterior facet (types I-IV depending on the number of fragments).

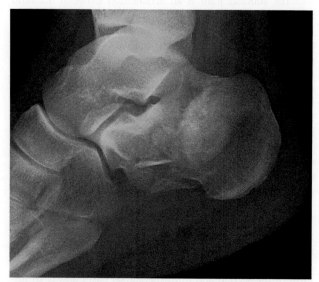

**Figure 24.4.** Severely comminuted intraarticular calcaneus fracture. Lateral radiograph of the calcaneus shows a severely comminuted intraarticular calcaneal body fracture with posterior subtalar joint extension and flattening of Böhler angle.

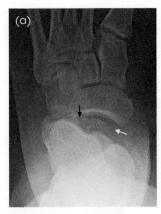 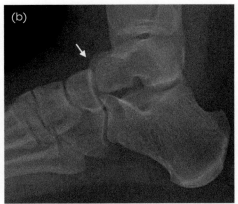

**Figure 24.5.** Talar subluxation. AP (*A*) and lateral (*B*) radiographs of the foot show dorsal and lateral subluxation of the talus (*white arrows*) with a displaced talar head fracture (*black arrow*).

- Essex-Lopresti classification of extraarticular calcaneal fractures is based on their location.
  - Type A fractures involve the anterior process of the calcaneus.
  - Type B fractures involve the mid calcaneus including the body and sustentaculum tali.
  - Type C fractures involve the posterior calcaneal tuberosity, including avulsion fractures of the Achilles tendon.
- Essex-Lopresti classification of the calcaneal fractures can also be divided into tongue-type and joint depression-type.

## Talar Neck Fractures

- Fractures of the talar neck are associated with talar dome ON, with increased risk related to the degree of displacement and dislocation as described by the Hawkins classification:
  - Type I is nondisplaced.
  - Type II is displaced with subtalar dislocation.
  - Type III is displaced with subtalar and tibiotalar displacement.
  - Type IV is displaced with subtalar, tibiotalar, and talonavicular displacement.

## Other Talar Fractures

- Talar head fractures are frequently associated with dislocation or subluxation (Figure 24.5).
- Talar body fractures may be coronal or sagittal shear fractures or severely comminuted crush fractures, which are associated with increased risk of ON.
- Lateral talar process fractures (snowboard injury) most commonly involve a single fracture line but may also be comminuted.
- Dorsal talar capsular avulsion fractures appear as a flake of bone adjacent to the anterosuperior talar neck (Figure 24.6).

## Navicular Fractures

- Navicular dorsal avulsion fractures appear as a flake of bone dorsal to the navicular.

- Medial tuberosity fractures can also occur at the attachment of the posterior tibialis tendon.
- Navicular body fractures are commonly associated with dislocation or subluxation and other foot fractures.

## Lisfranc Joint Injuries

- A Lisfranc fracture or dislocation will appear as greater than 2 mm of widening between the first and second metatarsal bases, or malalignment of the first and second tarsometatarsal joints (Figure 24.7).
- A small fleck of bone is often seen between the first and second metatarsal bases, termed the *fleck sign.*
- Additional fractures at the tarsometatarsal joints may be seen and are well-depicted on CT examination.

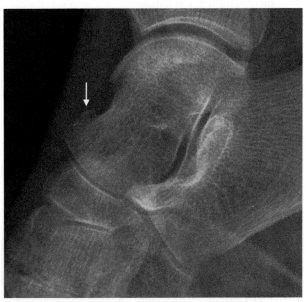

**Figure 24.6.** Talar head capsular avulsion injury. A lateral radiograph of the ankle shows a dorsal talus capsular avulsion fracture (*arrow*).

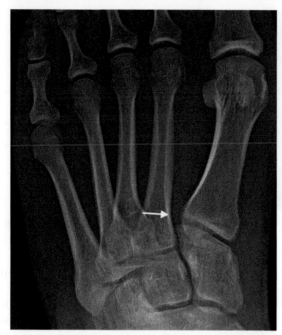

**Figure 24.7.** Subtle Lisfranc injury. AP radiograph of the foot shows mild widening of the Lisfranc interval in this patient with Lisfranc sprain (*arrow*).

- There is often dorsal subluxation of the metatarsals, because the dorsal Lisfranc ligament is the weakest (Figure 24.8).
- A cuboid compression fracture may also be seen.
- A *homolateral* Lisfranc fracture-dislocation involves shift of all metatarsals laterally (Figure 24.9).
- A *divergent* Lisfranc fracture-dislocation is less common and classically involves lateral displacement of the second through fifth metatarsals and medial displacement of the first metatarsal.

**Metatarsal and Phalangeal Fractures**
- A fifth metatarsal base avulsion fracture may be extraarticular or intraarticular (Figure 24.10).
- Fractures of the metatarsals apart from the fifth are classified as head, neck, shaft, or base fractures, which are typically transverse and more commonly involve the metatarsal shaft or neck.

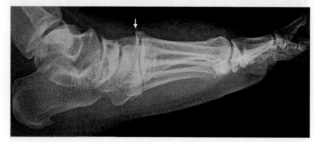

**Figure 24.8.** Lisfranc fracture/subluxation. A lateral radiograph of the foot shows a Lisfranc injury with dorsal subluxation of the second metatarsal base (*arrow*).

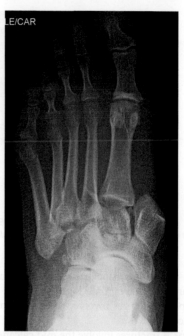

**Figure 24.9.** Homolateral Lisfranc fracture-dislocation. AP radiograph of the foot shows a homolateral Lisfranc fracture-dislocation. Note lateral displacement of all metatarsal bases with scattered small fracture fragments.

- Phalangeal fractures are usually transverse or oblique (Figure 24.11) and can be subtle and seen only on one image.
- Crush fractures of the phalanges usually have a stellate appearance.

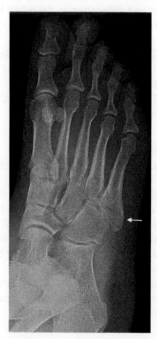

**Figure 24.10.** Fifth metatarsal base fracture. An oblique radiograph of the foot shows a mildly comminuted nondisplaced intraarticular avulsion fracture of the fifth metatarsal base (*arrow*).

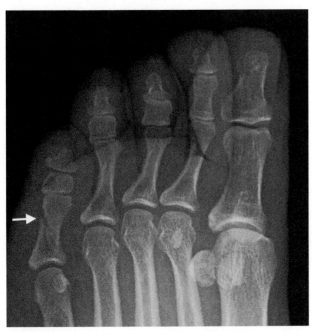

**Figure 24.11.** Intraarticular fracture of the fifth proximal phalanx. AP radiograph of the forefoot shows an oblique and comminuted fifth proximal phalangeal shaft and base fracture (*arrow*) with intraarticular extension.

## Treatment Options

### Calcaneal Fractures
- Conservative management for nondisplaced intraarticular fractures and extraarticular fractures
- Surgery for displaced intraarticular fractures and open fractures

### Talar Fractures
- Conservative management for nondisplaced talar head, neck, and body fractures and avulsion fractures
- ORIF for displaced fractures

### Navicular Fractures
- Conservative management for avulsion fractures and navicular body fractures with less than 1 mm of displacement
- Surgical treatment for medial tuberosity and navicular body fractures with more than 1 mm of displacement

### Lisfranc Injury
- Nondisplaced injuries are treated conservatively in a non-weight-bearing cast.
- Displaced injuries require surgical fixation.

### Fifth Metatarsal Fractures
- Fifth metatarsal base avulsion fractures heal well with conservative management.
- Jones fractures have slower healing because of poor vascular supply but usually heal with conservative management.
- Proximal diaphyseal metatarsal stress fractures have poor healing and may require surgical fixation.

### Other Metatarsal Fractures
- Other metatarsal fractures that are nondisplaced or minimally displaced can be treated with conservative management.
- With greater displacement, operative management with pinning or ORIF is recommended.

### Phalangeal Fractures
- Almost always conservative management with buddy taping and padding and rigid sole shoe

### Key Points
- For calcaneal fractures, degree of comminution and displacement is important to note as this can affect surgical management.
- Displaced talar neck fractures and severely comminuted talar body fractures predispose to ON.
- It is important to evaluate for subtle malalignment at the Lisfranc interval to not miss a Lisfranc injury.
- Fifth metatarsal base fractures are common, and this region should be evaluated in the setting of ankle trauma.
- Phalangeal fractures may be subtle and visible on only one projection.

### Recommended Reading
Mitchell MJ, Ho C, Resnick D, Sartoris DJ. Diagnostic imaging of lower extremity trauma. *Radiol Clin North Am.* 1989;27:909–28.

### References
1. Armagan OE, Shereff MJ. Injuries to the toes and metatarsals. *Orthop Clin North Am.* 2001;32:1–10.
2. Badillo K, Pacheco JA, Padua SO, Gomez AA, Colon E, Vidal JA. Multidetector CT evaluation of calcaneal fractures. *Radiographics.* 2011;31:81–92.
3. Daftary A, Haims AH, Baumgaertner MR. Fractures of the calcaneus: a review with emphasis on CT. *Radiographics.* 2005;25:1215–26.
4. Ha AS, Porrino JA, Chew FS. Radiographic pitfalls in lower extremity trauma. *AJR Am J Roentgenol.* 2014;203:492–500.
5. Melenevsky Y, Mackey RA, Abrahams RB, Thomson NB 3rd. Talar fractures and dislocations: a radiologist's guide to timely diagnosis and classification. *Radiographics.* 2015;35:765–79.
6. Pinney SJ, Sangeorzan BJ. Fractures of the tarsal bones. *Orthop Clin North Am.* 2001;32:21–33.
7. Polzer H, Polzer S, Mutschler W, Prall WC. Acute fractures to the proximal fifth metatarsal bone: development of classification and treatment recommendations based on the current evidence. *Injury.* 2012;43:1626–32.
8. Rammelt S, Heineck J, Zwipp H. Metatarsal fractures. *Injury.* 2004;35(suppl 2):Sb77–86.
9. Siddiqui NA, Galizia MS, Almusa E, Omar IM. Evaluation of the tarsometatarsal joint using conventional radiography, CT, and MR imaging. *Radiographics.* 2014;34:514–31.

# 4

# Trauma Miscellaneous

Edited by Mihra S. Taljanovic and Tyson S. Chadaz

# CHAPTER 25

# Stress Fracture

Jack Porrino and Alvin R. Wyatt II

## Mechanism of Injury

Fatigue-type stress injuries are related to repetitive overuse of normal bone resulting in an imbalance of bone formation and resorption. Insufficiency type stress injuries occur as a result of normal stress to weakened (osteopenic or osteoporotic) bones.

The force involved in the formation of a stress fracture is less than that tolerated by the bone, however, the repetitive nature of the force results in disruption of the bone.

Stress fractures account for more than 10% of all sports-related injuries and are particularly common in running sports. The most common sites of stress fracture include the pelvis (eg, pubic rami), femur, patella, tibia, fibula, medial malleolus, calcaneus, tarsal navicular, metatarsal (most commonly the second and third, known as *march fractures*), and great toe sesamoid bones. A stress reaction is considered an early form of stress fracture, in which abnormality is identified on bone scan or MRI, but no discrete fracture line is present.

Athletes and military recruits are particularly susceptible to femoral stress fractures occurring in the proximal and distal femur, respectively. The proximal, subtrochanteric femur is a vulnerable site because of the tubular shape and bowed morphology of the bone at this level.

Tibial stress fractures are common in long-distance runners, and may be transverse or longitudinal (vertical) involving the tibial diaphysis. Fibular stress fractures usually involve the distal third of the bone and are also seen in runners training on hard surfaces.

Predisposing conditions include a sudden increase in exercise intensity, poor bone mineral density (influenced by diet, hormone levels and biomechanics), altered biomechanics (such as leg length discrepancy, foot misalignment and abnormal gait), and suboptimal training surfaces and/or footwear.

## Imaging Strategy and Findings

### Radiographs

- Although radiographs are nearly always obtained in the initial workup of a stress fracture, their reported sensitivity in the literature is variable and often low with a range of 10-70%.
- They may demonstrate a stress fracture obviating the need for more advanced imaging or identify an alternative cause for pain.
- In the anterior tibial cortex, numerous stress fractures may be present as a series of radiolucent lines that are perpendicular to the long axis of the bone (Figure 25.1).

### Technetium Bone Scan

- The 3-phase technetium-99m bone scan is the nuclear diagnostic study of choice for the diagnosis of stress fractures, however, the sensitivity (74-84%) and specificity (33%) are inferior to MRI.
- A positive bone scan includes increased radiotracer uptake on all 3 phases of the study (Figure 25.2).
- The bone scan findings, however, are nonspecific and should be correlated with the clinical presentation, as tumor and infection can have a similar appearance.
- Additionally, differentiation of stress reaction from stress fracture can be difficult, and abnormal tracer uptake can occur in asymptomatic subjects in up to 40% of cases.

### Computed Tomography

- CT is a useful modality in the identification of stress fractures involving the pelvis or sacrum (Figure 25.3) and can be used to differentiate stress reaction from a stress fracture (Figure 25.4).
- This modality, however, has a limited role in clinical practice because of low sensitivity.

### Ultrasound

- Although not routinely performed in the diagnosis of stress fracture, US is a noninvasive modality that may identify a stress fracture, which is usually an incidental finding on an US study performed for other reasons.
- Imaging features include soft-tissue edema and/or fluid collections, periosteal thickening, and hyperemia.

### Magnetic Resonance Imaging

- MRI plays an important role in the diagnosis of stress fracture.
- Because of its outstanding sensitivity (86-100%) and specificity (100%), MRI is predominately the imaging modality of choice for the diagnosis of stress fractures. Imaging findings vary based on severity.
- On FS fluid-sensitive sequences, low-level stress reactions manifest as periosteal edema.
- As the injury progresses, BME becomes apparent followed by a discrete fracture line (Figures 25.5 and 25.6).

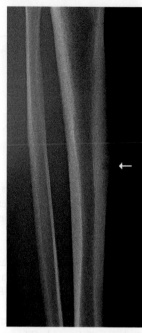

**Figure 25.1.** Tibial stress fracture on radiography. Lateral radiograph of the left tibia in an athlete demonstrates a lucent fracture line (*arrow*) disrupting the anterior cortex of the mid tibial diaphysis.

## Imaging Findings and Classifications

Classification or grading of stress fractures has been described with radiography, bone scan, CT, and MRI (Table 25.1). However, severity grades from one imaging modality may not

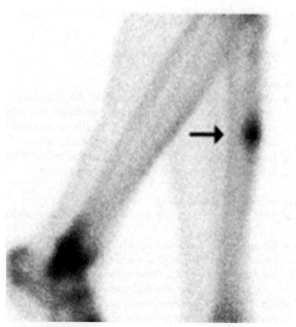

**Figure 25.2.** Tibial stress fracture on nuclear 3-phase bone scan. Spot image from the delayed phase of a technetium 99m methylene diphosphonate (MDP) whole body bone scan in an athlete demonstrates abnormal radiotracer accumulation at the site of a stress fracture involving the anterior cortex of the mid tibial diaphysis (*arrow*). Notably, abnormal radiotracer uptake was also apparent on the blood flow and blood pool images.

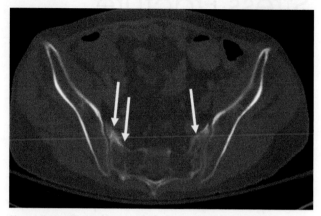

**Figure 25.3.** Bilateral sacral alar insufficiency fractures. Unenhanced axial CT image of the pelvis demonstrates osteopenia with bilateral zone I sacral alar insufficiency fractures with associated sclerosis (*arrows*).

correlate with grades from another imaging modality. Beck et al demonstrated that only MRI bears any relationship to clinical severity or time to healing.

## Treatment Options

With stress fractures, in particular in the athlete with aspirations of a speedy return to full activity, early diagnosis is paramount, as those with a delayed diagnosis take longer to return to their respective sport.

**Conservative Treatment**

- A return to activity may require months depending on the location of the stress fracture.
- Premature return to activity prior to complete bony union may result in delayed or nonunion.
- For femoral stress fractures, removal from the offending activity is the primary conservative treatment strategy.
- Deconditioning in the low-risk category of femoral stress fractures can be avoided by engaging in alternative activities, such as water running, swimming, or cycling.
- A gradual return to activity is used to avoid setback.

**Surgical Treatment**

- Surgical management, such as intramedullary nail fixation or ORIF, of the stress fracture is typically instituted when the injury has progressed to a displaced fracture of a weight-bearing bone, such as the femur, or when the stress fracture is on the tension side of the femoral neck.

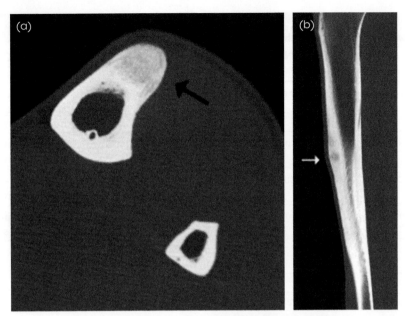

**Figure 25.4.** Tibial stress fracture on CT. Unenhanced axial (*A*) CT image of the leg in an athlete demonstrates focal cortical thickening of the anterior tibial diaphysis (*arrow*). In a sagittal reformatted image (*B*), note a faint fracture line (*arrow*) involving the anterior cortex of the mid tibial diaphysis. This should be differentiated from an osteoid osteoma which can have a similar imaging appearance.

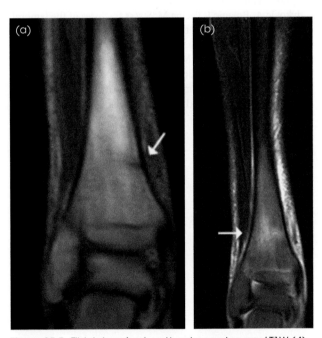

**Figure 25.5.** Tibial stress fracture. Unenhanced coronal T1W (*A*) and T2W FS (*B*) MR images of the leg in a middle-aged man with recent increase in exercise demonstrate BME with patchy decreased signal on T1W and high signal on T2W FS (*arrow*) images as well as a discrete hypointense fracture line in (*A*) (*arrow*).

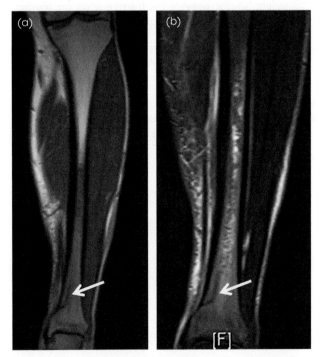

**Figure 25.6.** Longitudinal tibial stress fracture in a 53-year-old man with diabetes. Unenhanced coronal T1W (*A*) and STIR (*B*) MR images of the leg show a low signal intensity longitudinal (vertically oriented) fracture line (*arrow*) in the distal tibial diametaphysis. Note associated BME of low signal intensity in (*A*) and high signal intensity in (*B*).

**Table 25.1. Imaging Grading of Stress Fractures**

| GRADE | RADIOGRAPHY | BONE SCAN | COMPUTED TOMOGRAPHY | MAGNETIC RESONANCE IMAGING |
|-------|-------------|-----------|---------------------|----------------------------|
| I | Hazy gray cortex | Mild uptake at cortex | Soft-tissue thickening adjacent to periosteum | Periosteal edema on fluid-sensitive sequence with normal bone marrow |
| II | Acute periosteal reaction | Small focus of uptake | Increased attenuation of marrow space | Bone marrow edema (BME) on fluid-sensitive sequences |
| III | Cortical lucency | Medium focus of uptake | Osteopenia, resorption cavity of cortex, cortical striation | BME on T1-weighted (T1W) and fluid-sensitive sequences |
| IV | Fracture line | Large focus of uptake | Fracture line | Low signal intensity fracture line on all pulse sequences |

## Key Points

- Stress/fatigue fractures are the result of a repetitive stress on normal bone.
- Insufficiency type stress injuries occur as a result of normal stress to weakened (osteopenic or osteoporotic) bones.
- Although radiography is obtained commonly in the workup, MRI has come to the forefront for the diagnosis and management of stress fractures.
- Management of stress fractures is typically conservative, however, when there is a displaced stress fracture of a weight-bearing bone or the fracture is on the tension side of the femoral neck, surgical management may be necessary.

## Recommended Reading

Beck BR, Bergman AG, Miner M, et al. Tibial stress injury: relationship of radiographic, nuclear medicine bone scanning, MR imaging, and CT severity grades to clinical severity and time to healing. *Radiology*. 2012;263(3):811–18.

## References

1. Beck BR, Bergman AG, Miner M, et al. Tibial stress injury: relationship of radiographic, nuclear medicine bone scanning, MR imaging, and CT severity grades to clinical severity and time to healing. *Radiology*. 2012;263(3):811–8.
2. Behrens SB, Deren ME, Matson A, Fadale PD, Monchik KO. Stress fractures of the pelvis and legs in athletes: a review. *Sports Health*. 2013;5(2):165–74.
3. Ivkovic A, Bojanic I, Pecina M. Stress fractures of the femoral shaft in athletes: a new treatment algorithm. *Br J Sports Med*. 2006;40(6):518–20.
4. Niva MH, Sormaala MJ, Kiuru MJ, Haataja R, Ahovuo JA, Pihlajamaki HK. Bone stress injuries of the ankle and foot: an 86-month magnetic resonance imaging-based study of physically active young adults. *Am J Sports Med*. 2007;35(4):643–49.

# CHAPTER 26

# Physeal Injury

Jack Porrino and Alvin R. Wyatt II

## Mechanism of Injury

Because the ligamentous and capsular support of the joint is 2-5 times stronger than the cartilage, the epiphysis and physis are the sites most prone to injury in skeletally immature individuals. The epiphysis develops as a mass of 3 forms of hyaline cartilage at the articular end of the bone, *articular* at the outermost layer, *epiphyseal* in the center, and *physeal*, located between the epiphyseal cartilage and metaphysis. With time, one or more secondary ossification centers form within the epiphyseal cartilage, while the physeal cartilage is responsible for the synthesis of new longitudinal bone via endochondral ossification.

In children, 15-30% of fractures affect the physis, with potential of the injury to result in growth abnormalities/length discrepancy, joint surface deformities, or angular deformities. The growth disturbance is the result of direct damage to the physeal cartilage and/or formation of physeal bony bridging (Figure 26.1) stunting growth. Bony bridging develops because of abnormal communication of the epiphyseal and metaphyseal vessels. In the elite adolescent athlete, chronic physeal trauma can occur. Chronic trauma alters the metaphyseal vessels, disrupts endochondral ossification, and results in physeal chondrocytes remaining in the metaphysis. More common sites of chronic physeal injury include the proximal humerus in baseball players; wrist in gymnasts (Figure 26.2); and knees in soccer, tennis, and football players. As with acute physeal injuries, chronic physeal trauma can lead to growth disturbances and deformity if the stressor is not removed.

## Imaging Strategy and Findings

### Radiographs

Radiographs serve as the mainstay for the initial diagnosis of physeal injuries (Figures 26.2–26.4). Diagnosis can be challenging, however, because of either no or incomplete ossification of the epiphysis. If the diagnosis cannot be made on conventional radiography, a comparison view of the contralateral extremity can be obtained. Stress radiographs are controversial because of the potential of injury propagation. Any one of several alternative forms of imaging can be used, including radiographic tomography, US, CT, and MRI.

- Physeal injuries isolated to the physis manifest as abnormal widening of the affected physis with or without

displacement of the affected epiphysis on radiography (Figure 26.3).

### Technetium Bone Scan

Bone scan plays a limited role in the evaluation of the physeal injury, in that the normal physis already exhibits increased radiotracer uptake relative to surrounding bone.

### Computed Tomography

CT has demonstrated a high sensitivity and specificity for the detection of radiographically occult elbow fractures in the pediatric population, takes only seconds to perform, and requires no sedation. However, radiation exposure must be considered.

- In isolated shear injuries of the physis, CT may demonstrate abnormal widening of the physis with sclerotic margins.
- Fracture comminution and displacement may be best depicted on CT (Figure 26.5).
- Perhaps the most useful role of CT in physeal injury is in delineating the extent of growth arrest in planning for a bar resection.

### Ultrasound

US has the ability to provide useful information regarding surrounding soft tissue injury and potentially identify a radiographically occult fracture, however, it is highly operator dependent and also limited by the acoustic window.

### Magnetic Resonance Imaging

MRI has the ability to provide more detailed information regarding the extent of injury to the physeal growth plate, unmask radiographically occult injuries (Figure 26.6), and provide improved detail of developing bony bridging. Depending on patient age, sedation may be required.

- On MRI, the primary physis demonstrates a trilaminar appearance, with intermediate to high signal intensity in the resting and hypertrophic zones, low signal intensity in the zone of provisional calcification, and intermediate to high signal intensity in the metaphyseal spongiosa.
- Acute physeal injuries on MRI demonstrate a linear fracture line with surrounding BME with hyperintense signal on fluid-sensitive sequences and hypointense signal on T1W imaging (Figure 26.7).
- As the fracture line disrupts the physis, the normal trilaminar appearance is lost and replaced by edematous signal within the physis.

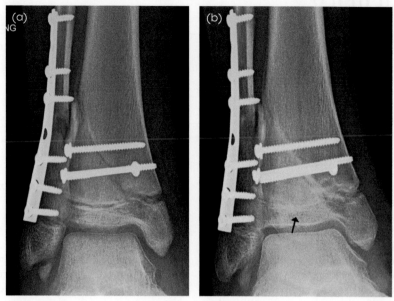

**Figure 26.1.** Bony bridging with physeal injury. Mortise radiograph (*A*) of the ankle shows surgical fixation of a Salter-Harris type II fracture of the distal tibia and fracture of the distal fibular diaphysis. At 2 month follow-up (*B*), the distal tibial physis is effaced suggestive of developing bony bridging (*arrow*).

- Focal loss of the normal physeal signal, most conspicuous on gradient recalled echo (GRE) imaging sequences, implies bony bridge development. Specifically, the normal hyperintense signal of the physis is replaced by a focus of hypointense signal that is isointense to the cortex.
- Chronic physeal injuries on MRI demonstrate irregularity and widening of the physis with abnormal increased fluid-sensitive signal.

## Classification
Physeal injuries are classified by the Salter-Harris classification model (Table 26.1).

**Specific Entities**
- Slipped capital femoral epiphysis (SCFE) reflects a Salter-Harris type I fracture through the physis of the femoral head and neck. The epiphysis becomes displaced and is susceptible to ON.
- The juvenile Tillaux fracture involves the anterolateral aspect of the distal tibia in the adolescent, extending through the physis and epiphysis (Salter-Harris type III injury) and exiting through the articular surface of the distal tibia.
- The triplane fracture is a Salter-Harris type IV injury involving the distal tibia with the fracture line typically sagittal within the epiphysis, axial through the lateral physis, and coronal within the posterior metaphysis.

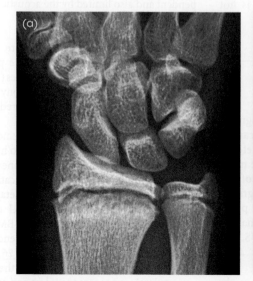
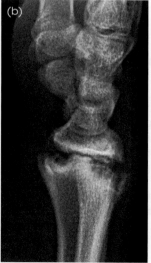

**Figure 26.2.** Gymnast wrist. PA (*A*) and lateral (*B*) radiographs of a wrist of a young, skeletally immature gymnast demonstrates abnormal distal radial physeal widening and subjacent cystlike changes related to a chronic Salter-Harris type I stress injury.

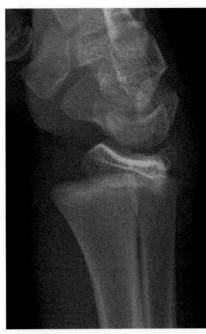

**Figure 26.3.** Displaced Salter-Harris type I fracture. Lateral radiograph of the wrist demonstrates a displaced Salter-Harris type I fracture of the distal radius.

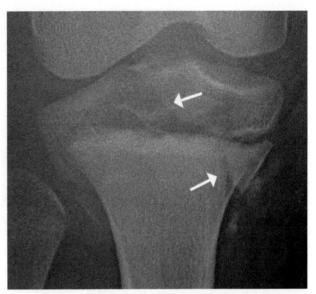

**Figure 26.4.** Salter-Harris type IV fracture. AP radiograph of the knee demonstrates a Salter-Harris type IV fracture of the proximal tibia with the fracture disrupting the epiphysis, physis and metaphysis (*arrows*).

■ The *focal periphyseal edema* (FOPE) zone on MRI of the adolescent knee may be seen around the time of expected skeletal age of maturation, likely relating to the early stages of physiologic physeal fusion. On knee MRI, the FOPE zone demonstrates periphyseal BME. It may be associated with pain, particularly when no other MRI abnormalities are present, and does not require treatment or imaging follow-up (Figure 26.8).

## Treatment Options

### Conservative Treatment

■ With acute physeal trauma, Salter-Harris type I injuries have an excellent prognosis with reduction and immobilization.

■ In general, Salter-Harris types IV (Figure 26.4) and V fractures have a poorer prognosis then types I-III, with a higher incidence of bony bridge formation,

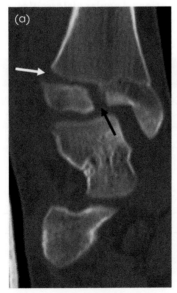
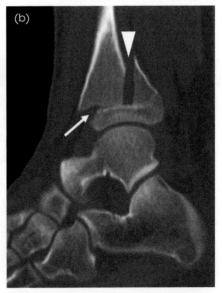

**Figure 26.5.** Triplane fracture in a 15-year-old adolescent. (*A*) Coronal and (*B*) sagittal reformatted CT images of the ankle show a triplane fracture with a vertical component through the epiphysis (*black arrow*), horizontal component through the lateral physis (*white arrow*), and oblique component through the posterior metaphysis (*arrowhead*). Note mild to moderate displacement at fracture sites.

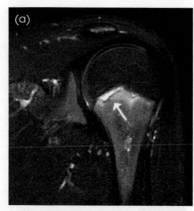
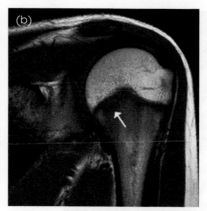

**Figure 26.6.** Salter-Harris type I injury in a 12-year-old girl. Coronal T2 W FS (*A*) and T1 W (*B*) MR images of the shoulder show high (*A*) and low (*B*) signal within the proximal humeral physis (*arrows*) consistent with a Salter-Harris type I injury.

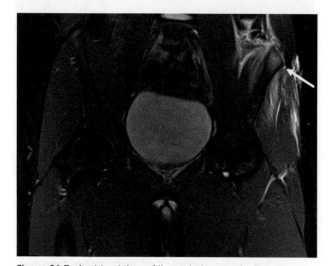

**Figure 26.7.** Avulsion injury of the anterior superior iliac spine. Coronal STIR MR image of the pelvis shows an apophyseal avulsion fracture of the left anterior superior iliac spine (*arrow*) with attachments of the sartorius and tensor fascia lata muscles. Note associated physeal edema, BME in the adjacent iliac crest and associated soft tissue edema.

leading to growth arrest, angulation, and/or limb length discrepancy.

- With chronic repetitive physeal injuries, management is predicated on a change to the inciting activity and rehabilitation prior to the development of permanent deformity.

**Surgical Treatment**

- Salter-Harris type III and IV injuries often require ORIF to minimize articular incongruity and to reduce the risk of physeal arrest by facilitating reduction of the physis.
- Although small bony bridging developed across the physis may resolve spontaneously, larger bony bridging most often seen with Salter-Harris type IV and V injuries may require surgery, such as resection or various forms of epiphysiodesis.
- Although there are no established guidelines, children with 2 years or 2 cm of remaining growth should be considered for bony bridging resection. Angular deformities may require correction osteotomy.

## Table 26.1. Salter-Harris Classification Model

| SALTER-HARRIS TYPE | FRACTURE INVOLVEMENT | OCCURRENCE(%) | FORMATION OF BRIDGE(%) |
|---|---|---|---|
| I | Isolated shear injury of the physis | 8.5 | 25 |
| II | Physis and metaphysis | 73 | 25 |
| III | Physis and epiphysis | 6.5 | 75 |
| IV | Physis, metaphysis and epiphysis | 12 | 75 |
| V | Compression injury of the physis | | |

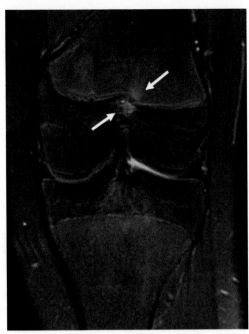

**Figure 26.8.** FOPE zone. Coronal T2W FS MR image of the knee shows focal BME (*arrows*) about the closing part of the distal femoral physis consistent with a FOPE zone. Courtesy of Tal Laor, MD.

## Key Points

- Classification of physeal injury is based on the Salter-Harris classification scheme.
- If there is a high clinical index of suspicion for a physeal injury in the context of normal radiographs, MRI can serve as a confirmatory study.

- Although Salter-Harris type I and II injuries typically are managed with reduction and immobilization, Salter-Harris type III through V injuries may require surgery in order to reduce the risk of physeal arrest or for the management of a bony bridging.

## Recommended Reading

Jaimes C, Chauvin NA, Delgado J, Jaramillo D. MR imaging of normal epiphyseal development and common epiphyseal disorders. *Radiographics*. 2014;34(2):449–71.

## References

1. Gufler H, Schulze CG, Wagner S, Baumbach L. MRI for occult physeal fracture detection in children and adolescents. *Acta Radiol*. 2013;54(4):467–72.
2. Jaimes C, Chauvin NA, Delgado J, Jaramillo D. MR imaging of normal epiphyseal development and common epiphyseal disorders. *Radiographics*. 2014;34(2):449–71.
3. Little JT, Klionsky NB, Chaturvedi A, Soral A, Chaturvedi A. Pediatric distal forearm and wrist injury: an imaging review. *Radiographics*. 2014;34(2):472–90.
4. Shi DP, Zhu SC, Li Y, Zheng J. Epiphyseal and physeal injury: comparison of conventional radiography and magnetic resonance imaging. *Clin Imaging*. 2009;33(5):379–83.
5. Wuerz TH, Gurd DP. Pediatric physeal ankle fracture. *J Am Acad Orthop Surg*. 2013;21(4):234–44.
6. Zbojniewicz AM, Laor T. Focal periphyseal edema (FOPE) zone on MRI of the adolescent knee: a potentially painful manifestation of physiologic physeal fusion? *AJR Am J Roentgenol*. 2011;197(4):998–1004. doi:10.2214/AJR.10.6243.

# CHAPTER 27

# Fracture Fixation

Jack Porrino and Alvin R. Wyatt II

## Introduction

Although many fractures can be treated nonoperatively, others require operative fixation, with the goal to stabilize the fractured bone, enable fast healing, and return early mobility and function of the injured extremity. Operative fixation is categorized as either internal or external.

## Conservative Management

Conservative treatment entails closed reduction for restoration of anatomic alignment, followed by stabilization through the use of traction or external splinting. A percutaneous Steinman pin or Kirschner wire can be placed through the bone with traction applied (Figure 27.1). The traction device is applied along the long axis of the bone providing temporary stability. External slings, splints, and casts can also be used and may be composed of plaster, synthetic casting material, plastic, or metal.

## External Fixation

The external fixator device consists of a scaffold of pins or wires that are placed percutaneously into the bone above and below the fracture and attached to an external rod, ring, or framed construct, which provides fracture fixation based on the principle of splinting (Figure 27.2). It is often used in the setting of open fractures with significant soft tissue injury or with fractures that are excessively comminuted, making ORIF challenging.

## Internal Fixation

ORIF has been used since the 1950s, restoring normal anatomy and allowing early mobilization. Internal fixation hardware is traditionally composed of stainless steel or elastic titanium. Internal fixation hardware includes pins/wires, screws, plates, and intramedullary nails/rods.

### Pins and Wires

- The most commonly used pins and wires are Steinman pins and Kirschner wires (Figure 27.3).
- Pins and wires are available in a variety of diameters and sizes and can be smooth or threaded/braided.
- In addition to internal fixation, they are used for temporary fixation of a fracture during reduction, can be used to attach traction devices, or serve as a guide for placement of a larger cannulated screw.

### Screws

- Orthopedic screws can be divided into 2 types: *cortical* or *cancellous*.
- Cortical screws are used in the diaphysis, and cancellous screws are designed to fix cancellous bone (Figure 27.4).
- Screws can be fully or partially threaded with the distance between threads referred to as the *pitch*. They come in a variety of diameters and sizes and can be hollow (cannulated) or solid. The cannulated screw can be placed over a guide pin.
- Screws are often used in combination with plates or intramedullary rods.
- A screw crossing a fracture line in effort to provide compression of the fracture fragments, either through a fixation plate or freestanding, is referred to as an *interfragmentary* or lag screw.

### Plates

- Plates are most commonly used for fixation of long bones and most are composed of stainless steel or titanium.
- They provide secure fixation without protruding pins/wires.
- Plates are used in combination with screws and come in a variety of forms such as the dynamic compression plate (DCP), low-contact DCP (LCDCP), tubular plates, blade plates, reconstruction plates, bridge plates and less-invasive stabilization system (LISS) plate (Figure 27.5).
- Particular note is made of the locking plate in which locking screws mate with the threaded plate holes, negating the need for double cortex fixation necessary with traditional compression plates. A large number of plates are combo (combination) plates and allow placement of both locking and bicortical screws (part of the screw holes have threads that accommodate placement of locking screws).

### Intramedullary Nails and Rods

- The placement of an intramedullary nail/rod is the standard treatment approach for diaphyseal fractures of the femur and tibia, permitting early weight-bearing (Figure 27.6).
- Most intramedullary nails are applied percutaneously, either in an antegrade or retrograde fashion.
- Some nails/rods require reaming the bone to enlarge the intramedullary canal.
- Cannulated forms of nails/rods can be placed over a guidewire under fluoroscopic guidance.

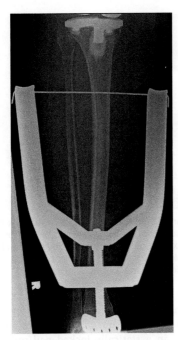

**Figure 27.1.** Skeletal traction. AP radiograph of the tibia and fibula of an elderly man demonstrates a Steinman pin across the proximal tibial diaphysis, placed under traction for management of a periprosthetic fracture of the distal femur at the site of total knee arthroplasty.

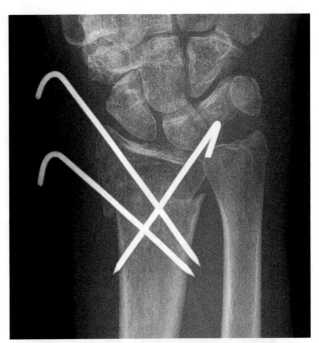

**Figure 27.3.** Kirschner wires/pins. PA radiograph of the wrist shows 3 percutaneous Kirschner wires transfixing the distal radius fracture in a middle-aged man.

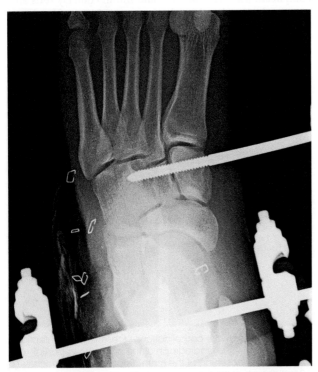

**Figure 27.2.** Uniplanar external fixator. AP radiograph of the foot of a young man with an open fracture-dislocation injury of the ankle demonstrates pins of an external fixator construct traversing the calcaneus and cuneiform bones.

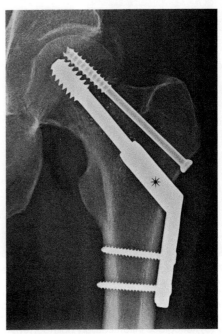

**Figure 27.4.** Dynamic hip screw device (DHS). AP radiograph of the hip of a middle-aged man demonstrates a DHS with a large cancellous screw within a barrel (*asterisk*) attached to a plate with 2 cortical screws for femoral neck fracture stabilization. An additional, smaller cancellous cannulated screw also fixes the femoral neck fracture, placed above the DHS.

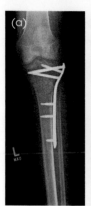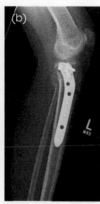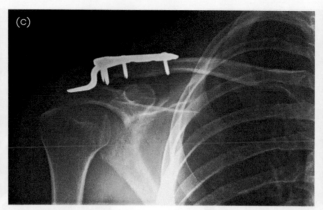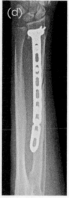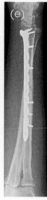

**Figure 27.5.** Various surgical plates. (*A*) AP and (*B*) lateral radiographs of the tibia and fibula show LISS plate used for fixation of a proximal tibial metaphyseal fracture (a type of precontoured periarticular locking plate that does not need to be completely opposed to bone). (*C*) AP radiograph of the clavicle shows a clavicular hook plate used for fixation of the distal clavicle fracture. (*D*) AP and (*E*) lateral radiographs of the forearm show an LCDCP, T-shaped, locking combo plate placed for fixation of radial mid shaft fracture. Note figure-of-eight configuration of proximal screw holes allowing placement of both bicortical and locking screws.

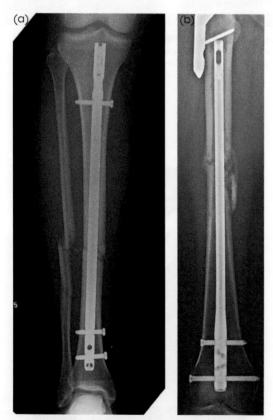

**Figure 27.6.** Intramedullary nails. (*A*) Antegrade intramedullary nail/rod. AP radiograph of the tibia and fibula shows an antegrade intramedullary nail with 1 proximal and 2 distal interlocking screws transfixing a healing tibial diaphyseal fracture site. Note a healing segmental fracture of the fibular diaphysis. (*B*) Retrograde intramedullary nail/rod, revision ORIF. AP radiograph of the femur in a young woman with fracture of the mid femoral diaphysis demonstrates a dynamic retrograde intramedullary nail without proximal interlocking screws and with 2 distal interlocking screws transfixing the fracture site. Additional hardware is incidentally noted in the proximal femoral metaphysis. Note screw tracts in the distal femur related to removed hardware.

- Proximal and distal interlocking screws are placed through the nail/rod to control rotational forces, resulting in a statically locked nail/rod. If locked at only one end, the nail/rod is considered dynamically locked.

**Hardware Complications**

With external fixation, as well as pins and wires used for internal fixation, wound or pin-track infection, pin/wire loosening, and pin/wire breakage are all possible complications. Plates, screws, and intramedullary rods and pins can loosen, break, and migrate. All forms of hardware can become infected or develop a periprosthetic fracture (Figure 27.7).

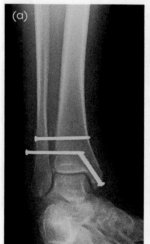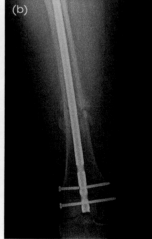

**Figure 27.7.** Hardware complications—loosening and infection. (*A*) Mortise (oblique) radiograph of the ankle shows partial extrusion and loosening of the more distal syndesmotic screw. (*B*) AP radiograph of the femur shows a retrograde intramedullary nail transfixing a distal femoral diaphyseal fracture. The more proximal of 2 distal interlocking screws is broken. Note periosteal reaction about the fracture site consistent with infected hardware, which was proven.

## Key Points

- Fracture fixation can be conservative or surgical.
- When surgical intervention is used, hardware ranges from external fixation to a variety of forms of internal fixation, including pins/wires, plates, screws, and intramedullary nails/rods.
- Complications of hardware include infection, loosening, breakage, and migration.

## Recommended Reading

Taljanovic MS, Jones MD, Ruth JT, Benjamin JB, Sheppard JE, Hunter TB. Fracture fixation. *Radiographics*. 2003;23(6):1569–90.

## References

1. Petscavage JM, Ha AS, Khorashadi L, Perrich K, Chew FS. New and improved orthopedic hardware for the 21st century: part 1, upper extremity. *AJR Am J Roentgenol*. 2011;197(3):W423–33.
2. Petscavage JM, Ha AS, Khorashadi L, Perrich K, Chew FS. New and improved orthopedic hardware for the 21st century: part 2, lower extremity and axial skeleton. *AJR Am J Roentgenol*. 2011;197(3):W434–44.
3. Porrino JA, Maloney E, Scherer K, Mulcahy H, Ha AS, Allan C. Fractures of the distal radius: postmanagement radiographic characterization. *AJR Am J Roentgenol*. 2014;203(4):846–53.

# CHAPTER 28

# Muscle Injury

Jack Porrino and Alvin R. Wyatt II

## Mechanism of Injury

Muscle injuries include contusion (related to a direct blow), laceration (following a penetrating injury), strain (as a result of distraction or shearing forces typically during eccentric contraction), and delayed-onset muscle soreness (caused by overuse). Strains most often occur at the myotendinous junction and frequently involve the hamstring, rectus femoris, biceps brachii, and gastrocnemius muscles. The resultant hemorrhage and inflammatory response result in predictable imaging abnormalities.

## Imaging Strategy

The role of radiography and CT examination is limited in the setting of muscle injury. Although muscle injury is often diagnosed clinically, US and MRI can aid in providing detailed information regarding the location, extent, and severity of injury in the early phase, influencing management. Additionally, MRI can depict complications of muscle trauma, including hematoma and seroma, scarring, and myositis ossificans (Figure 28.1).

## Imaging Findings and Classifications

### Ultrasound

- With contusion, the affected muscle may appear swollen and echogenic, with or without an associated hematoma, with imaging features dependent on the time the injury occurred relative to scanning.
- With muscle strain, US is useful in assessing the longitudinal extent of the injury, assessing the size of an associated hematoma, and detecting compression of adjacent structures.
- Muscle strain can be divided into 3 grades based on US appearance.
    - In a grade I strain, less than 5% of the muscle is damaged, with the affected muscle appearing hyperechoic.
    - In a grade II strain, greater than 5% of the muscle is damaged, but not the entire muscle, with discontinuity of the perimysium at the myotendinous or myofascial junction (Figure 28.2A).
    - In grade III strain, there is complete rupture at the myotendinous junction with hematoma.

- Color or power Doppler US can be used to assess neovascularization, inflammation, and healing of the muscle injury.

### Magnetic Resonance Imaging

- MRI provides detailed information pertaining to the location, extent, and severity of muscle injury (Figure 28.2B, C; Figures 28.3 and 28.4).
- T1W images provide excellent anatomic detail and assist with characterization of hemorrhage (Figure 28.3).
- Fat-suppressed, fluid-sensitive sequences such as T2W and STIR imaging are best for evaluating muscle edema or hemorrhage related to injury. Muscle strains often result in extracellular edema and hemorrhage, which appears brighter than the myofibers on fluid-sensitive sequences, often producing a *feather-like* or *feathery* appearance.
- Hemorrhage results in *blooming* artifact on GRE sequences as a result of the paramagnetic effects of hemosiderin.
- With contusion, there is focal but indistinct edema within the muscle, with or without an accompanying hematoma.
- Laceration results in a well-demarcated region of muscle fiber discontinuity with muscle edema and often hematoma.

There are a variety of grading systems for muscle strain. One proposed system is divided into 3 grades based on severity.

- Grade I strain is a microscopic injury without identifiable muscle disruption, resulting in focal, feathery edema (Figure 28.4).
- Grade II strains result in a partial-thickness macroscopic tear with muscle edema and hematoma (Figure 28.2B, C).
- Grade III strains result in complete disruption of the muscle at the myotendinous junction, with or without retraction, and a fluid gap at the site of muscle fiber discontinuity. Significant hematoma is often present with a grade III strain.

*Delayed-onset muscle soreness* is muscle pain and swelling that occurs several hours after vigorous activity, lasting for 2 to 3 days.

- MRI demonstrates edema within the affected muscle, similar to a grade I muscle strain.

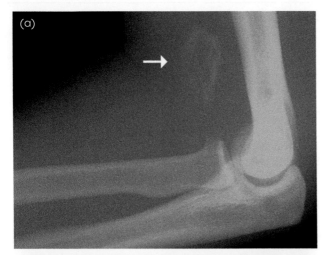

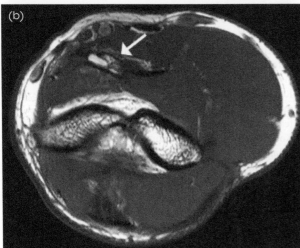

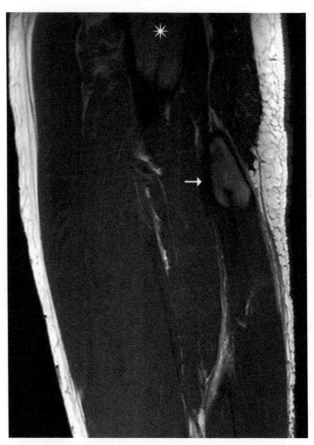

**Figure 28.3.** Intramuscular hematoma in a young female runner with acute injury of the hamstring. Sagittal T1W MR image demonstrates a circumscribed masslike intramuscular lesion (*arrow*) within the hamstring. Hyperintense signal on the T1W MR image within the lesion is compatible with an intramuscular hematoma and was seen in combination with diffuse muscle edema and tendon thickening. Note proximal femur (*asterisk*).

**Figure 28.1.** Myositis ossificans in a young man 2 years post elbow dislocation. Lateral radiograph of the elbow (*A*) demonstrates a calcified appearing mass (*arrow*) within the anterior soft tissues. Axial T1W MR image (*B*) through the level of the mass demonstrates a well-circumscribed mass (*arrow*) with signal characteristics comparable to the adjacent humeral bone marrow, findings consistent with myositis ossificans.

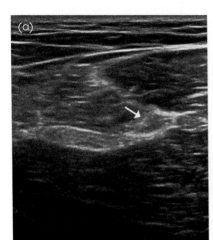
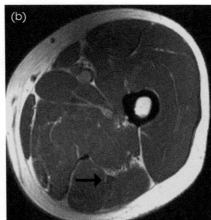
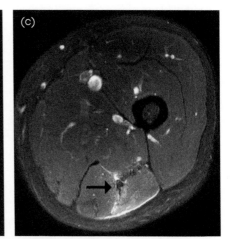

**Figure 28.2.** Grade II muscle strain in a young man with pain following an audible pop while exercising. (*A*) Transverse US image with corresponding axial T1W (*B*) and T2W FS (*C*) MR images at the same level, demonstrate focal thickening of the proximal myotendinous junction of the thigh biceps femoris muscle (*arrow*) with surrounding edema (*C*) and increased echogenicity (*A*). The findings are compatible with a grade II strain.

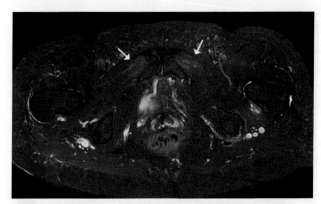

**Figure 28.4.** Grade I muscle strain in an 81-year-old woman. Axial T2W FS MR image of the lower pelvis shows bilateral adductor musculature edema, consistent with a grade I strain (*arrows*).

## Treatment Options

### Conservative

- Most grade I and II muscle strains respond to conservative therapy, aimed at symptom relief.
- For the high-profile athlete, further intensive physical therapy may be required in order to avoid reinjury.

### Surgical Treatment

- Grade III strains may require early surgical intervention to avoid permanent retraction and scar formation.

## Key Points

- Muscle injury can be the result of blunt or penetrating external trauma or distraction-type forces that occur with activity.
- Both US and MRI are useful imaging modalities in determining the location, extent, and severity of muscle injury.

### Recommended Reading

Shelly MJ, Hodnett PA, MacMahon PJ, Moynagh MR, Kavanagh EC, Eustace SJ. MR imaging of muscle injury. *Magn Reson Imaging Clin N Am*. 2009;17(4):757–73, vii.

Draghi F, Zacchino M, Canepari M, Nucci P, Alessandrino F. Muscle injuries: ultrasound evaluation in the acute phase. *J Ultrasound*. 2013;16(4):209–14.

### References

1. Draghi F, Zacchino M, Canepari M, Nucci P, Alessandrino F. Muscle injuries: ultrasound evaluation in the acute phase. *J Ultrasound*. 2013;16(4):209–14.
2. Gyftopoulos S, Rosenberg ZS, Schweitzer ME, Bordalo-Rodrigues M. Normal anatomy and strains of the deep musculotendinous junction of the proximal rectus femoris: MRI features. *AJR Am J Roentgenol*. 2008;190(3):W182–86.
3. Koulouris G, Connell D. Hamstring muscle complex: an imaging review [Erratum in: *Radiographics*. 2005;25(5):1436]. *Radiographics*. 2005;25(3):571–86.
4. Shelly MJ, Hodnett PA, MacMahon PJ, Moynagh MR, Kavanagh EC, Eustace SJ. MR imaging of muscle injury. *Magn Reson Imaging Clin N Am*. 2009;17(4):757–73, vii.

# CHAPTER 29

# Foreign Bodies

Jack Porrino and Alvin R. Wyatt II

## Mechanism of Injury

A foreign body, by definition, is any object originating from outside the body. Retained foreign bodies can occur in a variety of clinical settings, such as motor vehicle accidents, explosions, or gunshot injuries. The retained foreign body is a common reason for emergency department visits. The composition of the foreign body can vary (metal, glass, wood, stone, acrylic, graphite, Bakelite, thorns, sand, etc), as can the local response, which can include inflammation and infection.

## Imaging Strategy

### Radiographs

Radiographs are often acquired during the initial diagnosis of the foreign body (Figure 29.1A). Although metal, glass, and stone are radiopaque, other compositions, such as wood and plastic, may be radiolucent. Only 15% or less of wooden foreign bodies are apparent on radiographs.

### Computed Tomography

Most foreign bodies are apparent on CT, with metal generating artifact that does not typically limit accurate localization (Figure 29.1B). Those objects that are too deep for detection by way of US can be elucidated by way of CT. CT does, however, involve ionizing radiation and typically comes at a higher cost and lower availability when compared to US.

### Ultrasound

US provides real-time imaging without radiation exposure and is relatively inexpensive. For those foreign bodies composed of radiolucent materials, US provides an excellent and readily accessible alternative for diagnosis and has been shown to accurately demonstrate the size, shape, and location of the soft tissue foreign body (Figure 29.2).

US is particularly helpful in identifying superficial foreign bodies, as well as assessment of an associated soft tissue abscess, neurovascular abnormality, or tendon or ligament disorder. However, US is limited in the detection of deep foreign bodies or those adjacent to bone or gas. Additionally, it may potentially be difficult to distinguish foreign bodies from calcification, scar, acute hematoma, or soft tissue gas.

### Magnetic Resonance Imaging

If the composition of the foreign body is unknown, MRI should not be used as the initial modality for diagnosis because of the possibility of heating, migration, and artifact in those objects that are metallic. Additionally, MRI may not be able to reliably distinguish a foreign body from other structures that may appear hypointense, such as a scar, tendon, or calcification. As such, MRI has a limited role in the diagnosis and management of soft tissue foreign bodies (Figure 29.3).

## Imaging Findings and Classifications

### Radiography

- Depending on composition, a soft tissue foreign body may be radiopaque on conventional radiography.
- Radiographs may not permit determination of exact foreign body composition, its relationship to surrounding structures, or the degree of associated soft tissue injury.
- Radiolucent materials, such as plastic and wood, are typically not visualized by radiography.

### Ultrasound

- On US, all soft tissue foreign bodies are initially hyperechoic, however, wood may become less echogenic with time.
- The object is often surrounded by a hypoechoic halo composed of granulation tissue, edema, or hemorrhage.
- Posterior acoustic shadowing and reverberation artifact of the foreign body, the direct result of the surface characteristics and not object composition, aids in the identification of a foreign body.
- A smooth and flat surface creates a dirty shadow or reverberation artifact, whereas an irregular surface or those objects with a small radius of curvature creates a clean shadow.

## Treatment Options

### Conservative and Surgical Treatment

- Superficial foreign bodies are typically easy to remove percutaneously.
- The penetrating foreign body poses increased challenges, as the objects may reside adjacent to a vital structure requiring a more comprehensive surgical technique.

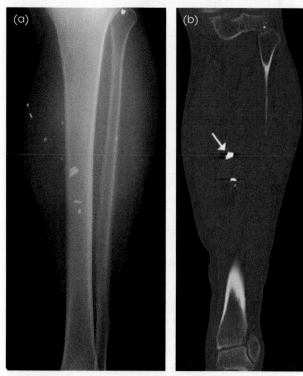

**Figure 29.1.** Metallic foreign bodies on radiograph and CT. Frontal radiograph (*A*) and unenhanced coronal reformatted CT image (*B*) of the leg demonstrate metallic foreign bodies/ shrapnel (*arrow*) scattered throughout the soft tissues.

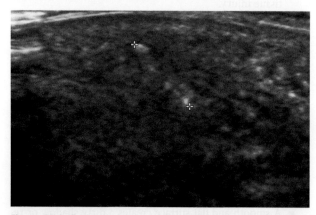

**Figure 29.2.** Foreign body on US. Transverse US image through the forefoot demonstrates an echogenic, nonshadowing foreign body (*between calipers*) within the plantar soft tissues at the level of the first and second toes interspace.

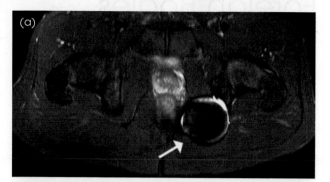

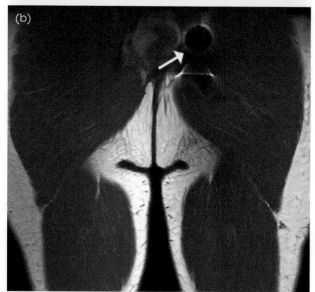

**Figure 29.3.** Foreign body on MRI. Axial STIR (*A*) and coronal T1W (*B*) MR images demonstrate a large focus of susceptibility artifact within the left gluteal soft tissues related to retained soft tissue metallic foreign body (*arrows*).

## Recommended Reading

Horton LK, Jacobson JA, Powell A, Fessell DP, Hayes CW. Sonography and radiography of soft-tissue foreign bodies. *AJR Am J Roentgenol.* 2001;176(5):1155–159.

## References

1. Aras MH, Miloglu O, Barutcugil C, Kantarci M, Ozcan E, Harorli A. Comparison of the sensitivity for detecting foreign bodies among conventional plain radiography, computed tomography and ultrasonography. *Dentomaxillofac Radiol.* 2010;39(2):72–78.
2. Boyse TD, Fessell DP, Jacobson JA, Lin J, van Holsbeeck MT, Hayes CW. US of soft-tissue foreign bodies and associated complications with surgical correlation. *Radiographics.* 2001;21(5):1251–56.
3. Horton LK, Jacobson JA, Powell A, Fessell DP, Hayes CW. Sonography and radiography of soft-tissue foreign bodies. *AJR Am J Roentgenol.* 2001;176(5):1155–59.

## Key Points

- Conventional radiography is often performed first during the diagnostic workup for a soft tissue foreign body, however, some materials, such as plastic and wood, are typically radiolucent.
- For the radiolucent foreign body in soft tissues, US is an excellent imaging modality for identification.
- On US, all foreign bodies appear hyperechoic and exhibit variable shadowing and reverberation as a result of surface characteristics and not composition.

# Section Two

# Arthritis

Edited by Kevin B. Hoover

# Inflammatory Arthritis

# CHAPTER 30

# Rheumatoid Arthritis

Kevin B. Hoover

## Introduction

Rheumatoid arthritis (RA) is a clinical syndrome that results in the inflammation of synovial tissues with secondary articular cartilage and bone damage. Damage is routinely assessed on radiographs, which can detect the characteristic erosions, joint-space narrowing, and joint swelling of RA. Ultrasound and MRI are useful for evaluating the soft tissue findings of RA, such as tenosynovitis and synovitis, and these modalities show superior sensitivity in detecting erosions to radiography.

## Pathophysiology and Clinical Findings

In developed countries, 0.5-1% of adults suffer from RA, with prevalence rising with age. RA is threefold more prevalent in women than men and is most prevalent in women older than 65 years. Fifty percent of the risk of developing RA is considered genetic. This risk is primarily because of alleles of the HLA-DRB1 gene that result in antibodies to citrullinated proteins (anti-citrullinated protein or peptide antibodies [ACPA]; anti-cyclic citrullinated peptide [anti-CCP]). Smoking is the most important environmental risk factor for RA and it doubles the risk, but only in ACPA-positive patients. The acute-phase reactants C-reactive protein (CRP) and erythrocyte sedimentation rate (ESR), may be abnormal in patients with RA. Rheumatoid factor (RF) and ACPA are more specific serum markers; one or both of which are elevated in 50-80% of RA patients. ACPA may be a more specific, sensitive, and better predictor of joint erosions and destruction than RF.

RA primarily involves the synovial joints of the extremities (peripheral skeleton), especially the small joints of hand and feet, but also the wrist, knee, elbow, and shoulder joints. Inflammation of the tendon sheath (tenosynovitis) and tendon most commonly involves the extensor tendons of the hands, fingers, and feet. Tendinosis of the Achilles, patellar, and rotator cuff tendons may occur because these tendons do not have a tendon sheath. When the spine (axial skeleton) is involved, it most often affects the synovial uncovertebral and apophyseal (facet) joints of the cervical spine. Symptoms of early RA are usually bilateral, including joint stiffness for longer than 1 hour and pain and swelling of the wrists and hands lasting longer than 6-12 weeks. Extraarticular findings may also be present, especially in more chronic disease, along with disability related to pain and immobility, fatigue, and depression. The 2010 European League Against Rheumatism/American College of Rheumatology classification (Table 30.1) scores the clinical and serologic findings with a score of 6 or more diagnostic of RA.

## Imaging Strategy

Radiography of the hands and feet is the standard initial imaging study in RA, which can detect characteristic erosions, joint-space narrowing, and malalignment rapidly and inexpensively. It also demonstrates characteristic proliferative findings of OA and the chondrocalcinosis of calcium pyrophosphate dihydrate deposition (CPPD) arthropathy, which are differential diagnoses (Table 30.2).

MRI is a useful secondary imaging modality because of its ability to detect the characteristic soft tissue and bone findings of early RA, especially BME, which can result in earlier diagnosis and treatment than radiography. The following MRI sequences in 2 orthogonal planes are routinely used in evaluation: T1W spin echo (SE) or fast spin echo (FSE) sequences; fluid-sensitive, fat-suppressed (T2W FSE with FS or STIR) sequences, and postcontrast T1W FS sequences acquired 5-10 minutes after injection. For commonly performed hand and wrist MRI, using a dedicated extremity coil with the patient in the "superman" position, with the hand extended overhead into the isocenter of the magnet, is optimal.

Like MRI, US is an appropriate secondary imaging modality in RA with the benefit of lower cost than MRI and the ability to evaluate multiple joints and body parts. In an initial patient evaluation of both hands and wrists, it can be used to confirm a new diagnosis of RA, revise a previous diagnosis, and help identify specific sites of disease involvement.

## Imaging Findings

### Radiography

- Earliest detectable (acute) joint findings
  - Periarticular soft tissue swelling
  - Periarticular osteoporosis
  - Diffuse joint-space loss
- Chronic joint findings
  - Marginal, cortical bone erosions most commonly involving
    - Hand and wrist
      - MCP joints (Figure 30.1)
      - PIP joints and characteristically sparing the DIP joints
      - Ulnar styloid process
      - Narrowing and erosions of intercarpal, radiocarpal, and the distal radioulnar joints
      - Fibrous or osseous fusion and/or ankylosis
    - Foot
      - Metatarsophalangeal (MTP) and PIP joints

### Table 30.1. 2010 American College of Rheumatology/European League Against Rheumatism Classification Criteria for Rheumatoid Arthritis[a]

| CATEGORY | TYPE | SCORE |
|---|---|---|
| Joint involvement | 1 large joint | 0 |
| | 2-10 large joints | 1 |
| | 1-3 small joints (± large joints) | 2 |
| | 4-10 small joints | 3 |
| | >10 joints (≥1 small) | 5 |
| Serology (at least 1) | Neg RF and Neg ACPA | 0 |
| | Low pos RF or ACPA | 2 |
| | High pos RF or ACPA | 3 |
| Acute-phase reactants (at least 1) | Normal CRP and ESR | 0 |
| | Abnormal CRP or ESR | 1 |
| Duration of symptoms | <6 weeks | 0 |
| | >6 weeks | 1 |

Abbreviations: ACPA, anti-citrullinated protein/peptide antibodies; CRP, C-reactive protein; ESR, erythrocyte sedimentation rate; neg, negative; pos, positive; RF, rheumatoid factor.
[a] A score of >6 is diagnostic of rheumatoid arthritis.

- Tarsal and subtalar joints (Figure 31.2A)
- Characteristic sparing of the DIP joints
- Fibrous or osseous fusion and/or ankylosis
- Erosions virtually diagnostic of RA in the correct clinical context

- Joint subluxations and deformities of the hands, often multiple digits
  - Swan-neck deformity (hyperextension of the PIP and hyperflexion of the DIP joint)
  - Boutonniere deformity (hyperflexion of the PIP and hyperextension of the DIP joint; Figure 30.1)

### Table 30.2. Inflammatory Arthropathies Features

| TYPE | RA | PSA/REA | AS/IBD-PSA |
|---|---|---|---|
| **Locations and symmetry** | ■ All joints except SIJ, symmetric | ■ Hands and feet<br>■ SIJ<br>■ Discontinuous spine involving all 3 columns<br>■ Large joints<br>■ Asymmetric early disease | ■ Continuous spine involvement of all 3 columns<br>■ SIJ<br>■ Large joints<br>■ Symmetric |
| **Imaging** | ■ Erosions, lacking bone production<br>■ Osteoporosis<br>■ Synovitis/tenosynovitis<br>■ Subluxations<br>■ Less severe enthesitis<br>■ Ankylosis | ■ Peripheral > axial erosions<br>■ Bone production and sclerosis<br>■ Tenosynovitis<br>■ Enthesitis<br>■ Course/thick syndesmophytes<br>■ Ankylosis<br>■ Less severe facet involvement | ■ Spine and SIJ fusion<br>■ Large joint inflammation<br>■ Enthesitis<br>■ Thin syndesmophytes |
| **Serology** | ■ 50-80% RF or ACPA pos | ■ HLA-B27 increases severity, but not specific | ■ HLA-B27 |

Abbreviations: ACPA, anti-citrullinated protein/peptide antibodies; AS, ankylosing spondylitis; HLA-327, human leukocyte antigen 327; IBD-SpA, inflammatory bowel disease-related seronegative spondyloarthropathy; pos, positive; PsA, psoriatic arthritis; RA, rheumatoid arthritis; ReA, reactive arthritis; RF, rheumatoid factor; SIJ, sacroiliac joint.

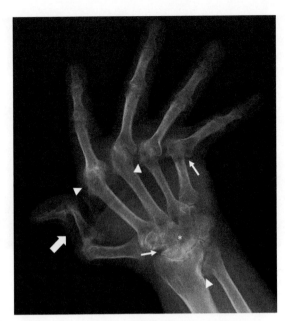

**Figure 30.1.** RA in a 65-year-old, seropositive woman on methotrexate. An AP hand radiograph demonstrates changes of chronic RA, including ulnar drift at the MCP and radiocarpal joints (*thin arrows*), boutonniere deformity of the first digit (*block arrow*), fusion of the carpus (*asterisk*), and chronic erosions of distal metacarpal heads and the distal radioulnar joint (*arrowheads*).

- Ulnar deviation and/or drift of the MCP joints and the carpus (Figure 30.1)
- Cystlike bone lesions (cysts)
- Joint and bone remodeling
  - Medially positioned femoral head (acetabular protrusion)
  - Eroded, attenuated olecranon and dens
- Diffuse osteoporosis
- Secondary OA in patients in remission
- Soft tissue rheumatoid nodules identified in 20-35% of RA patients between the skin and bone

- Rarely calcify
- Can be seen prior to the onset of arthritis
- Associated with seropositive and more severely erosive disease
- Multicentric reticulohistiocytosis (rare, non-Langerhans cell histiocytosis mimic of RA)
  - Narrows and erodes any joint, especially the DIP joints
  - Pruritic skin nodules with DIP involvement distinguish from RA

**Magnetic Resonance Imaging**
- Characteristic findings of RA detected with great sensitivity
  - Erosions (Figure 30.2B,C)
    - Cortical breaks detected in 2 imaging planes
    - Three to 7.7 fold more sensitive than radiographs in detecting erosions
  - Synovitis and tenosynovitis
    - Increased synovial fluid volume (Figure 30.2C) with a thickened synovium is most apparent on postcontrast sequences.
    - They may occur with or without joint inflammation.
    - Involved tendons may weaken and rupture.
  - BME
    - BME is a somewhat ill-defined region of increased fluid signal within the trabecular bone (Figure 30.2B,C and Figure 30.3C).
    - BME represents inflammatory cellular infiltrates, or osteitis, and is a reliable predictor of future erosion.
    - MRI is the only imaging modality proven to detect BME.
    - BME and synovitis can be detected in patients in clinical remission.
  - Rheumatoid nodules
    - Nonspecific imaging characteristics
    - Hypointense T1W signal (relative to muscle)
    - Intermediate to hyperintense signal on fluid-sensitive (T2W or STIR) sequences
    - Diffuse or heterogeneous enhancement on the postcontrast sequences

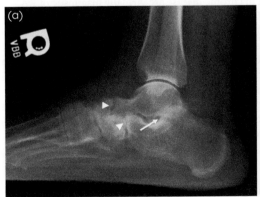
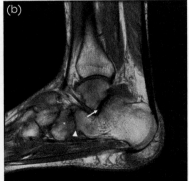
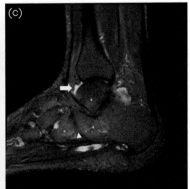

**Figure 30.2.** RA in a 48-year-old seropositive woman on methotrexate. (*A*) Lateral foot radiograph demonstrates narrowing of the posterior subtalar joint (*thin arrow*) with narrowing and erosion of the talonavicular and calcaneocuboid joints (*arrowheads*). (*B*) Sagittal T1W and (*C*) STIR MR images redemonstrate narrowing of the posterior subtalar joint (*thin arrow*) and a narrowed, eroded calcaneocuboid joint (*arrowhead*) with periarticular BME (*asterisks*). (*C*) The STIR image also clearly demonstrates cortical indistinctness (*arrowhead*) and a tibiotalar joint effusion (*block arrow*).

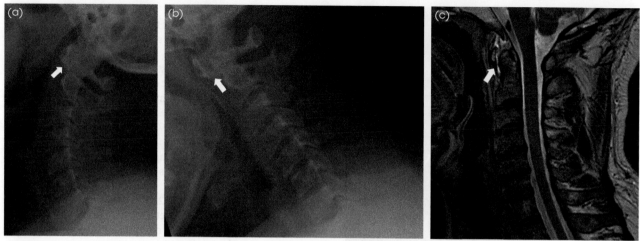

**Figure 30.3.** RA in a 45-year-old seropositive man treated with a biologic and hydroxyquinoline. (*A*) Extension radiograph of the cervical spine demonstrates normal alignment, including the atlantodens interval (*block arrow*). (*B*) Flexion radiograph demonstrates subluxation of the atlantodens interval (*block arrow*). (*C*) A sagittal T2W MR image demonstrates abnormal fluid signal interposed between the anterior arch of C1 and the dens caused by ligament destruction with periarticular erosion, irregularity, and edema (*block arrow*).

- Synovial cysts
  - Likely represent abnormal distention of a bursa that communicates with the adjacent joint (eg, popliteal or Baker cysts)
  - Synovitis also found in bursae, sometimes with secondary adjacent bone erosion
    - Especially the olecranon, subacromial-subdeltoid, and retrocalcaneal bursae

### Ultrasound
- Findings detected on MRI are reproducibly identified on US with notable exceptions of BME (osteitis) and joint-space loss because of cartilage thinning.
- Power Doppler signal is especially valuable in evaluating synovitis.
  - It correlates with the histologic severity of synovitis.
  - Elevated signal within at least 1 joint in a patient in clinical remission may be predictive of disease relapse.
- Discussed in more detail in Chapter 127, "Ultrasound for Rheumatologic Diseases."

### Other Imaging Modalities
- CT and nuclear medicine are less commonly used or indicated.
- CT is the gold standard for detecting erosions, but limited by the number of joints evaluated and sensitivity to soft tissue findings in RA, such as synovitis.
- Periarticular uptake on technetium bone scan is similar to osteitis on MRI.

## Treatment Options
- Disease-modifying antirheumatic drugs (DMARDs; most commonly methotrexate, sulfasalazine, and leflunomide) decrease the severity of RA symptoms and improve outcomes, including the necessity for joint fusion and replacement.

- Biologics, especially anti-tumor necrosis factor (TNF) antibodies, are added to DMARDs when there is an incomplete response.
- Biologics are discontinued when patients are in clinical remission, but DMARDs are continued.
- Glucocorticoid treatment is ideally limited to periods of DMARD adjustment and for use in intraarticular injection.
- Joint arthroplasty or fusion for painful joints is recommended, despite medical treatment.
- Surgical stabilization of atlantoaxial subluxation for patients with secondary neurologic impairment or pain can be offered.

### Key Points
- Early radiographic findings of RA are soft tissue swelling, periarticular osteoporosis and diffuse joint-space loss.
- The characteristic marginal erosions of the hands and feet of chronic disease are virtually diagnostic of RA.
- MRI and US are useful in identifying soft tissue findings and complications of RA, including synovitis, tenosynovitis, and tendon rupture.
- MRI is the only modality proven to identify BME, which is characteristic of early RA and predictive of future erosions.
- Early RA diagnosis and treatment with DMARDs has resulted in a trend toward less severe imaging findings, fewer physical limitations, and improved outcomes.

**Recommended Reading**

Narvaez JA, Narvaez J, De Lama E, De Albert M. MR imaging of early rheumatoid arthritis. *Radiographics.* 2010;30:143–163; discussion 163–65.

Tan YK, Conaghan PG. Imaging in rheumatoid arthritis. *Best Pract Res Clin Rheumatol.* 2011;25:569–84.

## References

1. Aletaha D, Neogi T, Silman AJ, et al. 2010 Rheumatoid arthritis classification criteria: an American College of Rheumatology/European League Against Rheumatism collaborative initiative. *Arthritis Rheum.* 2010;62(9):2569–81.

2. Arnett FC, Edworthy SM, Bloch DA, et al. The American Rheumatism Association 1987 revised criteria for the classification of rheumatoid arthritis. *Arthritis Rheum.* 1988;31:315–24.

3. Gandjbakhch F, Haavardsholm EA, Conaghan PG, et al. Determining a magnetic resonance imaging inflammatory activity acceptable state without subsequent radiographic progression in rheumatoid arthritis: results from a followup MRI study of 254 patients in clinical remission or low disease activity. *J Rheumatol.* 2014;41:398–406.

4. Kung TN, Bykerk VP. Detecting the earliest signs of rheumatoid arthritis: symptoms and examination. *Rheum Dis Clin North Am.* 2014;40:669–83.

5. Lard LR, Visser H, Speyer I, et al. Early versus delayed treatment in patients with recent-onset rheumatoid arthritis: comparison of two cohorts who received different treatment strategies. *Am J Med.* 2001;111:446–51.

6. Machold KP, Stamm TA, Eberl GJ, et al. Very recent onset arthritis—clinical, laboratory, and radiological findings during the first year of disease. *J Rheumatol.* 2002;29:2278–87.

7. McQueen FM. Imaging in early rheumatoid arthritis. *Best Pract Res Clin Rheumatol.* 2013;27:499–522.

8. Narvaez JA, Narvaez J, De Lama E, De Albert M. MR imaging of early rheumatoid arthritis. *Radiographics.* 2010;30:143–163; discussion 163–65.

9. Ostergaard M, Pedersen SJ, Dohn UM. Imaging in rheumatoid arthritis—status and recent advances for magnetic resonance imaging, ultrasonography, computed tomography and conventional radiography. *Best Pract Res Clin Rheumatol.* 2008;22:1019–44.

10. Scott DL, Wolfe F, Huizinga TW. Rheumatoid arthritis. *Lancet.* 2010;376:1094–108.

11. Tan YK, Conaghan PG. Imaging in rheumatoid arthritis. *Best Pract Res Clin Rheumatol.* 2011;25:569–84.

# CHAPTER 31

# Juvenile Idiopathic Arthritis

Kevin B. Hoover

## Introduction

Juvenile idiopathic arthritis (JIA) has a variety of clinical presentations that mirror those of the adult seropositive and seronegative arthropathies. JIA develops before age 16 and is characterized by prolonged synovial inflammation with joint pain, tenderness, loss of function, and sometimes joint destruction. Although the knee is the most commonly involved joint, temporomandibular joint (TMJ) and spine involvement are also commonly identified in both symptomatic and asymptomatic patients. Imaging, in association with clinical examination and serologic findings, is critical in diagnosis.

## Pathophysiology and Clinical Findings

JIA may be transient and self-limiting, however, 10-33% of children remain disabled into adulthood. In developed countries, it affects 0.016-0.15% of children. JIA has 7 subtypes, which develop before the age of 16, have symptoms persisting for at least 6 weeks, and involve a variable number of joints (Table 31.1). Cervical spine imaging findings are found in 60% of patients, especially in *polyarticular and systemic arthritis*. Sacroiliitis is also identified in 30% of *enthesitis-related arthritis* patients, but may not be detectable on radiographs until 5-10 years after onset of clinical symptoms. TMJ involvement is seen in 17-87% of JIA patients, who may remain asymptomatic, and is best assessed by MRI. Retrognathia and jaw asymmetry may be detected on physical examination, but only after irreversible condylar damage has occurred. The presence of anti-citrullinated protein antibody (ACPA) and antinuclear antigen (ANA), can be helpful in distinguishing the rheumatoid factor *(RF)-positive* and *oligoarthritis* subtypes, respectively.

## Imaging Strategy

Baseline radiographs of clinically suspicious joints are useful at initial patient evaluation to determine the presence of inflammatory changes and to exclude other causes of joint inflammation. Radiographs are more useful in detecting the late rather than early joint changes of JIA, but repeat imaging should be used sparingly because of radiation dose. Contrast-enhanced MRI and Doppler US have greater sensitivity for the detection of synovitis and findings of inflammation that are radiographically occult. Although US is useful for evaluating multiple joints in the extremities, contrast-enhanced MRI is the preferred imaging modality, especially for the evaluation of complex joints that are frequently affected and potentially asymptomatic: the TMJ and SI joints.

A high field strength MRI of 1.5 T or higher should be used with a coil that is size-matched to the area of concern. T1W SE or FSE sequences; fluid-sensitive, FS (T2W FSE or STIR) sequences in 2 orthogonal planes; and postcontrast T1W FS sequences acquired in 2 orthogonal planes 5-10 minutes after injection should be obtained. A larger field of view for MRI of the pelvis should be used to include both hip joints, which may be involved.

## Imaging Findings

### Radiography

- Radiography is useful for excluding noninflammatory causes of joint pain and swelling.
- Radiology has limited sensitivity in detecting the early changes of JIA because of the large amount of epiphyseal cartilage in pediatric patients and the potential for repair caused by cartilage vascularization.
- Early radiographic findings are as follows:
  - Soft tissue swelling, joint effusions, and periarticular osteopenia, such as in RA
- Later radiographic findings are as follows:
  - Growth disturbances
    - Epiphyseal enlargement (Figure 31.1A), widening of the intercondylar notch, lower patella squaring, hypoplastic vertebrae, and small intervertebral discs are seen. (Figure 31.1B).
    - Limb length discrepancies and malalignment can be detected.
    - Premature growth plate closure caused by hyperemia can also be detected, including advanced bone age on hand radiographs.
  - Ankylosis can be detected within 3-5 years of JIA onset of the carpal and tarsal bones and apophyseal joints of the cervical spine (Figure 31.1).
  - Odontoid erosion and atlantodens interval widening and instability on flexion-extension radiographs can be seen.

### Magnetic Resonance Imaging

- MRI is the optimal imaging technique for comprehensive evaluation of involved joints:
  - TMJ, especially in children younger than 4 years old, who may be asymptomatic even in severe erosive disease
    - Active inflammation shows BME, synovial enhancement, and joint effusion.

**Table 31.1.** Juvenile Idiopathic Arthritis Subtypes

| SUBTYPE | DEFINING CHARACTERISTICS | FREQUENT PRESENTATION |
|---|---|---|
| Oligoarthritis | 1-4 joints | Positive ANA, most common subtype, knees and ankles, preschool-aged girls, 30% suffer from iridocyclitis |
| Polyarthritis: RF-positive | 5 or more joints | ACPA, small joint erosions of the hands, adolescent girls |
| Polyarthritis: RF-negative | 5 or more joints | RF and ACPA negative, ANA variable, more heterogeneous joint involvement |
| Systemic arthritis | Recurrent daily fevers | Rashes, lymphadenopathy, hepatosplenomegaly and multi-organ failure. Symmetric and polyarticular joint involvement may occur late in disease course. |
| Enthesitis-related arthritis | Enthesitis | Boys older than 6 years, enthesitis most commonly of the mid- and hind-foot, asymmetric arthritis of lower extremities including hip. Spine rarely involved until adulthood |
| Juvenile psoriatic arthritis | Heterogeneous | Large or small joint involvement and dactylitis that may occur before skin changes |
| Undifferentiated arthritis | None of the above | |

Abbreviations: ACPA, anti-citrullinated protein antigen; ANA, antinuclear antigen; RF, rheumatoid factor.

- Sacroiliitis
  - Subchondral or periarticular BME, erosions, and synovial enhancement are seen.
  - Ankylosis is a rare late manifestation of JIA.
- MRI is the most sensitive technique to evaluate for bone erosions:
  - Areas of cortical irregularity with low signal on T1W sequences and high signal on fluid-sensitive sequences with well-defined margins (Figures 31.2 and 31.3)

- Visible in 2 planes with cortical disruption in 1 plane adjacent to the capsule or ligament attachments
- Twice as sensitive in detecting erosions compared to radiographs
- Synovitis and tenosynovitis show abnormally increased water signal in a joint or in the tendon sheath (Figure 31.2B and 31.3C).
  - Contrast enhancement is the most sensitive technique for detecting thickened, avidly enhancing synovium (Figure 31.3D).

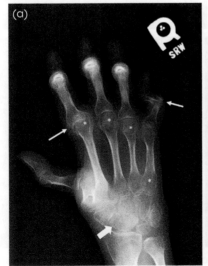 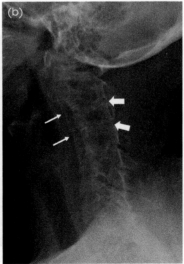

**Figure 31.1.** JIA in a 44-year-old man. Radiographs of the hand and the cervical spine show end-stage disease. (*A*) PA radiograph of the hand shows boutonniere deformities of all the digits with second MCP and fifth PIP joint subluxations (*thin arrows*), along with epiphyseal overgrowth (*asterisks*) with fusion of the scaphoid and capitate bones (*thick arrow*). (*B*) Lateral radiograph of the cervical spine shows ankylosis of the C2-C5 facet joints with narrowed intervertebral discs, partial fusion of the vertebral bodies (*thin arrows*), and facet joints (*thick arrows*) with abnormal kyphosis.

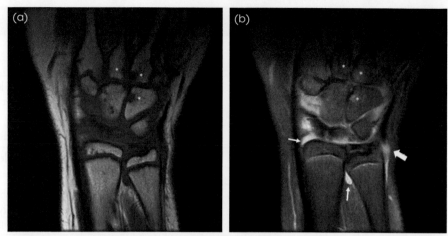

**Figure 31.2.** JIA in a 12-year-old RF and ACPA positive, untreated boy with wrist pain. (*A*) T1W coronal MR image demonstrates focal areas of abnormal fat replacement involving the hamate and base of the second through fourth metacarpals consistent with erosions (*asterisks*) with more diffuse low signal involving the lunate and scaphoid largely related to volume averaging. (*B*) Coronal T2W FS MR image demonstrates edema at the sites of low T1 signal (*asterisks*) as well radiocarpal, midcarpal, and distal radioulnar joint effusions (*thin arrows*) and extensor carpi ulnaris tenosynovitis (*thick arrow*).

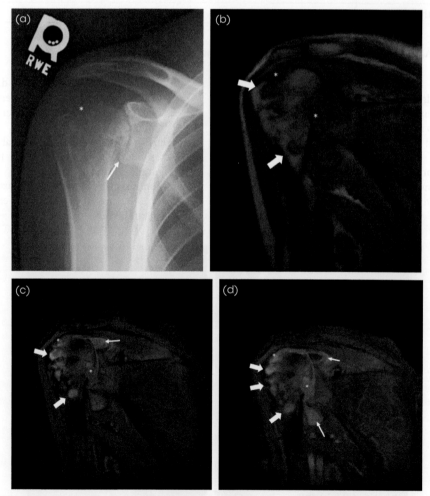

**Figure 31.3.** JIA in a 17-year-old seropositive untreated girl with shoulder pain. (*A*) An AP radiograph demonstrates osteopenia with glenohumeral joint narrowing and erosion (*thin arrow*) with erosion at the greater tuberosity near the rotator cuff attachment (*asterisk*). Coronal (*B*) T1W, (*C*) T2W FS, and (*D*) T1W FS postcontrast MR images redemonstrate erosive changes in the same regions (*asterisks*), heterogeneous joint effusion with enhancing synovitis, and low T1 and high T2 signal cystlike changes in the humeral head (*thick arrows*). In (*C*), note low signal intensity foci probably related to rice bodies (*thin arrows*) and in (*D*), contrast enhancement of the intraosseous cystlike changes (*thick arrows*).

- Synovitis and tenosynovitis can progress to more chronic frondlike pannus and rice bodies (Figure 31.3D).
- They are often detected in asymptomatic patients.
- MRI can show enthesitis at tendon or ligament attachments:
  - Soft tissue edema, increased tendon or ligament intrasubstance fluid signal or thickening, BME, and bursitis
  - Most common at the Achilles tendon insertion
- BME in JIA, like in RA, is related to osteitis with inflammatory cellular infiltrate:
  - Ill-defined fluid signal, dark signal on T1W sequences and enhancement on T1W postcontrast images

### Ultrasound

- US has similar sensitivity to MRI in evaluating peripheral disease except it cannot detect osteitis.
- US is especially useful in the hands and feet.
- Multiple peripheral joints can be quickly assessed to aid in JIA subtype classification.
- US can facilitate intraarticular injection, determine patient response to intraarticular therapy, and can be used for serial examinations to monitor disease.
- See Chapter 127, "Ultrasound for Rheumatologic Diseases."

## Treatment Options

- Intraarticular steroid injection of involved joints is a standard and valuable treatment that helps prevent deformity secondary to joint contractures.
- Disease-modifying antirheumatic drugs (DMARDs) and methotrexate are the standard and effective systemic treatment.
- Although promising in randomized controlled trials, antibodies such as anti-tumor necrosis factor (TNF) and anti-interleukin compounds are not as widely used and still being investigated.

## Key Points

- Radiographs of involved joints are useful for initial, baseline assessment of JIA, but should be used sparingly because of ionizing radiation risks and the often chronic nature of the disease.
- Radiographs are sensitive to late findings of JIA such as erosions, abnormal bone growth, and ankylosis, but not early changes of JIA.
- MRI is sensitive in detecting the early findings of JIA, including synovitis and BME, which occur even in asymptomatic joints.
- US can be useful in evaluating multiple joints for JIA diagnosis, guiding intraarticular injections, and serial monitoring.

### Recommended Reading

Sheybani EF, Khanna G, White AJ, Demertzis JL. Imaging of juvenile idiopathic arthritis: a multimodality approach. *Radiographics*. 2013;33:1253–73.

### References

1. Munir S, Patil K, Miller E, et al. Juvenile idiopathic arthritis of the axial joints: a systematic review of the diagnostic accuracy and predictive value of conventional MRI. *AJR Am J Roentgenol*. 2014;202:199–210.
2. Nusman CM, Hemke R, Schonenberg D, et al. Distribution pattern of MRI abnormalities within the knee and wrist of juvenile idiopathic arthritis patients: signature of disease activity. *AJR Am J Roentgenol*. 2014;202:W439–46.
3. Prakken B, Albani S, Martini A. Juvenile idiopathic arthritis. *Lancet*. 2011;377:2138–49.
4. Sheybani EF, Khanna G, White AJ, Demertzis JL. Imaging of juvenile idiopathic arthritis: a multimodality approach. *Radiographics*. 2013;33:1253–73.

# CHAPTER 32

# Ankylosing Spondylitis

Kevin B. Hoover

## Introduction

AS is a potentially debilitating disease that progresses to anky-losis of the axial skeleton if not appropriately diagnosed and treated. Because early symptoms may be subtle and nonspe-cific, imaging of the axial skeleton is important and may be ac-quired for other reasons (eg, trauma). Radiographs can detect later findings, which are fairly specific, but MRI is the most sensitive imaging technique to detect the characteristic early inflammatory changes at ligament and tendon attachments. It has the added benefit that it does not use radiation, which is important as patients are often young when first diagnosed and may require repeat imaging.

## Pathophysiology and Clinical Findings

AS is an idiopathic inflammatory disease with an estimated incidence of 0.55-1.4% in the population. It primarily affects white boys and men with a 2:1-9:1 male-to-female ratio. AS typically presents in late adolescence to early adulthood and rarely after 40 years. Compared to 5-6% of the white North American population, 80-90% of patients are human leu-kocyte antigen (HLA)-B27 positive. However, HLA-B27 is identified in other seronegative spondyloarthritides (SpA) and its presence alone is not indicative of disease.

The diagnosis of AS and the other SpA, starts with Assessment of SpA International Society (ASAS) classification criteria. Axial SpA is defined as either sacroiliitis on imaging, plus 1 clinical feature (Box 32.1), or HLA-B27 positivity, plus 2 clinical features. Peripheral SpA is defined by arthritis, enthesitis, or dactylitis plus 2 clinical features. Some clinical features (eg, psoriasis, dactylitis) are useful in distinguishing AS from other SpA. Inflammatory bowel disease (IBD)-related SpA is indistin-guishable from AS based on musculoskeletal imaging. Because of the nonspecific nature of the symptoms, the time to diagnosis of AS after symptoms onset averages 7 years. The most common presenting symptoms of AS are morning stiffness and pain of the low back (inflammatory back pain). Younger patients may experience more peripheral symptoms. Approximately 20% of patients progress to severe debilitation because of extraskeletal pathology (eg, pulmonary fibrosis). Other complications in-clude spine instability caused by discovertebral (Andersson) lesions and cauda equina syndrome caused by dural ectasia with associated bowel, bladder, and sexual dysfunction.

## Imaging Strategy

The appropriate first step for patients with possible AS is radi-ography of the pelvis and spine to look for inflammation and ankylosis. Pelvis radiographs need to include the hip joints, which may also be involved. In clinically suspected patients without characteristic erosions or sclerosis on radiography, MRI of the pelvis should be obtained using axial and coronal T1W and fluid-sensitive (T2W with FS or STIR) sequences and postcontrast T1W FS sequences in axial and coronal planes with a large enough field of view to include the hip joints. Spine MRI may also be helpful in identifying the char-acteristic enthesitis of the vertebral corners. CT is a useful al-ternative if MRI is unavailable or unsafe for the patient. It is especially useful to exclude discovertebral (Andersson) lesions in the setting of modest to severe trauma in fused spine.

## Imaging Findings

### Radiography

- Radiography of the pelvis is the most common initial study.
    - SI joint erosions and marginal sclerosis may progress to ankylosis (Figures 32.1 and 32.2).
    - Hip and other large joint involvement occurs espe-cially when symptoms begin prior to 21 years.
- Small joint involvement in AS is rare.
- Spine radiographs may be useful in distinguishing AS from other SpA.
    - Of AS patients, 50% have spondylitis.
    - Enthesitis may be detected:
        - Erosion and reactive sclerosis ("shiny corners") at insertion of the annulus fibrosus of the inter-vertebral disc on the ring apophysis of vertebral endplate
        - Often progressing to outer annulus fibrosus os-sification with fine, symmetric syndesmophytes bridging vertebral bodies (Figure 32.1)
- Fusion often begins in the thoracolumbar or lumbar spine and progresses cranially, compared to more random involvement of other SpA.
- Isolated cervical spine involvement in AS is rare.
- Vertebral squaring, loss of the normal vertebral concavities, occurs with progressive fusion.
- Apophyseal joints, paraspinous ligaments, and spinous processes also ossify and fuse, giving rise to the characteristic *bamboo spine* and *dagger sign* (Figure 32.2).
    - The bamboo spine is a radiographic feature seen in AS that occurs as a result of vertebral body fusion by marginal syndesmophytes.

**Box 32.1.** Assessment of SpondyloArthritis International Society: Spondyloarthropathy Features

Inflammatory back pain
Arthritis
Enthesitis (heel)
Uveitis
Dactylitis
Psoriasis
Crohn disease and colitis
Good response to NSAIDs
Family history of SpA
HLA-B27
Elevated CRP
Sacroiliitis on imaging

- The dagger sign is a radiographic feature seen in AS characterized with a single central radiodense line on frontal radiographs of the spine related to ossification of supraspinous and interspinous ligaments. It is most common at the thoracolumbar or cervicothoracic junctions.
- Flexion and extension radiographs may be useful in identifying atlantoaxial subluxation in AS.
- Progressive lung disease is the most common extraskeletal manifestation, and includes bullous emphysema and fibrosis, which may be detectable on spine radiographs.

### Magnetic Resonance Imaging
- MRI is highly sensitive for the inflammatory changes of the SI joints and spine.

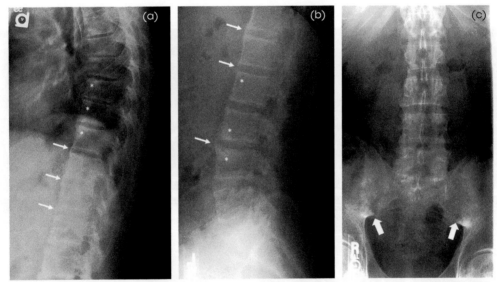

**Figure 32.1.** IBD-related seronegative spondyloarthropathy in an untreated 51-year-old man. (*A, B*) Lateral thoracic and lumbar spine radiographs demonstrate multilevel bridging syndesmophytes (*thin arrows*) with sclerosis at the corners of the vertebrae (shiny corners, *asterisks*) with continuous involvement from the lumbosacral junction cranially. (*C*) Frontal radiograph of the lumbar spine demonstrates complete ankylosis of the SI joints (*arrows*).

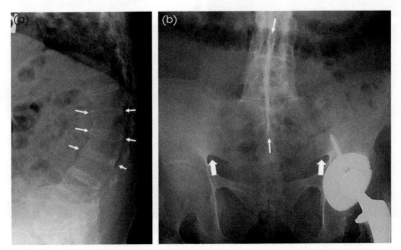

**Figure 32.2.** Chronic AS. (*A*) A lateral thoracolumbar spine radiograph in a 58-year-old woman with chronic, untreated disease shows complete ankylosis of the lumbar spine from the L1-L4 levels with a bamboo spine appearance with thin paravertebral syndesmophytes (*arrows*). (*B*) Frontal radiograph in a 71-year-old woman with chronic AS shows the dagger sign (*thin arrows*) and complete, symmetric fusion of the SI joints (*block arrows*).

- Because of the lack of ionizing radiation, it is used for serial imaging.
- Fluid-sensitive sequences readily detect BME, joint widening, joint fluid, and synovitis.
- AS may present as asymmetric sacroiliitis, but it inevitably progresses to bilateral, symmetric SI joint involvement (Figures 32.3 and 32.4).
- MRI has superior soft tissue contrast, but subtle erosions may be better seen on CT.
- Contrast may increase the sensitivity in distinguishing active from inactive disease and detect response to treatment, if enhancement decreases from baseline (Figure 32.4).
- Spine MRI may detect the following:
  - Dural ectasia with widening of the thecal sac and posterior vertebral scalloping
  - Atlantoaxial widening or subluxation
- Discovertebral lesions with fluid signal extending through all 3 vertebral columns with adjacent, degenerative bone and marrow signal depending on acuity

**Computed Tomography**
- CT is more sensitive than radiography and an alternative to MRI when it is unavailable or contraindicated.
  - It is not optimal for repeated imaging because of dosage of ionizing radiation.
  - Active inflammation is not easily distinguished from chronic disease.
  - Typical changes are as follows:
    - Serrated erosions on the iliac side of the SI joint caused by thinner cartilage (Figure 32.3)
    - Progressive enthesitis with sclerosis, ligamentous ossification and ankylosis, with eventual resolution of sclerosis

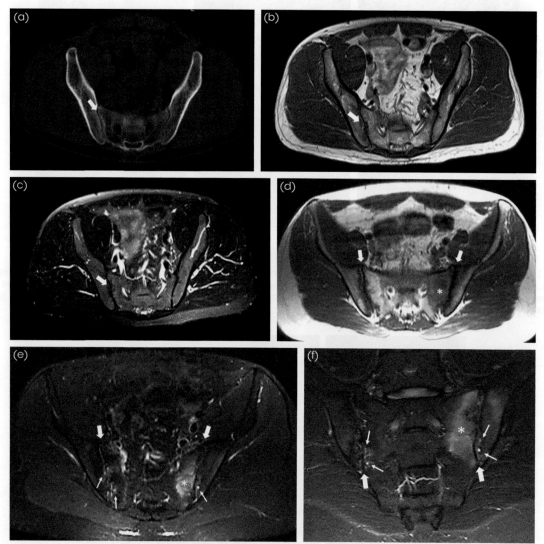

**Figure 32.3.** Sacroiliitis. (*A*) An axial CT image of a 30-year-old man with IBD-related spondyloarthropathy demonstrates subtle asymmetric erosion and sclerosis involving the right SI joint (*arrow*). (*B*) Axial T1W and (*C*) T2W FS MR images demonstrate subtle sclerosis and cortical irregularity of the right SI joint (*B*) with periarticular erosions and subtle adjacent BME (*C*) (*arrow*). (*D*) Axial T1W, (*E*) STIR, and (*F*) oblique coronal STIR MR images of a 32-year-old man with untreated AS demonstrate asymmetric, bilateral sacroiliitis on the left greater than the right (*thick arrows*) with associated periarticular edema (*asterisks*), left-side joint-space narrowing and small fluid signal erosions (*thin arrows*).

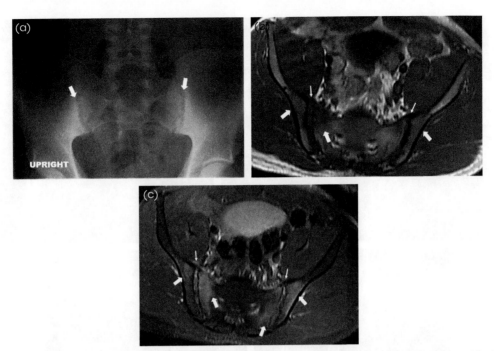

**Figure 32.4.** Sacroiliitis in an untreated 23-year-old man with newly diagnosed AS. (*A*) Frontal radiograph of the pelvis shows extensive sclerosis surrounding patent SI joints with indistinct margins (*arrows*). (*B*) Axial T1W and (*C*) T2W FS MR images demonstrate periarticular replacement of marrow fat signal (*B*) with inflammatory marrow edema (*C*) (*thick arrows*). SI joint widening with intraarticular fluid signal (*thin arrows*) is also consistent with sacroiliitis.

- Discovertebral or Andersson lesions are a pseudoarthrosis through all 3 spine columns caused by erosion or fracture through syndesmophytes or incomplete fusion between long fused segments (Figures 32.5 and 32.6).

### Ultrasound
- US is not as useful as radiography or other cross-sectional imaging for evaluation of the axial skeleton, but can be used to guide therapeutic injections.

- US of inflammatory arthritis is reviewed in Chapter 127, "Ultrasound for Rheumatologic Diseases."

### Treatment Options
- Exercise and early and continuous NSAIDs are cornerstone treatments.
- Tumor necrosis factor (TNF) inhibitors can halt joint destruction in active, refractory disease.

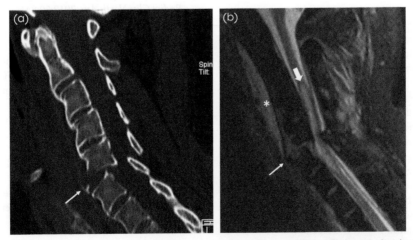

**Figure 32.5.** Spinal fracture in a 77-year-old man with AS status post motor vehicle collision with hyperextension injury. (*A*) Sagittal CT reformatted image of the cervical spine demonstrates fracture and posterior subluxation at the C5-C6 level. Note fracture through anterior syndesmophytes at the intervertebral disc and anterior inferior corner of C5 (*arrow*) and associated severe spinal canal stenosis. (*B*) Sagittal STIR MR image demonstrates high signal at the same level deep to the ossified ALL (*thin arrow*). Note prevertebral soft tissue hematoma (*asterisk*) in the mid and upper cervical spine and extensive cervical cord edema (*block arrow*) consistent with severe cord contusion resulting in quadriplegia.

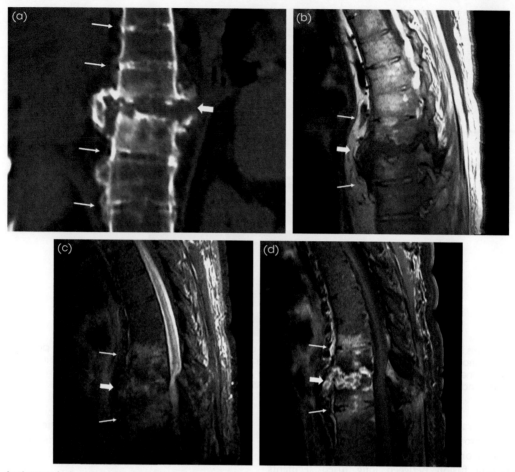

**Figure 32.6.** Andersson lesions in a 44-year-old paraplegic with chronic AS. (*A*) Coronal reformatted CT image demonstrates a discovertebral (Andersson) lesion at T10-T11 with pseudoarthrosis and hypertrophic bony margins (*thick arrow*). There is diffuse vertebral fusion with bridging syndesmophytes (*thin arrows*). (*B*) Sagittal T1W, (*C*) STIR, and (*D*) T1W FS postcontrast MR images demonstrate multiple Andersson lesions. Although the most severe lesion is at T10-T11 (*thick arrow*), marginal edema and enhancement is also seen at the T9-T10 and T11-T12 intervertebral disc levels (*thin arrows*) consistent with active inflammation.

■ Surgical treatment may be required for unstable spine fractures.

**Recommended Reading**

Amrami KK. Imaging of the seronegative spondyloarthropathies. *Radiol Clin North Am.* 2012;50:841–54.

**References**

1. Amrami KK. Imaging of the seronegative spondyloarthropathies. R*adiol Clin North Am.* 2012;50:841–54.
2. Dougados M, Baeten D. Spondyloarthritis. *Lancet.* 2011;377:2127–37.
3. Mease P. Psoriatic arthritis and spondyloarthritis assessment and management update. *Curr Opin Rheumatol.* 2013;25:287–96.
4. Rudwaleit M, van der Heijde D, Landewe R, et al. The Assessment of SpondyloArthritis International Society classification criteria for peripheral spondyloarthritis and for spondyloarthritis in general. *Ann Rheum Dis.* 2011;70:25–31.

## Key Points

■ The axial skeleton is predominantly involved with large joint involvement demonstrated in younger AS patients.

■ Pelvis and spine radiographs are a useful first study to identify the characteristic chronic findings of AS in the SI joints and spine.

■ MRI is useful to evaluate acute, preradiographic changes, distinguish active from chronic AS, and evaluate response to therapy.

■ Although CT is useful to evaluate subtle erosive and productive joint changes of AS, use is limited by radiation dose and insensitivity in distinguishing active from chronic inflammation.

■ IBD-related SpA and AS have indistinguishable imaging findings.

# CHAPTER 33

# Psoriatic Arthritis

Kevin B. Hoover

## Introduction

Psoriatic arthritis (PsA) is characterized by enthesopathy, joint erosions, destruction, and fusion in either a symmetric or asymmetric pattern. Peripheral disease often precedes axial skeleton involvement, and disease may be exclusively peripheral. Radiographic evaluation of symptomatic joints is the first step in imaging evaluation. MRI and US of symptomatic joints and/or MRI of the SI joints may be useful in clinically challenging cases.

## Pathophysiology and Clinical Findings

Psoriasis is an inflammatory, cutaneous disease affecting approximately 2% of the population with characteristic raised, erythematous skin plaques with a silver scale. It is a heritable, polygenic disease associated with multiple major histocompatibility complex (MHC) alleles, including human leukocyte antigen (HLA)-B27, bacterial infections, inflammatory bowel disease, mechanical stress, and obesity. PsA occurs in approximately 30% of psoriasis patients and precedes the skin changes of psoriasis in approximately 50% of patients. The strongest predictors for the development of PsA are nail disease, obesity, and the HLA-B27 allele. There are no diagnostic autoimmune markers. PsA onset is usually between ages 30 and 50 years with an equal frequency in men and women. It can occur in children and accounts for 6-8% of all juvenile arthritis.

The signs and symptoms of PsA include peripheral and axial arthritis, dactylitis, enthesitis, and skin and nail disease. Arthritis presents with joint and/or back pain and morning stiffness longer than 30 minutes that improve with activity, most commonly in the feet and hands, followed by knees, wrists, ankles, and shoulders. Axial arthritis is found in 40% of PsA patients and may be asymptomatic, but it is uncommon in the absence of peripheral disease. Arthritis mutilans is rapid bone and joint destruction seen in 5% of patients, more commonly in younger, HLA-B27 positive patients with axial disease and nail involvement. Approximately 50% of patients suffer from dactylitis, with a decreased range of motion, swelling, tenderness, and an often hot digit or digits, which is a presenting sign in 30% of patients. Dactylitis of the feet is more common than the hands and is associated with more severe radiographic disease. Enthesitis is inflammation at tendon and ligament attachments onto the bone, which may be the only manifestation of PsA. It is a presenting symptom in 35% of patients and present in approximately 50% of patients over

the course of disease. Findings of PsA may be indistinguishable from reactive arthritis (ReA), requiring clinical correlation to distinguish the diseases. The Assessment of SpA International Society (ASAS) classification criteria are also useful in diagnosing PsA and distinguishing it from other seronegative spondyloarthropathies (SpA) (see Chapter 32, "Ankylosing Spondylitis").

## Imaging Strategy

Radiography is the primary imaging technique used for clinical diagnosis and monitoring therapy of PsA. MRI of symptomatic joints can facilitate early diagnosis and classification in patients with undifferentiated arthritis and response to therapy in later disease stages, when radiographic findings may be severe. MRI is a preferred modality to US because it can detect the BME of active inflammation and evaluate the axial skeleton.

- Tailored field-of-view MRI of an affected peripheral joint using either a dedicated extremity coil or surface coil, or body coils for the axial skeleton, using the following sequences: at least one T1W sequence plane to evaluate tissue fat; two plane fluid-sensitive (T2W fat-suppressed or STIR) sequences to detect BME, tenosynovitis, joint effusions, bursitis and soft tissue edema; also useful are T1W FS postcontrast sequences (add T1W precontrast FS sequence) to help identify active inflammation and distinguish simple fluid from synovitis in joints and tendon sheaths

## Imaging Findings

### Radiography

- In early disease, radiographs are often normal or show subtle findings of enthesitis and soft tissue swelling.
  - The sclerosis and bone production of enthesitis is seen in all forms of SpA, including PsA.
    - Common sites are calcaneal attachments of the plantar fascia and Achilles tendon, iliac crests, femoral trochanters, humeral tuberosities, and anterior patella.
    - Fluffy periostitis and significant sclerosis at attachments (Figure 33. 1) may help distinguish enthesitis from benign bone production or enthesopathy of DISH and chronic stress changes.

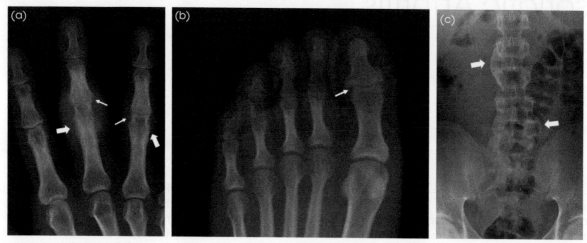

**Figure 33.1.** PsA in a 30-year-old woman. (*A*) An AP radiograph centered on the distal middle finger demonstrates periarticular soft tissue swelling with underlying erosions (*thin arrows*) and periostitis (*thick arrows*) most conspicuous at the third and fourth PIP joints. (*B*) An AP radiograph of the distal forefoot demonstrates erosion of the first IP joint (*thin arrow*) and overlying soft tissue swelling with multiple areas of periarticular fluffy bone proliferation. (*C*) An AP lumbar spine radiograph shows thick paravertebral ossifications (*thick arrows*) and bilateral sacroiliitis.

- MRI or US are more sensitive and specific in the detection of active inflammation.
- Soft tissue swelling most often of the interphalangeal (IP) joints of the fingers and toes may be subtle on radiography.
    - Diffuse digit swelling in dactylitis results in a *sausage digit* appearance.
- In more advanced disease, radiography may reveal erosions, hyperostosis, and fragmentation.
    - PsA is associated with both erosions and bone production and proliferative bone changes (Figures 33.1 and 33.2) unlike RA, which is primarily erosive and lacking bone production.
    - Characteristic radiographic findings are as follows:
        - Apparent small joint widening in the hands and feet

- *Mouse-ear* appearance from peripheral IP joint erosions and fluffy new bone production
- *Ivory* distal phalanx of a toe or finger with a sclerotic appearance and soft tissue swelling
- *Pencil-and-cup* deformity of the IP joints when the head of the proximal phalanx resembles a pencil tip and the base of the distal phalanx a cup (Figure 33.2)
- *Opera-glass hand* or *main en lorgnette* deformity caused by severe erosion and subluxation with digit-shortening relative to soft tissues
- Periostitis of the bones of hands, feet, and lower leg (Figure 33.1)
- Hand and foot involvement indistinguishable from OA, especially erosive OA, in approximately one-third of patients

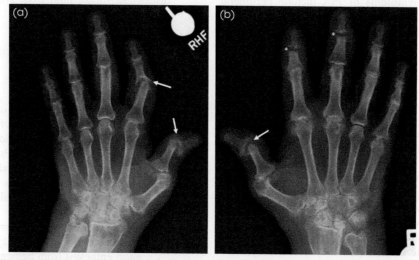

**Figure 33.2.** PsA in a 56-year-old woman with arthritis mutilans. AP radiographs of the (*A*) left and (*B*) right hands show pencil-in-cup deformities of the bilateral first IP and left second PIP joints (*thin arrows*) with both narrowing and widening (*B, asterisks*) of joint spaces, erosions, proliferative bone changes, and soft tissue swelling of the digits.

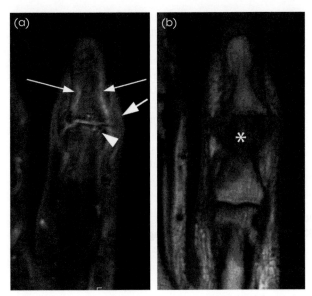

**Figure 33.3.** PsA of a finger on MRI. (*A*) Coronal T2W FS MR image of the index finger demonstrates soft tissue edema (*short arrow*) and periostitis (*thin arrows*) with interphalangeal joint cartilage destruction, central erosion (*arrowhead*), and periarticular BME. (*B*) T1W MR image shows marked bone marrow replacement in the region of BME consistent with osteitis (*asterisk*).

- Axial PsA
  - Bilateral and symmetrical sacroiliitis, but may be asymmetrical
    - Subchondral erosions and sclerosis predominantly on the iliac side of joint with eventual joint-space widening

- Ankylosis of the SI joints less common than in AS
- Spine disease uncommon in the absence of SI joint involvement
- Vertebral body bridging by asymmetric fluffy, thick, or curvilinear paravertebral ossifications (syndesmophytes)
- Relative facet joint sparing
- Complete bony bridging of the disc margins seen in approximately 25% of patients
  - May result in pseudoarthrosis formation across the disc space, called *discovertebral* or *Andersson lesions*
- Cervical vertebral, apophyseal, or spinous process erosions
- Imaging findings that may help distinguish axial PsA from AS and inflammatory bowel disease-related SpA (see Table 30.2 in Chapter 30, "Rheumatoid Arthritis")
  - Thicker, coarser-appearing syndesmophytes
  - Less common SI joint ankylosis than in AS
  - Comparatively less facet joint erosions or fusion

**Computed Tomography**
- Similar imaging findings to radiography with superior resolution in multiple planes
  - Gold standard for assessing bone structural damage
  - Primarily used to evaluate SI joint involvement
  - New bone formation seen on CT of psoriasis patients used to diagnose PsA
  - Active and chronic inflammation images not easily distinguished, unlike MRI
  - Because of high ionizing radiation dose, not frequently used

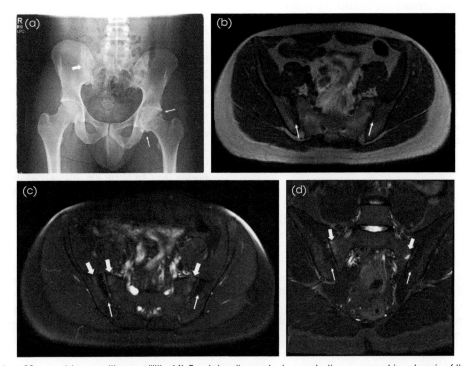

**Figure 33.4.** PsA in a 29-year-old man with sacroiliitis. (*A*) Frontal radiograph demonstrating asymmetric sclerosis of the right (*thick arrow*) greater than left SI joint. There is also asymmetric OA involving the left greater than right hip joint. Given the exuberant bone formation (*thin arrows*), this may be a manifestation of PsA. (*B*) Axial T1W, (*C*) axial T2W FS, and (*D*) coronal T2W FS images demonstrate asymmetric marginal sclerosis (*thin arrows*) and periarticular edema (*thick arrows*) involving the right greater than left SI joint.

### Magnetic Resonance Imaging

- MRI is useful to evaluate the inflammatory and structural changes of peripheral PsA.
  - BME is indicative of active inflammation or osteitis like in RA (Figures 33.3, 33.4).
    - PsA is seen at capsular attachments and entheses, whereas it is subchondral in OA.
    - BME is not predictive of future bone erosions, unlike in RA.
  - Bone erosions and proliferation can be detected on both T1W and fluid-sensitive sequences (Figures 33.3, 33.4).
  - BME and periostitis of DIP joints and distal phalanges often extends to the nail bed unlike other inflammatory arthritides (Figure 33.3).
  - In dactylitis, there is edema and enhancement of entheses, synovium, subcutaneous tissues, and tendon sheaths, especially the flexor tendons.
- MRI shows similar findings to the axial disease of other SpA, including:
  - Vertebral BME, enthesitis, fat infiltration, erosions, bone proliferation, ankylosis, and discovertebral lesions are seen.
  - Sacroiliitis is a sensitive indicator of early and active disease with BME and enhancement.
  - In more chronic disease, low bone signal intensity on all MRI sequences occurs from cortical sclerosis.
  - Involvement of the costotransverse, costovertebral, and facet joints is less common than in AS.

### Ultrasound

- US is a sensitive technique to evaluate the peripheral, but not the axial skeleton:
  - Similar findings are detected to MRI, but without sensitivity to bone marrow changes.
  - Discussed in more detail in Chapter 127, "Ultrasound for Rheumatologic Diseases."

## Treatment Options

- Disease-modifying antirheumatic drugs (DMARDs) are routinely prescribed in PsA despite lack of efficacy in published literature.
- Combination DMARD and tumor necrosis factor (TNF) inhibitor therapy is effective in moderate and severe disease.

## Key Points

- PsA is a challenging diagnosis because it often initially presents without psoriasis, lacks specific serologic markers, and resembles OA and other inflammatory arthropathies.
- PsA is associated with both bone erosions and proliferative bone changes.

- Radiography is the primary imaging modality for initial diagnosis and monitoring disease progression and treatment efficacy.
- Radiography is less sensitive in detecting the early changes of PsA and more sensitive in detecting the erosions and joint destruction of chronic disease.
- MRI is more sensitive than radiography in detecting early findings of PsA including BME and periarticular edema and enhancement.
- US is sensitive to early PsA changes of the peripheral joints, but limited by its inability to detect BME and evaluate the axial skeleton.

## Recommended Reading

Klecker RJ, Weissman BN. Imaging features of psoriatic arthritis and Reiter's syndrome. *Semin Musculoskelet Radiol.* 2003;7:115–26.

## References

1. Aleo E, Migone S, Prono V, Barbieri F, Garlaschi G, Cimmino MA. Imaging techniques in psoriatic arthritis: update 2012-2014 on current status and future prospects. *J Rheumatol Suppl.* 2015;93:53–56.
2. Barnas JL, Ritchlin CT. Etiology and pathogenesis of psoriatic arthritis. *Rheum Dis Clin North Am.* 2015;41:643–63.
3. Gladman DD. Clinical features and diagnostic considerations in psoriatic arthritis. *Rheum Dis Clin North Am.* 2015;41:569–79.
4. Helliwell PS, Ruderman EM. Natural history, prognosis, and socioeconomic aspects of psoriatic arthritis. *Rheum Dis Clin North Am.* 2015;41:581–91.
5. Jacobson JA, Girish G, Jiang Y, Sabb BJ. Radiographic evaluation of arthritis: degenerative joint disease and variations. *Radiology.* 2008;248:737–47.
6. Klecker RJ, Weissman BN. Imaging features of psoriatic arthritis and Reiter's syndrome. *Semin Musculoskelet Radiol.* 2003;7:115–26.
7. McHugh NJ. Early psoriatic arthritis. *Rheum Dis Clin North Am.* 2015;41:615–22.
8. Mease P. Psoriatic arthritis and spondyloarthritis assessment and management update. *Curr Opin Rheumatol.* 2013;25:287–96.
9. Ogdie A, Weiss P. The epidemiology of psoriatic arthritis. *Rheum Dis Clin North Am.* 2015;41:545–68.
10. Poggenborg RP, Bird P, Boonen A, et al. Pattern of bone erosion and bone proliferation in psoriatic arthritis hands: a high-resolution computed tomography and radiography follow-up study during adalimumab therapy. *Scand J Rheumatol.* 2014;43:202–208.
11. Soriano ER. Management of psoriatic arthritis: traditional disease-modifying rheumatic agents and targeted small molecules. *Rheum Dis Clin North Am.* 2015;41:711–22.
12. Spira D, Kotter I, Henes J, et al. MRI findings in psoriatic arthritis of the hands. *AJR Am J Roentgenol.* 2010;195:1187–93.

# CHAPTER 34

# Reactive Arthritis

Kevin B. Hoover

## Introduction

Reactive arthritis (ReA) is a postinfectious seronegative spondyloarthropathy (SpA), resulting in an inflammatory arthritis of the peripheral and axial skeleton. Lower extremity findings are more common than those of the upper extremity, which include enthesopathy, often fluffy periostitis and periarticular erosions. SI joint involvement is also common, which often initially has an asymmetric pattern that is indistinguishable from psoriatic arthritis (PsA). The arthritis and productive inflammatory changes of ReA may be identified using radiography, MRI and US.

## Pathophysiology and Clinical Findings

ReA is a SpA suspected in younger patients, especially those 25-30 years old, with inflammatory back pain, oligoarthritis, and extraarticular symptoms following infection, usually gastrointestinal (post-dysentery) or genitourinary (postvenereal). Usually the causative organism cannot be found because arthritis emerges after the infection has cleared. The term *Reiter syndrome* has been largely replaced by ReA, but when used, it is associated with the classic triad of large joint inflammation, urethritis in men and cervicitis in women, and eye inflammation, mainly uveitis or conjunctivitis. Incidence, prevalence, and percentage of patients developing disease after organism exposure varies between studies, but it is estimated that 5% of post-chlamydia patients develop ReA. The incidence in men is the same as women. By 6 months, 50% of patients are asymptomatic, and 20% develop chronic disease. Although the human leukocyte antigen (HLA)-B27 allele is not useful for the diagnosis of ReA, 20-25% of HLA-B27 positive patients develop chronic arthritis compared to 1-4% HLA-B27 negative patients.

The Assessment of SpA International Society (ASAS) classification criteria are useful in diagnosing ReA and distinguishing it from other SpA (see Chapter 32, "Ankylosing Spondylitis"). Axial skeletal involvement is found in up to 50% of patients with ReA in a similar pattern to the other spondyloarthropathies, especially PsA. Of those with chronic ReA, 40-60% have SI joint involvement, and radiography of the joints is often an initial diagnostic step. Approximately 30% of patients have spine involvement, and approximately 17% present with dactylitis, similar to PsA.

## Imaging Strategy

Peripheral disease is first evaluated by radiography, which is useful in identifying baseline structural damage and ongoing damage during treatment. US or MRI, however, are more useful to identify the enthesitis, tenosynovitis, and bursitis of active disease. Diagnosing axial ReA, such as the other SpA, starts with radiography of the SI joints. In young patients, those with short symptom duration, or nondiagnostic radiographs, MRI of the pelvis is valuable to evaluate the SI joints with a field of view large enough to include the hips, which are less commonly involved in ReA than AS or inflammatory bowel disease-related SpA. Axial and coronal T1W, fluid-sensitive (T2W FS or STIR) and postcontrast T1W FS sequences acquired with a body coil through the pelvis, and spine if symptomatic, are frequently sufficient. Coronal oblique sequences in the plane of the SI joints and sagittal images of the spine may be beneficial.

## Imaging Findings

### Radiography

- Radiography detects characteristic changes in an estimated 70% of patients with established disease, including the following:
  - Asymmetry
  - Lower extremity involvement more frequent and severe than the other SpA
    - Especially the small joints of the foot, in particular the PIP joints
    - Also the calcaneus, ankle, and knee
  - Soft tissue swelling resulting in a *sausage digit* radiographic appearance
  - Bony erosions with adjacent bony proliferation, periostitis, and fluffy enthesopathy (Figure 34.1*A, B*)
    - *Pencil in cup* and *ivory phalanx* deformities, such as in PsA
    - Erosions especially subjacent to inflamed bursae or tendon sheaths (Figure 34.1*A, B*)
      - May be present in the wrist
      - In 25-50% patients near the Achilles attachment on the calcaneus
- SI joint involvement may be unilateral or asymmetric with iliac erosions and apparent joint space widening (Figure 34.1*C*).
  - Early disease is difficult to detect on radiography.
  - It eventually becomes more symmetric, proliferative, and sclerotic.
  - It may result in ankylosis with continued active disease, but less commonly than in PsA.

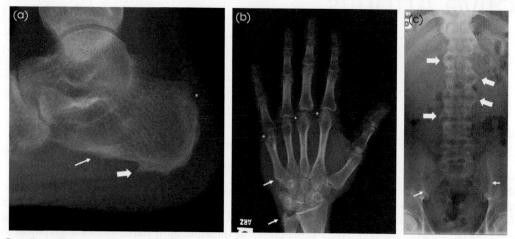

**Figure 34.1.** Reactive arthritis in a 35-year-old man following venereal (gonorrhea) disease. (*A*) Lateral radiograph of the calcaneus demonstrates plantar enthesopathy with possible adjacent erosion dorsally (*thick arrow*), plantar sclerosis (*thin arrow*), and subtle periostitis and erosion of the proximal tuberosity (*asterisk*) in the expected location of the retrocalcaneal bursa. (*B*) An AP hand radiograph shows erosions of the metacarpal heads (*asterisks*) and fluffy periostitis and erosion of the ulna aspect of the fifth metacarpal base and the ulnar styloid (*thin arrows*). (*C*) Frontal radiograph of the lumbar spine shows coarse paravertebral ossifications (bulky syndesmophytes) involving the T12-L3 levels (*thick arrows*) and bilateral SI joint erosive changes with subjacent sclerosis consistent with sacroiliitis (*thin arrows*).

- Spine involvement tends to spare anterior spine and cervical spine.
  - Asymmetric or unilateral bulky, comma-shaped paravertebral ossifications are more common than thinner syndesmophytes (Figure 34.1C).
  - Less commonly, sclerotic vertebral "shiny corners" similar to AS can be seen, because of enthesitis at the vertebral attachments of the intervertebral disc
  - Imaging findings are compared to other inflammatory arthropathies in Table 30.2 (see Chapter 30, "Rheumatoid Arthritis").

**Magnetic Resonance Imaging**
- MRI is the gold standard for the diagnosis of axial disease in ReA and the other SpA.

- MRI detects active inflammation without ionizing radiation.
  - Fluid-sensitive sequences show BME, joint fluid, and the joint space widening (Figure 34.2B, C).
  - Subtle erosions may be difficult to detect compared to CT.
  - Marginal vertebral body edema and enhancement may predict new syndesmophytes.
  - A decrease from baseline MRI in periarticular enhancement on postcontrast T1W FS imaging correlates with a response to treatment, even with persistent underlying BME.
- Characteristic peripheral skeleton findings (Figure 34.2) are as follows:
  - Periarticular edema
  - Erosions

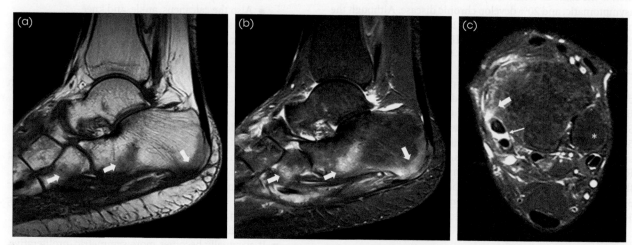

**Figure 34.2.** Reactive arthritis on MRI of the ankle in a 30-year-old patient following venereal (chlamydia) disease. (*A*) Sagittal T1W MR image shows areas of low T1 signal within the calcaneus corresponding to ligament and tendon entheseal attachments (*arrows*). (*B*) Sagittal STIR MR image shows more extensive BME in the same regions (*thick arrows*). (*C*) Axial T2W FS MR image shows high signal distended tibialis posterior and flexor digitorum tendon sheaths in keeping with tenosynovitis (*thin arrow*) with adjacent tibial BME (*thick arrow*). A small synovial-fluid complex is also seen in the peroneal tendon sheath posterior to the lateral malleolus (*asterisk*).

- Joint inflammation with effusion
- Bursitis
- Tendonitis and tenosynovitis

## Computed Tomography

- CT is more sensitive than radiography, but less sensitive than MRI in detecting the inflammatory changes of ReA.
- CT detects erosions and sclerosis in the complex anatomy of the SI joint and vertebral body shiny corners.
- Active inflammation is not well assessed, and sclerosis may be present in both active and inactive PsA.
- CT is not optimal for following younger patients because of radiation dose.

## Ultrasound

- US is most useful in identifying active inflammation in the peripheral skeleton rather than the SI joints.
- Enthesitis, erosions and tenosynovitis may be detected, especially in the feet.

## Treatment Options

- NSAIDs are standard treatment for articular symptoms, but are not proven to reduce radiographic progression.
- Steroid joint injections are useful for short-term relief.
- If symptoms are more severe, a disease-modifying antirheumatic drug (DMARD) can be used.
- Sulfasalazine treatment is the best-studied DMARD for ReA, and especially effective if given within the first 3 months of symptoms.
- Unlike the other SpA, tumor necrosis factor (TNF) inhibitors may not be appropriate especially in those with chronic chlamydia-induced venereal ReA.

## Key Points

- Radiographs of the SI joints are the standard first imaging test in diagnosis of ReA, then MRI if nondiagnostic.
- ReA imaging may be identical to other SpA, especially PsA.
- In addition to infectious disease history and younger age, asymmetry of symptoms, imaging findings, and lower extremity involvement are characteristic of ReA.

## Recommended Reading

Klecker RJ, Weissman BN. Imaging features of psoriatic arthritis and Reiter's syndrome. *Semin Musculoskelet Radiol.* 2003; 7:115–26.

## References

1. Amrami KK. Imaging of the seronegative spondyloarthopathies. *Radiol Clin North Am.* 2012;50:841–54.
2. Carter JD, Hudson AP. Reactive arthritis: clinical aspects and medical management. *Rheum Dis Clin North Am.* 2009;35:21–44.
3. Jacobson JA, Girish G, Jiang Y, Sabb BJ. Radiographic evaluation of arthritis: degenerative joint disease and variations. *Radiology.* 2008;248:737–47.
4. Klecker RJ, Weissman BN. Imaging features of psoriatic arthritis and Reiter's syndrome. *Semin Musculoskelet Radiol.* 2003;7:115–26.
5. Mandl P, Navarro-Compan V, Terslev L, et al. EULAR recommendations for the use of imaging in the diagnosis and management of spondyloarthritis in clinical practice. *Ann Rheum Dis.* 2015;74:1327–39.
6. Mathew AJ, Ravindran V. Infections and arthritis. *Best Pract Res Clin Rheumatol.* 2014;28:935–59.
7. Selmi C, Gershwin ME. Diagnosis and classification of reactive arthritis. *Autoimmun Rev.* 2014;13:546–49.

# 2

# Metabolic Arthropathies

Josephina A. Vossen

Crystal-induced arthritides (CIA) (Table 35.1) are a group of arthritides caused by deposition of crystals in articular and periarticular tissues. The most commonly seen crystalline deposition diseases include deposition of monosodium urate (MSU) resulting in gout, CPPD disease, and deposition of basic calcium phosphate (BCP) resulting in calcific periarthritis. Synovitis and soft tissue inflammation can develop in response to crystal deposition.

**Table 35.1. Clinical and Imaging Features of the Different Crystalline Arthropathies**

|  | GOUT | CPPD | HEMOCHROMATOSIS | ALKAPTONURIA |
|---|---|---|---|---|
| Age at onset | >50 y | >60 y | <50 y | >30 y |
| Chondrocalcinosis | Rare | Common | Very common | Rare |
| MCP involvement | Common | Common | Very common | Late stage |
| Synovitis |  | Episodic | Occasional |  |
| Marginal erosions | Very common | Very rare | Very rare | Rare |
| First site of disease | Frequently first MTP joint | Knee, symphysis pubis, and TFCC of the wrist | Second and third MCP joints | Spine, knee |

Abbreviations: CPPD, calcium pyrophosphate deposition; MCP, metacarpophalangeal; MTP, metatarsophalangeal; TFCC, triangular fibrocartilage complex.

# CHAPTER 35

# Gout

Josephina A. Vossen

## Introduction

Gout represents a group of metabolic conditions with deposition of monosodium urate (MSU) crystals in soft tissues and joints. These crystals form in the presence of elevated serum urate levels. Gout is considered to have 4 phases, characterized by asymptomatic hyperuricemia, recurrent attacks of acute arthritis, intercritical gout, and chronic tophaceous gout.

## Pathophysiology and Clinical Findings

Acute gout is usually monoarticular and characterized by an inflammatory response with influx of neutrophils into synovial fluid and membranes. Tophaceous gout is a chronic granulomatous tissue reaction with masslike deposits of MSU that can occur in synovium, cartilage, tendon, ligament, bone, and bursa.

Gout is the most common crystalline type of arthropathy, with a current prevalence in the United States of 3.9%. The disease has a male-to-female ratio of 8:1, and the classic presentation is a painful, red, hot, and swollen first MTP joint (podagra) in a middle-aged man. Acute gout can resemble cellulitis with swelling, warmth, erythema, and desquamation over the inflamed area.

Serum uric acid measurement and 24-hour urinary uric acid evaluation can be obtained. Hyperuricemia is defined as a serum urate concentration greater than 7 mg/dL. Daily uric acid excretion of more than 700 mg/day is considered overproduction. However, hyperuricemia is not diagnostic of gout.

The gold standard for gout diagnosis is joint aspiration and synovial fluid analysis with confirmation of needle-shaped negatively birefringent MSU crystals by polarized light microscopy. Imaging offers the potential for noninvasive diagnosis of gout.

## Imaging Strategy

Radiography is generally used in the initial evaluation of gouty arthritis to determine the presence of erosions and tophi. US and dual-energy CT (DECT) show particular promise in the assessment of gout, both for diagnosis and monitoring. DECT acquisitions at 80 kV and 140 kV are used for the evaluation of the affected site. MRI is not commonly used for the diagnosis or management of patients with gout.

## Imaging Features

### Radiography
- Acute gout
  - Nonspecific appearance
  - Asymmetric swelling and subcortical cystlike changes without erosions
- Chronic gout
  - Asymmetric erosions in a periarticular distribution
  - Strong predilection for distal joints, especially in the lower extremities
  - Bone erosions with *punched-out* appearance, sclerotic borders and *overhanging edges* (Figure 35.1)
  - Normal mineralization with relative preservation of the joint spaces until late in the disease
  - Soft tissue tophi appearing as nodular soft tissue masses with amorphous increased density or patchy calcification in periarticular and peritendinous locations (Figure 35.1)
    - *Lumpy, bumpy* appearance
  - Bursal involvement with the olecranon bursa most commonly involved

### Computed Tomography
- CT can visualize both bone erosions and tophi.
- DECT allows for differentiation of the chemical composition of the scanned tissue by analyzing the difference in attenuation of a material imaged simultaneously using 2 different photon energy levels (kVp) (Figure 35.2).
  - Post processing of the images enables color coding of the uric acid deposits.
  - DECT is superior for precipitated MSU crystals (tophi) compared to MSU dissolved in joint or bursal fluid.

### Ultrasound
- Hyperechoic linear foci overlying the surface of the anechoic joint cartilage (*double contour* sign; see Figure 127.12).
  - Believed to represent MSU crystals overlying articular cartilage
- MSU crystals in synovial fluid or tissue producing small bright echoes (*snowstorm* appearance)
- Detailed description of findings in Chapter 127, "Ultrasound for Rheumatologic Diseases"

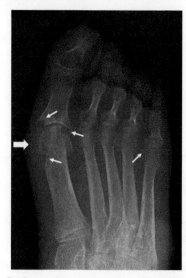

**Magnetic Resonance Imaging**
- Usually not used for primary diagnosis
- Can demonstrate synovitis, bone erosions, and/or tophi
- Characteristic appearance of tophi
    - Usually isointense to slightly hypointense to muscle on short echo time (TE) images
    - Variable T2W signal, possibly caused by differences in internal calcium concentrations
    - Relatively homogeneous postcontrast enhancement

---

**Treatment Options**
- Diet restrictions; avoiding high-purine foods such as organ meat, smelt, sardines, and mussels
- NSAIDs
- Urate-lowering agents (such as allopurinol)
- Colchicine
- Systemic and intraarticular glucocorticoids
- Biologic agents that inhibit the action of interleukin-1 beta

**Figure 35.1.** Radiographic appearance of gout. Dorsoplantar foot radiograph shows large marginal, punched-out juxtaarticular erosions with overhanging edges at the first MTP joint (*thin arrows*) with adjacent soft tissue swelling containing radiopaque foci consistent with tophaceous gout (*thick arrow*). Erosion of the fifth metatarsal head is also evident (*thin arrow*). The joint spaces are relatively preserved.

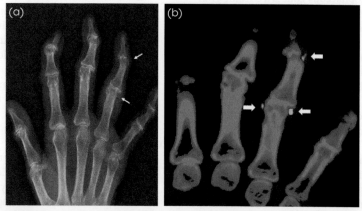

**Figure 35.2.** Gout in a 92-year-old woman. (*A*) A PA radiograph of the right hand demonstrates fourth-digit DIP and PIP periarticular and juxtaarticular erosions with adjacent soft tissue swelling (*thin arrows*). Note associated extensive degenerative changes of the interphalangeal joints. (*B*) DECT image of the same hand with color coding reveals green masses (*thick arrows*) at the fourth PIP and DIP joints, consistent with gout tophi. Given the distribution in the juxtaarticular soft tissues, rather than intraarticular, a joint aspiration might not have detected crystals.

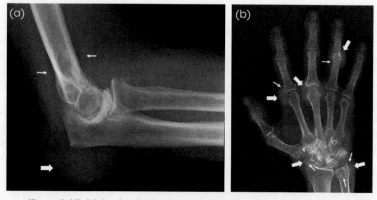

**Figure 35.3.** A 72-year-old man with gout. (*A*) A lateral radiograph of the right elbow demonstrates hyperdense soft tissue overlying the olecranon with swelling (*thick arrow*) consistent with tophaceous bursitis. There is also an elbow joint effusion with elevation of the anterior and posterior fat pads (*thin arrows*). (*B*) A PA radiograph of the right hand demonstrates hyperdense soft tissue tophi with associated swelling (*thick arrows*) and areas of juxtaarticular and periarticular erosion and intraosseous tophus (distal ulna) (*thin arrows*).

## Key Points

- Swelling and joint effusion in acute gout
- Spares the joint space until late in the disease
- Bone erosions with *punched-out* appearance, sclerotic borders and *overhanging edges* and soft tissue tophi resulting in a *lumpy, bumpy* appearance

## Recommended Reading

Chowalloor P, Siew T, Keen H. Imaging in gout: a review of the recent developments. *Ther Adv Musculoskelet Dis.* 2014;6(4):131–43.

## References

1. Taljanovic MS, Melville DM, Gimber LH, et al. High-resolution US of rheumatologic diseases. *Radiographics.* 2015;35(7):2026–48.
2. Desai MA, Peterson JJ, Garner HW, Kransdorf MJ. Clinical utility of dual-energy CT for evaluation of tophaceous gout. *Radiographics.* 2011;31(5):1365–75.

# CHAPTER 36

# Calcium Pyrophosphate Dihydrate Deposition Disease

Josephina A. Vossen

## Introduction

CPPD disease is characterized by intraarticular and periarticular deposition of calcium pyrophosphate crystals. This can result in an acute CPPD-induced synovitis with goutlike symptoms, formerly known as pseudogout, as well as structural joint inflammation and damage, commonly named *pyrophosphate arthropathy*. The pathologically or radiographically evident calcification in the hyaline or fibrocartilage is termed *chondrocalcinosis*. CPPD can be hereditary or sporadic.

## Pathophysiology and Clinical Findings

CPPD is a common crystalline type of arthropathy in the United States. CPPD disease is most often seen in middle-aged and elderly patients, and has no major sex predominance. The most specific test for CPPD diagnosis is visualization of weakly positively birefringent rhomboid calcium pyrophosphate dihydrate crystals in synovial fluid aspirate from an affected joint. Approximately 7% of the adult population has articular CPPD crystal deposits at the age of 70.

## Imaging Strategy

Conventional radiography is the main diagnostic tool for CPPD. Ultrasound can be useful to evaluate multiple joints, tendon and ligament calcification. Associated tissue inflammation can be seen as increased vascularity on color and power Doppler imaging. Dual-energy CT (DECT) is currently only used in the research setting.

## Imaging Features

### Radiography

- Chondrocalcinosis is most commonly seen at the knee, symphysis pubis, and triangular fibrocartilage of the wrist (Figures 36.1 through 36.3).
- Arthropathy resembling OA is seen, but with a distinctive distribution:
  - The patellofemoral compartment of the knee (Figure 36.2B) is preferentially involved.
  - At the wrist and hand, CPPD affects the triangular fibrocartilage, radiocarpal joint, and predominantly second and third MCP joints with hooked osteophytes. The appearance is similar to that seen in patients with hemochromatosis.
  - At the ankle and foot, CPPD commonly affects the first MTP joint involvement and talonavicular joint.
- Calcification surrounding the dens is seen, also referred to as *crowned dens*, which increases the risk for fractures.
- Calcification involving the enthesis and adjacent tendons (ie, proximal hamstrings) is seen.

### Computed Tomography

- Both chondrocalcinosis and tendon and ligament calcification can be visualized.

### Ultrasound

- CPPD deposits are hyperechoic and present in different patterns:
  - Thin hyperechoic bands, within the hyaline cartilage, fibrocartilage, tendons, and ligaments
  - A punctate pattern, composed of several small hyperechoic foci within the hyaline cartilage, fibrocartilage, tendons, and ligaments
  - Homogeneous hyperechoic nodular or oval deposits, frequently mobile, localized in bursae and articular recesses
- Findings are described in more detail in Chapter 127, "Ultrasound for Rheumatologic Diseases."

### Magnetic Resonance Imaging

- Because MRI findings are often nonspecific, this modality is not used for primary diagnosis.
- On knee MRI, the meniscus may appear enlarged with loss of normal homogeneously dark signal.
  - Meniscal fluid signal may result from calcium, which can mimic a meniscal tear.
- Dark appearance of the cartilage is seen on all sequences.

## Treatment Options

- Joint lavage with intraarticular steroid injection can be used.
- NSAIDs and low-dose oral colchicine are used when multiple joints are involved.

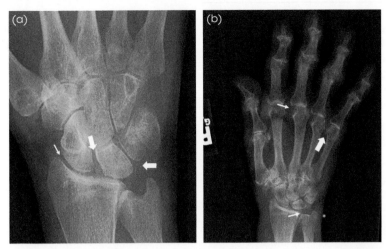

**Figure 36.1.** CPPD with chondrocalcinosis and arthropathy. (*A*) PA radiograph of the wrist demonstrates chondrocalcinosis of the scapholunate and lunotriquetral ligaments (*thick arrows*) and the hyaline cartilage (*thin arrow*). (*B*) PA radiograph of the hand demonstrates extensive chondrocalcinosis of the triangular fibrocartilage of the wrist and the MCP joints (*thin arrows*) with calcifications near the extensor carpi ulnar tendon with ulnar styloid erosions (*asterisk*). Diffuse OA is also evident most severe in the interphalangeal (IP) joints with fusion of the fourth PIP joint. A small hooklike osteophyte is seen at the distal fifth metacarpal (*thick arrow*).

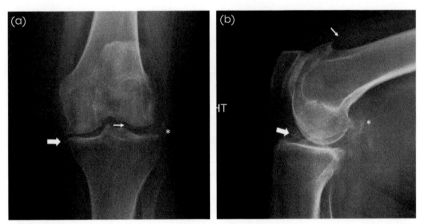

**Figure 36.2.** CPPD in a 69-year-old woman with chronic knee pain. (*A*) AP radiograph of the knee reveals meniscal fibrocartilage calcification (*thick arrow*, extruded meniscus) and hyaline cartilage calcification (*thin arrow*). There is also lateral capsular calcification (*asterisk*). (*B*) Lateral radiograph of the knee depicts meniscal calcification (*thick arrow*) and posterior capsular calcification (*asterisk*). There is advanced patellofemoral compartment OA with a suprapatellar joint effusion (*thin arrow*).

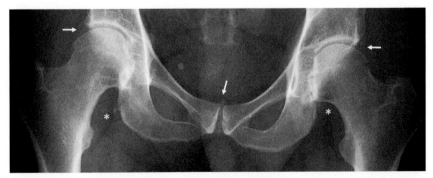

**Figure 36.3.** CPPD with chondrocalcinosis and soft tissue calcifications of the pelvis and hips. AP radiograph of the lower pelvis and hips demonstrates calcification of the acetabular labral fibrocartilage bilaterally and the symphysis pubis cartilage (*thin arrows*). Subtle calcifications near the right ischial tuberosity at the hamstring tendon origin and at the left hip joint are also visible (*asterisks*).

## Key Points

- Most commonly seen as chondrocalcinosis of the knee, symphysis pubis and triangular fibrocartilage of the wrist
- Normal bone mineralization
- Arthropathy in uncommon distribution, including the patellofemoral, radiocarpal, or talonavicular joints

## Recommended Reading

Miksanek J, Rosenthal A. Imaging of calcium pyrophosphate deposition disease. *Curr Rheumatol Rep*. 2015;17(3). doi:10.1007/s11926-015-0496-1.

# CHAPTER 37

# Calcium Hydroxyapatite Deposition Disease

Josephina A. Vossen

## Introduction

Hydroxyapatite (HA) crystal deposition disease (HADD) is clinically manifested by localized pain, swelling, and tenderness about the affected joint along with variable limitation of joint motion. However, not all patients with HADD are symptomatic. Radiographs may show calcifications of varying size and shape in the periarticular tendons, bursae, and joint capsule. The disease may be mono- or polyarticular in distribution. When intraarticular, HA crystals can cause joint destruction.

## Pathophysiology and Clinical Findings

Basic calcium phosphate crystals encompass several types of crystals, including carbonate apatite, octacalcium phosphate, and whitlockite crystals. HA is thought to be the most abundant crystal within this group. Calcium crystals can deposit in tendons, bursae, muscles, and periarticular structures. Crystal deposition may cause calcific tendinosis, periarthritis, bursitis, and bone erosion. The natural progression of calcific tendinosis has been described in 4 phases: precalcific, formative, resorptive, and postcalcific. The inflammatory resorptive phase is the most symptomatic phase, characterized by the appearance of leukocytes, lymphocytes, and giant cells forming calcium granulomas. Rupture of crystals into the shoulder joint can cause a secondary rapid destructive arthropathy known as *Milwaukee syndrome*. Crystal deposition occurring in the upper oblique fibers of the longus colli can result in severe pain with swallowing.

Calcium crystal deposition is asymptomatic in two-thirds of cases and often identified as an incidental radiographic finding. Most cases are seen between the ages of 30 and 60, with equal sex distribution. Depositions are often monoarticular and the shoulder (supraspinatus and infraspinatus tendons), hip (gluteal tendons), and wrist are the most commonly affected joints. HADD frequently has a distinct radiographic appearance; however, exact diagnosis of the disease is made by direct identification of calcium phosphate crystals collected from the affected tissue using electron microscopy.

## Imaging Strategy

Radiography is the main diagnostic tool for HADD. CT scanning is not commonly used but can provide additional information about location of the crystal deposition. US can be useful in evaluation and image-guided treatment of calcific tendinitis. MRI is not usually acquired, however, routine imaging of joints can detect low signal calcium deposits and sometimes adjacent soft tissue or bone inflammation, when symptomatic.

## Imaging Findings

### Radiography

- Presence of calcifications in the periarticular soft tissues
- Early crystal deposits are cloudy, amorphous densities, without trabeculation or cortication.
- More mature deposits are denser, homogeneous, and well circumscribed (Figure 37.1A).
- The shoulder is the most commonly involved joint, with calcifications often occurring near the insertion of supraspinatus tendon on the greater tuberosity (Figure 37.1A).
- Erosion of bone adjacent to calcification at the insertion site of the tendons can be visualized.
- Radiographs of Milwaukee shoulder syndrome show the following (Figure 37.2):
  - Disuse osteoporosis, bony destruction, malalignment.
  - Intra- and periarticular calcifications.
  - Loss of the normal acromiohumeral interval caused by superior subluxation of the deformed humeral head is often present because of chronic rotator cuff tendon rupture.
  - The syndrome can resemble a neuropathic joint.

### Computed Tomography

- Calcific tendinitis may be detected in a similar distribution to radiographs with great sensitivity (Figure 37.3).
- Subtle osseous erosions can be shown.

### Ultrasound

- Tendon calcification is seen as a hyperechoic focus, with or without posterior acoustic shadowing (Figure 37.1C).
  - In the formative phase, the calcifications are often hard deposits. On US, the superficial border is sharply marginated, and there is relatively clean posterior acoustic shadowing.

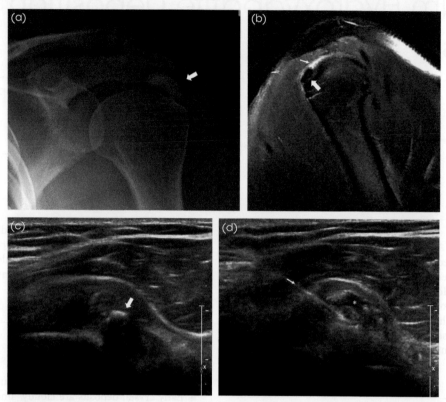

**Figure 37.1.** HADD of the rotator cuff in a 51-year-old woman with acutely increased shoulder pain. (*A*) AP shoulder radiograph shows large, dense, but amorphous (*toothpaste*) calcification without trabeculation in the supraspinatus tendon (*thick arrow*). (*B*) A sagittal T2W MR image demonstrates low signal HA within the anterior supraspinatus at the footplate (*thick arrow*) with adjacent subacromial-subdeltoid bursitis (*thin arrow*). (*C*) US shows a calcification with posterior acoustic shadowing at the rotator cuff footplate (*thick arrow*). (*D*) US image obtained during lavage shows a needle (*thin arrow*) extending to the calcification with decreased acoustic shadowing and fluid distension of the calcification (*asterisk*). Residual calcifications often persist immediately after barbotage with a delay until partial or complete resolution.

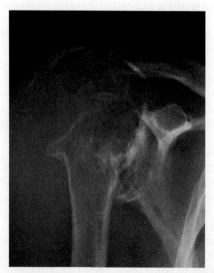

**Figure 37.2.** Milwaukee shoulder in a 77-year-old woman with worsening chronic shoulder pain. An AP shoulder radiograph reveals partial collapse of the humeral head, with cephalic migration of the proximal humerus, joint-space narrowing and erosion of the distal clavicle, acromion, humeral head, and glenoid. Soft tissue swelling with amorphous calcifications are observed.

- In the resorptive phase, the lesions become soft and appear on US as more amorphous and ill-defined. There is decreased posterior acoustic shadowing.
- Increased vascularity seen on color and power Doppler imaging may indicate active inflammation.
- US is useful in evaluation of calcific tendinitis, particularly in the shoulder, and to guide treatment (Figure 37.1*D*).

**Magnetic Resonance Imaging**
- Calcifications appear as focal areas of low signal on all pulse sequences, typically located in or near the tendon in an adjacent bursa (Figure 37.1*B*).
- Fluid-sensitive MR images can show surrounding areas of increased signal intensity compatible with edema.
- Enhancement on T1W FS postcontrast imaging often indicates active inflammation.
- Calcifications may erode into the adjacent bone and mimic infection or tumor.

**Treatment Options**
- Usually conservative management with analgesics, NSAIDs, and physical therapy
- Image-guided needle aspiration and/or lavage of the calcification, often performed with US, also called

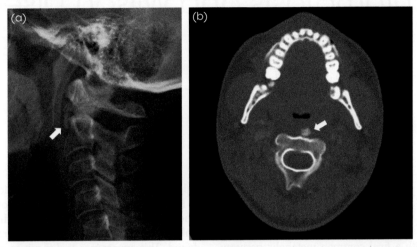

**Figure 37.3.** HADD of the Longus colli tendon in the neck of a 53-year-old woman with retropharyngeal pain. (*A*) Lateral radiograph of cervical spine reveals calcification anterior to C1-C2 (*thick arrow*). (*B*) An axial CT image shows this calcification located in the left longus colli muscle (*thick arrow*).

*barbotage* (Figure 37.1*D*; see Chapter 128, "Ultrasound-Guided Musculoskeletal Procedures")
- Local steroid injections
- Surgical evacuation of the calcification if needed
- Newer approaches, including extracorporeal shock wave therapy

- Calcific tendinitis, calcific bursitis, and sometimes osseous erosions can be seen.
- HADD most frequently involves the supraspinatus tendon and/or subacromial-subdeltoid bursa of the shoulder, followed by the gluteal tendons of the hip.
- The adjacent joint is usually normal.

## Key Points
- Calcium crystal deposition usually involves the tendons or bursa around a single joint.

## Recommended Reading
Siegal DS, Wu JS, Newman JS, Del Cura JL, Hochman MG. Calcific tendinitis: a pictorial review. *Can Assoc Radiol J.* 2009;60(5):263–72.

# CHAPTER 38

# Hemochromatosis and Wilson Disease

Josephina A. Vossen

## Introduction

### Hemochromatosis

Hemochromatosis is an iron-storage disease with genetic heterogeneity, but with a final common metabolic pathway resulting in an increase in intestinal absorption and excessive deposition of iron in parenchymal cells. This eventually results in tissue damage and organ failure. Primary hemochromatosis is an autosomal recessive inherited disorder. Secondary hemochromatosis results from increased intake and accumulation of iron of known cause, such as alcoholic cirrhosis, multiple blood transfusions, and chronic hemolytic anemia.

### Wilson Disease

Wilson disease, also known as *hepatolenticular degeneration*, is a rare autosomal recessive inherited disorder of copper metabolism that is characterized by excessive deposition of copper in the liver, brain, kidneys and other tissues.

## Pathophysiology and Clinical Findings

### Hemochromatosis

Excessive storage of iron in the liver, skin, pancreas, heart, bones, joints, and testes may result in abdominal pain, weakness, lethargy, and weight loss. Additional symptoms include cirrhosis, increase in skin hyperpigmentation, diabetes mellitus, congestive heart failure, and/or arrhythmias, arthritis, and hypogonadism. Hemochromatosis is more common in men than women. The diagnosis of hemochromatosis is based on clinical symptoms and elevated transferrin-iron saturation (45% or higher) and serum ferritin concentration above the upper limit of normal (ie, >300 ng/mL in men and >200 ng/mL in women). Definitive diagnosis is made by liver biopsy to document histologic evidence of iron overload.

Arthropathy develops in up to 80% of patients with primary hemochromatosis and appears to be related to the deposition of small amounts of iron or hemosiderin within the affected joints. The arthropathy is progressive and irreversible. Men tend to become symptomatic between ages 40 and 60. Women develop symptoms approximately 15 years after the date of last menstrual cycle. Symptoms include mild joint pain, swelling, and stiffness, initially affecting the MCP joints. Involvement is usually symmetric. At a later stage, arthropathy of the large joints, such as the wrists, elbows, hips, knees, and shoulders, is common. Acute arthralgia may be secondary to calcium pyrophosphate crystal deposition. Chondrocalcinosis is found in 30-50% of patients, most often in the wrists and knee joints. In the large joints, including the hip, knee and ankle joints, typical signs of degenerative arthritis can be found. This appearance is difficult to differentiate from that of CPPD arthropathy. Osteopenia and osteoporosis are also common with a prevalence of 25-35%.

### Wilson disease

Wilson disease can manifest as hepatic, neurologic, hematologic, or psychiatric disturbances, or a combination of these, in individuals ranging in age from 3 years to older than 60 years. The prevalence of Wilson disease is estimated at 1 in 30,000 in most populations. A pathognomonic sign is the presence of greenish brown Kayser-Fleischer rings at the corneal limbus. Wilson disease is often fatal if not recognized and treated.

The arthropathy of Wilson disease is a degenerative process that resembles OA. Symptomatic joint disease occurs in 20-50% of patients and usually arises late in the disease, frequently after 20 years. The arthropathy generally involves the spine and large appendicular joints, such as knees, wrists, and hips.

## Imaging Strategy

Radiography is the standard method for detecting structural changes associated with hemochromatosis arthropathy and Wilson disease. CT can further depict osseous changes. US and MRI are not routinely used in diagnosis.

## Imaging Findings

### Hemochromatosis
### Radiography

- Hemochromatosis typically affects the hands and wrists with predominant involvement of the MCP joints, especially the second and third MCP joints.
  - Uniform joint-space narrowing, subchondral cysts, and formation of hooklike osteophytes at the radial aspect of the metacarpal heads (Figure 38.1) is seen.
  - Joint involvement in the hands is strongly symmetric.
  - Wrist involvement includes the carpometacarpal (CMC) and midcarpal compartments.
- Chondrocalcinosis is found in 30-50% of the patients, most often seen in the wrist and knee joints.

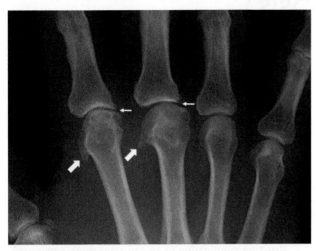

**Figure 38.1.** Hemochromatosis in a 29-year-old man. A coned-down, frontal radiograph of the hand shows narrowing of the MCP joints (*thin arrows*) with hooked osteophytes at the radial aspect of the second and third metacarpal heads (*thick arrows*). Bone mineralization remains normal.

- In the large joints, including the hip, knee, shoulder, and ankle joints, typical signs of OA can be found.
- Osteopenia can be detected.

**Computed Tomography**
- Joint-space narrowing, subchondral cysts, hook-like osteophytes, and chondrocalcinosis can be visualized.
- Increased radiodensity of the liver is often seen.

**Wilson Disease**
**Radiography**
- Osseous changes related to Wilson disease include osteoporosis and osteomalacia (rickets, fractures, deformities).
- Additional findings include the following:
  - Subchondral bone fragmentation
  - OA advanced for chronologic age
  - Calcification of the joint capsule and tendon insertion, subarticular cysts, and osteochondritis
- Arthropathy is often seen in the hand, wrist, foot, hip, shoulder, elbow, and knee.

**Computed Tomography**
- Can visualize OA and calcifications

## Treatment Options

**Hemochromatosis**
- Therapeutic phlebotomy throughout the patient's life to keep the ferritin level between 25 and 50 ng/mL
- Dietary modifications, including the restriction of medicinal iron, mineral supplements, excess vitamin C, and uncooked seafood

**Wilson Disease**
- The mainstay of therapy for Wilson disease is lifelong use of copper chelating agents (eg, D-penicillamine, trientine).
- Dietary modifications, including the restriction of substances high in copper (liver, brain, chocolate, mushrooms, shellfish, and nuts)
- Transjugular intrahepatic shunting (TIPS) is reserved for recurrent or uncontrolled variceal bleeding unresponsive to standard conservative measures.
- Orthotopic liver transplantation is curative.

## Key Points
**Hemochromatosis**
- Iron-storage disease
- Typically affecting the second and third MCP joints
- Hooklike osteophytes at the metacarpal heads
- Symmetric joint involvement

**Wilson Disease**
- Autosomal recessive inherited disorder of copper metabolism
- Osteoporosis, osteomalacia, and OA advanced for chronologic age

## References
1. Adamson TC, Resnik CS, Guerra J, Vint VC, Weisman MH, Resnick D. Hand and wrist arthropathies of hemochromatosis and calcium pyrophosphate deposition disease: distinct radiographic features. *Radiology.* 1983;147:377–81.
2. Aksoy M, Çamli N, Dinçol K, Erdem Ş, Akgün T. Osseous changes in Wilson's disease. *Radiology.* 1972;102:505–10.
3. Cavallino R, Grossman H. Wilson's disease presenting with rickets. *Radiology.* 1968;90:493–94.
4. Mindelzun R, Elkin M, Scheinberg IH, Sternlieb I. Skeletal changes in Wilson's disease. *Radiology.* 1970;94:127–32.
5. Morais SA, du Preez HE, Akhtar MR, Cross S, Isenberg DA. Musculoskeletal complications of haematological disease. *Rheumatology (Oxford).* 2016;55:968–81.

# CHAPTER 39

# Alkaptonuria (Ochronosis)

Josephina A. Vossen

## Introduction

Alkaptonuria is an autosomal recessive inherited disorder caused by the deficiency of homogentisate 1,2-dioxygenase enzyme in the degradative pathway of aromatic amino acids such as phenylalanine and tyrosine. This results in accumulation of excess homogentisic acid and its oxide (named *alkapton*) in different intra- and extraarticular structures.

## Pathophysiology and Clinical Findings

Homogentisic acid accumulation causes damage to connective tissues. Pathologic brown-black pigmentation of connective tissues, such as cartilage, skin, and sclerae, is seen in patients with alkaptonuria, and termed *ochronosis*. Excreted homogentisic acid in the urine results in a characteristic dark brown or black color when the urine is alkalinized and oxidized. Other manifestations of alkaptonuria include renal, urethral, and prostatic calculi, arthropathy, and valvular disease.

Alkaptonuria is rare with a prevalence of less than 1:250,000 in most populations. Specific diagnosis of the disease is made by demonstrating homogentisic acid in urine using gas chromatography-mass spectrometry analysis. Early involvement of the intervertebral discs at the thoracic and lumbar levels is very common, occurring in approximately 50% of affected individuals. Typically, clinical symptoms of ochronotic arthropathy begin around the age of 30-40 with low back pain and stiffness. Premature arthritis in the large joints develops after the third decade and usually affects the large weight-bearing joints, mainly the hips, knees, and later the shoulders.

## Imaging Strategy

Radiography is the standard method for detecting changes associated with alkaptonuria. CT can aid in the detection of intervertebral disc calcification.

## Imaging Findings

### Radiography

- Radiographs of the spine show loss of intervertebral height, disc calcification, and vacuum phenomenon accompanied by vertebral body fusion, predominantly in the lumbar spine (Figure 39.1*A*).
- SI joints are spared.

- Radiographs of the large joints (predominantly hips, knees, and shoulders) may show joint-space narrowing, subchondral cystlike changes, and osteophyte formation.
- Ochronotic arthropathy can be aggressive, with rapid destruction culminating in an end-stage disease requiring arthroplasty.
- Tendon ochronotic pigment deposition can cause tendinopathy, rupture, and calcific tendinosis.

### Computed Tomography

- May be used to evaluate non-musculoskeletal systems (eg, nephrolithiasis) (Figure 39.1*B*)
- Can visualize intervertebral disc calcification and large joint OA

### Magnetic Resonance Imaging

- Not routinely used in ochronotic arthropathy
- Can show uniform loss of intervertebral disc height with central intradiscal low T1 and T2 signal, corresponding to intervertebral disc calcification

## Treatment Options

- Pain control and physical therapy
- Surgical treatment including lumbar fusion and joint replacement

## Key Points

- Rare autosomal recessive metabolic disease
- Deposition of homogentisic acid
- Ochronotic arthropathy is the articular manifestation of alkaptonuria
- Progressive degenerative arthropathy mainly affecting the spine and knee joints
- Calcification of intervertebral discs

## Recommended Reading

Ventura-Ríos L, Hernández-Díaz C, Gutiérrez-Pérez L, et al. Ochronotic arthropathy as a paradigm of metabolically induced degenerative joint disease. A case-based review. *Clin Rheumatol.* 2016;35(5):1389–95.

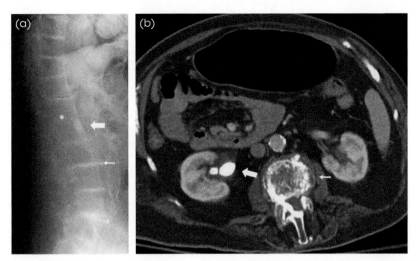

**Figure 39.1.** Alkaptonuria with nephrolithiasis and spinal ochronosis. (*A*) A lateral radiograph of the lumbar spine shows advanced degenerative changes with extensive disc height loss and disc calcification involving the visualized thoracic and lumbar spines (*thin arrow* at representative level). Vertebral fusion at the L1-L2 level is evident (*asterisk*). Note a calculus overlying the L2 vertebra (*thick arrow*). (*B*) Axial CT image in soft tissue window shows large calculi in the right renal collecting system (*thick arrow*) and degenerative changes of the lumbar spine (*thin arrow*).

# Connective Tissue Diseases

# CHAPTER 40

# Systemic Lupus Erythematosus

Josephina A. Vossen

## Introduction

Systemic lupus erythematosus (SLE) is a chronic multisystem autoimmune disease that follows a relapsing and remitting course. The clinical manifestations are highly variable, ranging from indolent to fulminant. SLE likely has a multifactorial etiology involving genetic susceptibility, age, hormonal factors, and environmental triggers. Imaging of the musculoskeletal system is used primarily to evaluate the potentially painful sequelae of SLE.

## Pathophysiology and Clinical Findings

In the U.S. population, the overall incidence of SLE is 5.1 per 100,000 per year and the prevalence is 52.2 per 100,000. Incidence and prevalence are substantially higher in individuals of African American or African Caribbean descent. More than 90% of cases of SLE occur in women, frequently starting at childbearing age. The initial diagnosis is based on history and physical examination, along with selected laboratory tests. Antinuclear antibody (ANA) testing and other specific antibodies such as dsDNA, anti-Sm, Ro/SSA, La/SSB, and U1 ribonucleoprotein (RNP) form the mainstay of serologic testing.

Arthritis is one of the most common manifestations of SLE, occurring in approximately 90-95% of the patients, and involvement of 2 or more peripheral joints constitutes one of the American College of Rheumatology criteria for the classification of the disease. Joint involvement in SLE is often characterized by arthralgia. Joint tenderness, swelling, and effusions can be transient, migratory, and reversible. Persistent arthropathy, preferentially involving the small joints, is often associated with tenosynovitis and swelling. A subset of patients have a chronic, reducible nonerosive deforming arthropathy (called *Jaccoud arthropathy*) caused by inflammation of the joint capsule and tendons and subsequent fibrosis. A minority of patients have an arthropathy with clinical and imaging findings similar to RA (called *rhupus*). Additional findings in SLE include tendon weakening, tendon rupture, and soft tissue calcification. Approximately 10-13% of patients present with tenosynovitis, including epicondylitis, rotator cuff tendinopathy, Achilles tendinopathy, posterior tibial tendinopathy, and plantar fasciitis. ON occurs in up to 40% of patients with SLE, likely caused by a combination of steroid treatment and vasculitis. Although myalgia is a common symptom, true myositis is less common.

## Imaging Strategy

The initial imaging evaluation of SLE arthropathy is with radiographs of the symptomatic joints, usually the hands. Modalities such as US and MRI are used particularly when assessing the degree of synovitis or destructive change, which will influence diagnosis and management. MRI of the hands should use a small field of view (FOV) with a dedicated hand and wrist coil and T1W and fluid-sensitive imaging. MRI of the lower extremities using large FOV and a body coil may be useful in patients with proximal muscle weakness to detect myositis.

## Imaging Findings

### Radiography

- Articular deformities, especially of the hand including
  - Ulnar deviation at the MCP joints (Figure 40.1)
  - Swan neck deformity (hyperextension at the PIP and flexion at the DIP joints)
  - Z-deformity of the thumb (flexion at the first MCP and hyperextension of the interphalangeal [IP] joint; Figure 40.1)
  - Often without articular erosions
  - Deformities are often reducible, best seen on the oblique Nørgaard or *ball-catcher* view (Figure 40.1)
- Additional findings include
  - Soft tissue swelling
  - Periarticular osteopenia
  - Acral sclerosis (sclerosis of the tufts of the distal phalanges)
  - Acroosteolysis (resorption of the tufts of the distal phalanges)
  - Calcifications (calcinosis) of the subcutaneous and periarticular tissues
  - ON of the femoral head, humeral head, femoral condyle, tibial plateau, and talus (most common sites)
  - Discussed in more detail in Chapter 115, "Osteonecroses and Osteochondroses"

### Computed Tomography

- Acral sclerosis, acroosteolysis, and ON easily detected

### Ultrasound

- Sensitive modality for detecting effusions, synovial hypertrophy, tenosynovitis, and infrequent bone erosions

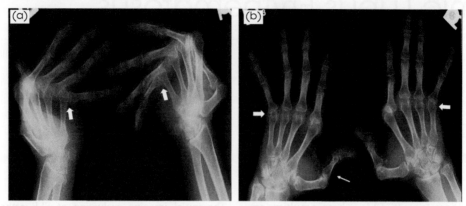

**Figure 40.1.** SLE in a 57-year-old woman with Jaccoud arthropathy. PA (*A*) and ball-catcher/Nørgaard (*B*) radiographs of the hand demonstrate the classic reduction of ulnar deviations and joint subluxations at the MCP joints (*thick arrows*) between both views without periarticular erosions. Z-deformity of the thumb is evident (*thin arrow*).

## Magnetic Resonance Imaging

- Most sensitive and specific modality for detecting ON
- Highly sensitive and specific for detecting synovitis, tenosynovitis, and rare erosions
- Myositis (uncommon) involving proximal muscles of limbs
  - Resembles, and may be masked by, steroid-induced myopathy
  - Characteristic signal changes
    - Increased signal on T1W images compared to normal skeletal muscle
    - T2W FS images accentuating areas of high signal inflammation surrounding low signal fat
    - Inflamed muscle enhancement detected on postcontrast T1W FS imaging relative to normal or atrophic muscle

## Treatment Options

- Given the episodic and limited nature of the arthritis flares, intermittent salicylates and NSAIDs are frequently used.
- Low-dose glucocorticoids have been a mainstay in the management of SLE.
- Disease-modifying antirheumatic drugs (DMARDs) are used preventively to reduce the incidence of flares and the progress of the disease. DMARDs commonly in use are antimalarials such as hydroxychloroquine and immunosuppressants (eg, methotrexate and azathioprine).

## Key Points

- SLE is an autoimmune connective tissue disorder with multisystem involvement.
- Arthropathy results in reducible deformities especially of the hands.
- Subtypes include Jaccoud arthropathy (a chronic nonerosive reducible arthropathy) and rhupus (arthropathy with findings similar to RA).
- Complications include ON, tendon rupture, calcinosis, and myopathy.

## Recommended Reading

Grossman JM. Lupus arthritis. *Best Pract Res Clin Rheumatol.* 2009;23(4):495–506.

## References

1. Goh YP, Naidoo P, Ngian GS. Imaging of systemic lupus erythematosus. Part II: gastrointestinal, renal, and musculoskeletal manifestations. *Clin Radiol.* 2013;68:192–202.
2. Grossman JM. Lupus arthritis. *Best Pract Res Clin Rheumatol.* 2009;23:495–506.
3. Kolasinski SL, Chi AS, Lopez-Garib AJ. Current perspectives on imaging for systemic lupus erythematosus, systemic sclerosis, and dermatomyositis/polymyositis. *Rheum Dis Clin North Am.* 2016;42:711–32.
4. Lalani TA, Kanne JP, Hatfield GA, Chen P. Imaging findings in systemic lupus erythematosus. *Radiographics.* 2004;24:1069–86.

# CHAPTER 41

# Scleroderma

Josephina A. Vossen

## Introduction

Scleroderma, or systemic sclerosis (SSc), is a systemic connective tissue disease characterized by vascular, autoimmune, and fibrotic changes affecting the skin and internal organs, with an overproduction of collagen. Although not used in the classification of SSc, imaging of the musculoskeletal system is commonly obtained because of symptomatic involvement. Imaging findings overlap with other connective tissue diseases and erosive arthritides.

## Pathophysiology and Clinical Findings

The pathogenesis of SSc is complex and remains incompletely understood. SSc is a heterogeneous disease with subsets of presentation, including limited skin involvement (limited cutaneous SSc), diffuse skin sclerosis with severe, progressive internal organ involvement (diffuse cutaneous SSc), and internal organ involvement only (SSc sine scleroderma). The diagnosis of SSc, and classification by the American College of Rheumatology, is based on clinical criteria including skin changes, central and peripheral vascular manifestations, including Raynaud phenomenon, interstitial lung disease, and the detection of specific autoantibodies. Characteristic, bilateral skin thickening of the fingers, or sclerodactyly, extending proximal to the MCP joints is diagnostic. Involvement of the tips of digits (acral) with Raynaud phenomenon, sclerodactyly, soft tissue thinning, pitting, and acroosteolysis is likely secondary to vascular disease.

SSc affects women more than men and frequently becomes apparent in the fourth to sixth decades of life. The prognosis of the disease mainly depends on the amount of visceral involvement, however, musculoskeletal involvement is a major cause of pain and disability. Joint involvement has been reported to occur in up to 96% of SSc patients. An overlap syndrome of SSc with RA has been described in 5% of patients. The earliest manifestations of diffuse cutaneous SSc are swelling of the hands, arthralgia, myalgia, and fatigue. Joint pain, immobility, and contractures develop because of fibrosis around tendons and other periarticular structures. Contractures can be associated with palpable and/or audible deep tendon friction rubs. Muscle involvement results in myopathy or less frequently, in myositis. Frank inflammatory arthritis is less common.

## Imaging Strategy

Radiographs of symptomatic body parts, most commonly the hands, are the standard initial imaging assessment of the musculoskeletal system. The radiographic detection of calcinosis and acral bone and soft tissue findings help in narrowing the differential diagnosis. Gray-scale and Doppler ultrasound is sometimes used for evaluating tendon and articular abnormalities. MRI using dedicated extremity coils with small FOV imaging, T1WI and fluid-sensitive sequences are used primarily in evaluating symptomatic soft tissues, especially of the hands. MRI of the lower extremities using large FOV and a body coil is useful to evaluate patients with hip girdle weakness and pain to detect myositis and chronic myopathy.

## Imaging Features

### Radiography

- Hands are routinely imaged and may show the following:
    - Acral soft tissue resorption
    - Acroosteolysis with distal phalanx tuft resorption, sharpening and eventual loss (Figure 41.1A).
    - Subcutaneous, juxtaarticular, and capsular calcinosis (Figure 41.1A, B)
    - Joint-space narrowing
    - Periarticular osteopenia
    - Flexion contracture
- Erosive arthritis is less common:
    - MCP, DIP and, especially, first carpometacarpal (CMC) involvement (Figure 41.1A)
    - Resembles distribution of psoriatic arthritis and erosive osteoarthritis
    - Concurrent RA (overlap syndrome) with an erosive pattern more typical of RA, and commonly involves the wrist, MCP, and PIP joints

### Computed Tomography

- CT is not routinely acquired for evaluation of the musculoskeletal system.
- Findings are similar to radiography (Figure 41.1C).
- Symptomatic spinal and paraspinal calcifications can be localized.

### Magnetic Resonance Imaging

- Hand imaging can demonstrate inflammatory changes even without clinical evidence of synovitis, including the following:
    - Fluid signal surrounding the tendon (tenosynovitis) and within the joint (synovitis) with a thickened sheath or joint capsule from fibrosis
    - Periarticular erosions
    - BME

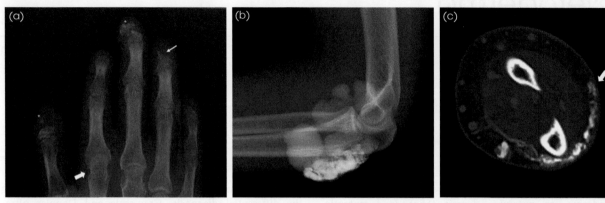

**Figure 41.1.** Scleroderma in a 40-year-old, rheumatoid factor (RF) negative man. (*A*) PA radiograph of the hand shows acroosteolysis of all the distal phalangeal tufts (*thin arrow*) and predominantly distal soft tissue calcinosis (*asterisk*). Second to third MCP joint marginal erosions are also evident resembling RA (*thick arrow*). (*B*) Lateral elbow radiograph demonstrates extensive periarticular calcinosis extending to the extensor skin surface. (*C*) Axial CT image of the forearm without contrast shows extensor surface, subcutaneous calcifications (*thick arrow*).

- Proximal lower extremity MRI may detect muscle changes indistinguishable from dermatomyositis:
  - Myositis shows increased signal on fluid-sensitive imaging (T2W FS, STIR) and subcutaneous edema.
  - High signal on T1WI from fatty atrophy is seen in chronic myositis or myopathy.
- Low signal soft tissue calcifications may be demonstrated.
- Focal and diffuse skin involvement can initially show localized high skin signal on fluid-sensitive sequences with subsequent replacement by dark, fibrous tissue.

### Ultrasound
- Sensitive in detection of the following:
  - Hypoechoic subcutaneous tissue thickening
  - Subcutaneous calcifications
    - Especially palmar fingertips and areas of chronic stress (eg, overlying olecranon)
    - With or without posterior acoustic shadowing
  - Tenosynovitis, more common in advanced disease
    - Fibrous deposits with tendon sheath thickening
    - Inflammatory hypervascular tenosynovitis (may indicate an overlap syndrome)
    - Associated with carpal tunnel syndrome
  - Decreased blood flow on Doppler US in fibrotic tissue

### Treatment Options
- Recommendations for treatment are targeted to specific symptoms
- Calcium channel blockers for milder cases and prostanoids in more severe cases of Raynaud phenomenon
- Acetaminophen and NSAIDs for arthralgias
- Steroids, methotrexate, or azathioprine for myopathy and myositis
- Steroid injections for tenosynovitis and carpal tunnel syndrome

### Key Points
- Scleroderma is a rare, autoimmune disease.
- Vascular, autoimmune, and fibrotic changes affect the skin, musculoskeletal system, and other internal organs.
- Musculoskeletal system involvement is common, especially involving the acral soft tissues and osseous structures.
- Bone and joint changes can often be identified on hand radiographs.
- US and MRI are commonly used to evaluate tenosynovitis and myopathy.

### Recommended Reading
Chapin R, Hant FN. Imaging of scleroderma. *Rheum Dis Clin North Am*. 2013;39:515–46.

### References
1. Boutry N, Hachulla E, Zanetti-Musielak C, Morel M, Demondion X, Cotten A. Imaging features of musculo-skeletal involvement in systemic sclerosis. *Eur Radiol*. 2007;17:1172–80.
2. Chapin R, Hant FN. Imaging of scleroderma. *Rheum Dis Clin North Am*. 2013;39:515–46.
3. Kolasinski SL, Chi AS, Lopez-Garib AJ. Current perspectives on imaging for systemic lupus erythematosus, systemic sclerosis, and dermatomyositis/polymyositis. *Rheum Dis Clin North Am*. 2016;42:711–32.
4. Lorand V, Czirjak L, Minier T. Musculoskeletal involvement in systemic sclerosis. *Presse Med*. 2014;43:e315–28.

# CHAPTER 42

# Polymyositis and Dermatomyositis

Josephina A. Vossen

## Introduction

Polymyositis and dermatomyositis are idiopathic inflammatory myopathies (IIMs). IIMs represent a heterogeneous group of muscle diseases, which, based on distinct clinical-pathological features comprise the following main subtypes: dermatomyositis, polymyositis, necrotizing myopathy, and inclusion body myositis. Most imaging modalities are sensitive in detecting soft tissue calcifications present in some subtypes. Definitive diagnosis is based on muscle biopsy. Treatment is primarily by immune suppression.

## Pathophysiology and Clinical Findings

This group of disorders is characterized by muscle inflammation, proximal muscle weakness, and elevated muscle enzymes. Diagnosis is based on clinical examination, muscle enzyme laboratory values, electromyography (EMG), and muscle biopsy. Both polymyositis and dermatomyositis are thought to be rare autoimmune disorders with a reported incidence between 3 and 6 cases per 100,000 in the United States. There is a female predominance. Dermatomyositis affects both children and adults, whereas polymyositis generally occurs after the second decade of life. The most common clinical signs are subacute reduction of the muscular strength in the proximal muscles, joint contractures, and muscular atrophy during the late stages of the disease. Arthralgia with multiple tender and/or swollen joints is common in more chronic disease with an estimated frequency of 33-53% of IIM patients. The symmetric hand involvement and distribution can be similar to rheumatoid arthritis.

### Polymyositis

Polymyositis is characterized by muscular manifestations and results in chronic muscle degeneration and atrophy. Polymyositis symmetrically affects the proximal muscles of the lower and upper extremities, especially the vastus lateralis, vastus intermedius, triceps, and brachioradialis muscles.

### Dermatomyositis

Dermatomyositis is primarily characterized by cutaneous signs, such as photosensitive erythematous rash, which can accompany or precede symmetric proximal muscle weakness. An acute inflammatory myopathy with relative sparing of the rectus femoris and biceps femoris muscles is seen. Soft tissue calcifications are most common in patients who develop dermatomyositis as a child, and seen in approximately 70% of pediatric patients, but are also seen in an estimated 11-20% of those who develop the disease in adulthood.

## Imaging Strategy

Radiography is often obtained during the initial disease evaluation and might demonstrate soft tissue calcifications. Both grayscale US and MRI have high sensitivity in depicting muscle involvement. MRI of the proximal lower extremities using body coils with large FOV is often performed, especially to guide muscle biopsy.

## Imaging Features

### Radiography

- Radiography is most useful in detecting soft tissue calcifications (calcinosis) (Figure 42.1A).
  - Calcifications are often linear or sheetlike in dermatomyositis, but may be nodular or reticular
- Nonspecific soft tissue swelling and/or edema may be detected.
- Chronic disease is associated with arthritis similar to SLE:
  - Nonerosive subluxations, especially of the first interphalangeal (IP) joint of the hand associated with the clinical finding of *floppy thumb*

### Computed Tomography

- Detects soft tissue findings with greater sensitivity than radiography
  - Muscle fatty atrophy from chronic myositis with decreased tissue attenuation and muscle size
  - Nonspecific soft tissue swelling and/or edema of subcutaneous tissues
  - Soft tissue calcinosis including involvement of the skin (calcinosis cutis)

### Ultrasound

- Able to evaluate the extent and location of muscle inflammation
- Chronic muscle degeneration, fatty infiltration, and atrophy associated with hyperechoic muscle and/or decreased muscle size and obscured fascia
  - Often more severe in polymyositis than dermatomyositis

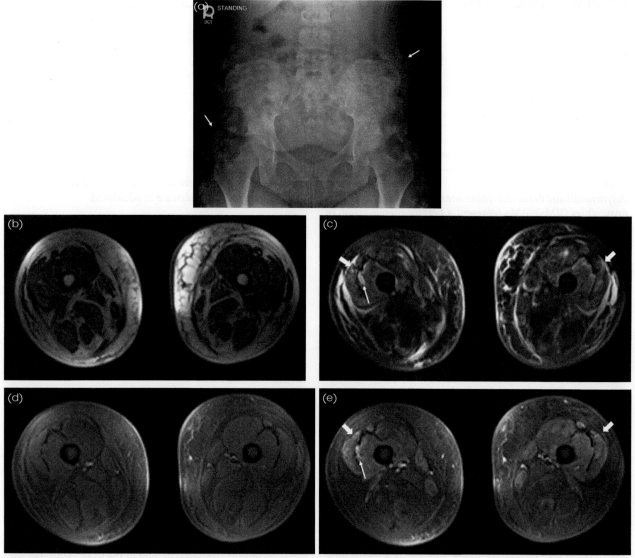

**Figure 42.1.** Dermatomyositis in a 27-year-old woman. (*A*) Frontal radiograph of the pelvis demonstrates diffuse, nodular, and reticular soft tissue calcifications with normal underlying bones and joints (*thin arrows*). (*B-E*) MRI images obtained 6 years prior to the radiograph. (*B*) Axial T1W image shows scattered low signal reticular subcutaneous soft tissue stranding and superficial fascial thickening with diffuse mild muscular atrophy. Areas of discrete (*thin arrow*) and more diffuse (*thick arrows*) intramuscular fluid signal on the T2W FS image (*C*) demonstrate enhancement comparing T1W FS image precontrast (*D*) and postcontrast (*E*) consistent with active myositis, which is most conspicuous among the anterior vastus muscles. Diffuse subcutaneous reticular and superficial fascial fluid signal and fluid signal dissecting through the deep intermuscular tissue planes (*C*) does not enhance (*E*), consistent with edema. This appearance of dermatomyositis on this MRI study is indistinguishable from polymyositis. No soft tissue calcifications were present at the time of MRI.

- Acute inflammatory myopathy associated with hypoechoic muscle caused by tissue edema often with a slight increase in muscle size

### Magnetic Resonance Imaging
- MRI is the most sensitive modality to visualize muscle edema, inflammation, and fasciitis.
  - Increased signal is seen on fluid-sensitive sequences (STIR or T2W with FS) (Figure 42.1*C*).
  - T1W images depict loss of normal striated muscle architecture and fatty atrophy in chronic disease.
  - Intravenous contrast does not increase examination sensitivity and is not routinely administered.

- MRI can distinguish subcutaneous edema from active inflammation (Figure 42.1*D*).
- MRI is the optimal technique to identify actively inflamed muscle, guiding muscle biopsy and avoiding sampling error.

### Treatment
- Exercise to maintain muscle strength and functionality
- Corticosteroids
- Immunosuppressive therapy, such as methotrexate, azathioprine, or mycophenolate mofetil

- Monoclonal antibodies, such as infliximab, etanercept, or rituximab
- Intravenous immunoglobulin (IVIG)

## Key Points
- Polymyositis and dermatomyositis are inflammatory myopathies.
- MRI is the most useful imaging modality to detect acute muscle inflammation and to guide biopsy.
- Radiographs and CT may detect calcinosis.

## Recommended Reading
Kuo GP, Carrino JA. Skeletal muscle imaging and inflammatory myopathies. *Curr Opin Rheumatol*. 2007;19:530–35.

## References
1. Day J, Patel S, Limaye V. The role of magnetic resonance imaging techniques in evaluation and management of the idiopathic inflammatory myopathies. *Semin Arthritis Rheum*. 2016;46(5):642–49.
2. Klein M, Mann H, Plestilova L, et al. Arthritis in idiopathic inflammatory myopathy: clinical features and autoantibody associations. *J Rheumatol*. 2014;41:1133–39.
3. Kolasinski SL, Chi AS, Lopez-Garib AJ. Current perspectives on imaging for systemic lupus erythematosus, systemic sclerosis, and dermatomyositis/polymyositis. *Rheum Dis Clin North Am*. 2016;42:711–32.
4. Kuo GP, Carrino JA. Skeletal muscle imaging and inflammatory myopathies. *Curr Opin Rheumatol*. 2007;19:530–35.
5. Walker UA. Imaging tools for the clinical assessment of idiopathic inflammatory myositis. *Curr Opin Rheumatol*. 2008;20:656–61.

# CHAPTER 43

# Mixed Connective Tissue Disease

Josephina A. Vossen

## Introduction

Mixed connective tissue disease (MCTD) is a generalized connective tissue disorder that includes clinical features commonly seen in SLE, scleroderma (systemic sclerosis [SSc]), and polymyositis. Arthritis and myositis are common features that may not be evident on radiographs, but may be apparent on US and MRI. Although diagnosis is based on clinical findings and laboratory values, imaging is useful to narrow the differential diagnosis.

## Pathophysiology and Clinical Findings

MCTD is rare entity, which is more common in women than in men. The peak incidence of MCTD is around 40 years. In the early stages, symptoms are nonspecific and include arthralgia, *puffy* hands, low-grade fever, and low-grade polymyositis. Characteristic clinical symptoms of MCTD eventually emerge, including Raynaud phenomenon, hand edema, arthritis, and prominent synovitis. The distinctive overlap features of SLE, SSc, and polymyositis commonly appear sequentially over time. Arthritis is a common feature with MCTD, most often presenting as polyarticular, nonerosive, and nondeforming. A broader spectrum of joint disease may occur, however, including a deforming arthritis and/or an erosive arthritis. Patients with MCTD are likely to develop interstitial lung disease and pulmonary hypertension. There is a relative low prevalence of serious renal and neurologic involvement. The presence of high titers of a distinctive autoantibody, called *anti-U1 ribonucleoprotein* (RNP), is required for the diagnosis of MCTD. Patients often have a positive antinuclear antibody (ANA) with a high titer speckled pattern.

## Imaging Strategy

Radiographs are standard in the initial evaluation of symptomatic extremities, often obtained of both hands. The detection of soft tissue calcifications is helpful in narrowing the differential diagnosis to a connective tissue disease. In cases where the presence of active disease is in question, US can evaluate multiple joints, especially the small joints of the hands. MRI is also useful to evaluate arthritis using a dedicated extremity coil. MRI is especially sensitive in the detection of myositis. Often the pelvis and proximal lower extremities are imaged to detect myositis using a body coil and large FOV. MRI findings can be used to guide muscle biopsy when needed.

## Imaging Features

### Radiography
- Can visualize the dermatologic findings of MCTD including digit and hand swelling, acrosclerosis, and calcinosis cutis (Figure 43.1)
- May demonstrate features of SSc, SLE, and RA to variable extents
- Features characteristic of SSc
  - Soft tissue atrophy
  - Soft tissue calcifications (calcinosis)
  - Distal phalanx tuft resorption (acroosteolysis)
  - DIP joint erosions
- Features characteristic of SLE
  - Nonerosive joint deformity (Jaccoud arthropathy)
  - ON
- Features characteristic of inflammatory arthritis resembling RA
  - Juxtaarticular osteoporosis
  - Joint-space narrowing
  - Marginal erosions
- Preferential ankylosis of the capitate to the trapezoid

### Ultrasound
- Rapid evaluation of multiple small joints of the hands can detect the extent and location of periarticular erosions.
- US can demonstrate myositis:
  - Discussed in Chapter 42, "Polymyositis and Dermatomyositis"

### Magnetic Resonance Imaging
- Detects features of polymyositis, especially in the proximal lower extremities
  - Muscle edema with T2 hyperintense fluid signal
  - Fasciitis with hyperintense signal best visualized on fluid-sensitive sequences (STIR, T2W FS)
  - Fatty replacement with increased T1 signal intensity
  - Muscle atrophy
  - Discussed in Chapter 42, "Polymyositis and Dermatomyositis"
- Highly sensitive in detection of early findings in inflammatory arthritis
  - BME
  - Erosions
  - Effusion with synovitis (Figure 43.1B, C)

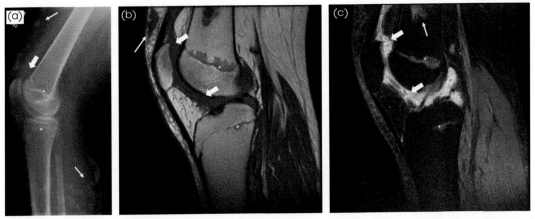

**Figure 43.1.** MCTD in a 25-year-old woman. (*A*) Lateral knee radiograph demonstrates soft tissue calcifications (*thin arrows*) and a small joint effusion (*thick arrow*) with delayed skeletally maturity with open physes (*asterisks*). (*B, C*) Sagittal T1W (*B*) and T2W (*C*) MR images show a joint effusion with rice bodies consistent with a chronic synovitis (*thick arrows*). Note open physes (*asterisks*). Soft tissue calcifications of intermediate to low signal intensity are also evident anterior to the quadriceps tendon (*B*) (*thin arrow*). Focal ON is partially visualized in the distal femur (*C, thin arrow*) likely related to chronic corticosteroid use.

## Treatment Options

- Targeted medical therapy to specific organ involvement and extent of disease activity
- NSAIDs and hydroxychloroquine for arthritis and arthralgia
- Low-dose oral corticosteroids or low-dose methotrexate is reserved for more refractory synovitis

## Key Points

- MCTD is a generalized connective tissue disorder that includes clinical features commonly seen in SLE, SSc, and polymyositis.
- Patients have high titers of anti-U1 RNP.
- Characteristic clinical symptoms include Raynaud phenomenon, swollen *puffy* hands, and arthritis.
- Imaging may detect evidence of nonerosive or erosive arthritis, calcinosis, and myositis.

## References

1. Gunnarsson R, Hetlevik SO, Lilleby V, Molberg O. Mixed connective tissue disease. *Best Pract Res Clin Rheumatol.* 2016;30:95–11.
2. Halla JT, Hardin JG. Clinical features of the arthritis of mixed connective tissue disease. *Arthritis Rheum.* 1978;21:497–503.
3. Pope JE. Other manifestations of mixed connective tissue disease. *Rheum Dis Clin North Am.* 2005;31:519–33, vii.
4. Schulze M, Kotter I, Ernemann U, et al. MRI findings in inflammatory muscle diseases and their noninflammatory mimics. *AJR Am J Roentgenol.* 2009;192:1708–16.
5. Udoff EJ, Genant HK, Kozin F, Ginsberg M. Mixed connective tissue disease: the spectrum of radiographic manifestations. *Radiology.* 1977;124:613–18.

# Degenerative Arthritis

# CHAPTER 44

# Osteoarthritis of the Upper and Lower Extremity Joints

Daichi Hayashi, Ali Guermazi, and Frank W. Roemer

## Introduction

OA is a major public health problem that primarily affects the elderly worldwide. For example almost 10% of the U.S. population suffers from symptomatic knee OA by age 60. Overall, the annual health care expenditures related to OA have been estimated at $186 billion. The most commonly involved joints are the knee and hip, the small joints of the fingers, the base of the thumb, and the great toe. Conventional radiography remains the gold standard imaging technique for the evaluation of OA. MRI can assess all structures of the joint, including the assessment of cartilage morphology and biochemical composition, which may be a target for intervention and marker of progression.

## Pathophysiology and Clinical Findings

OA, or degenerative joint disease, is considered a disease of the whole joint, involving osseous and nonosseous articular and periarticular tissues. Cartilage destruction is a central feature of OA that causes pain, swelling, and problems with joint movement. Other features of OA result from progressive joint destruction, including bone spurs called *osteophytes* caused by bone and ligament damage, subchondral sclerosis, or eburnation, which is a bone response to altered mechanics, and bone remodeling, including cystlike changes, caused by the absence of cartilage and *bone on bone* articulation. In general, patients suffer from limited range of motion or stiffness after inactivity that improves after movement, mild swelling around a joint, and pain that is worse after activity or toward the end of the day.

## Imaging Strategy

Radiography remains the gold standard imaging technique for the evaluation of OA in clinical practice. MRI can assess all joint structures, including cartilage, meniscus, ligaments, muscle, subchondral bone marrow, and synovium and is able to visualize the joint in a 3D fashion without the projectional limitations of radiography. MRI may be useful clinically in evaluating the cause of knee pain, especially in patients with subtle radiographic findings. Moreover, MRI enables the assessment of 3D cartilage morphology and biochemical composition that can guide treatment. Fluid-sensitive FSE sequences (eg, T2W or PD) with fat saturation are useful for identifying focal meniscal fibrocartilage

and hyaline cartilage defects and areas of focal BME, also termed *bone marrow lesions*. Utility of MRI is not limited for OA in the knee joint, but also other joints, including hands, shoulders, hips, and the spine. Diagnostic US is not a commonly used imaging tool for OA but can be used to evaluate synovitis, which may also be seen in OA. CT is excellent for detailed evaluation of the changes of OA such as subchondral bone sclerosis, subchondral cystlike changes, and osteophytes.

## Imaging Findings

### Radiography

Radiography is inexpensive and the most commonly used modality for imaging of OA and detects (Figure 44.1) the following:

- Osteophytes, which are diagnostic of OA on radiographs
- Subchondral sclerosis and cystlike changes
- Joint-space narrowing (JSN) the most commonly used criterion for the assessment of structural OA progression
  - Complete joint-space loss is a structural indicator for arthroplasty.
  - JSN is affected by changes in joint positioning on radiographs, including weight bearing.
- Joint remodeling and intraarticular ossific bodies
- Joint alignment that may affect disease progression in specific joint locations

The severity of radiographic OA can be assessed qualitatively as none, mild, moderate, and severe based on the number and severity of findings.

- The Kellgren and Lawrence (K&L) grading system is widely used to describe the structural severity of OA (Table 44.1).

Tomosynthesis is a radiographic technique that generates cross-sectional images from a single pass of the x-ray tube (Figure 44.2):

- More sensitive than radiography in the detection of osteophytes and subchondral cystlike changes

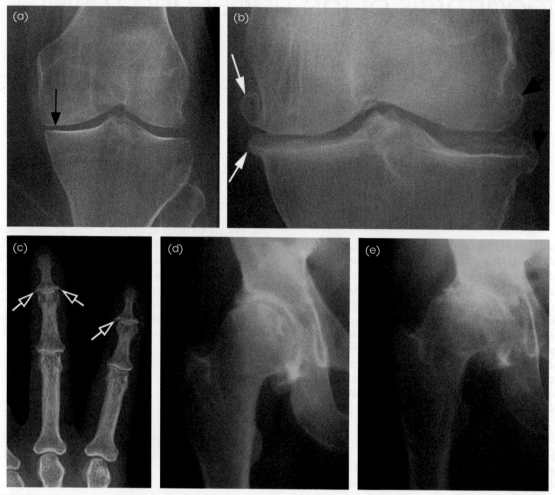

**Figure 44.1.** OA on radiographs. (*A*) AP radiograph of the knee shows definite JSN of the medial femorotibial compartment (*arrow*). This represents grade 3 femorotibial OA according to the K&L grading scheme. (*B*) AP radiograph of the knee shows large marginal osteophytes of the medial (*white arrows*) and lateral (*black arrows*) femorotibial compartments. Note additional JSN of the medial compartment. Image represents the hypertrophic phenotype of femorotibial OA and also represents grade 3 femorotibial OA according to K&L. (*C*) DIP joints of the third and fourth digits show characteristic radiographic signs of OA including marginal osteophyte formation (*arrows*) and asymmetric JSN. Soft tissue changes such as synovitis are only poorly visualized on radiograph and are depicted as increased soft tissue opacity reflecting soft tissue swelling. (*D, E*) Progressive OA of the hip over a 4-year period. Note progressive craniolateral migration of the right femoral head as well as sclerotic and cystlike changes in the acetabulum and femoral head.

## Magnetic Resonance Imaging

MRI detects abnormalities including meniscus or labrum tearing, hyaline cartilage defects with JSN, cystlike changes, osteophytes, malalignment, and preradiographic pathologic changes of OA, including bone marrow lesions and synovitis (Figure 44.3).

- Synovitis on non-contrast-enhanced MRI is indirectly depicted as edema and abnormal signal changes within the Hoffa fat pad and the presence of joint effusion. Contrast-enhanced MRI reveals synovial thickening and nodularity and enables direct visualization of synovitis.
- Synovitis severity and BME size are associated with knee pain, unlike other MRI imaging characteristics of OA.

Compositional MRI enables visualization of the biochemical properties of different joint tissues, which has been mostly applied for ultrastructural assessment of articular cartilage (Figure 44.4).

- Early degenerative cartilage matrix changes can be evaluated using advanced MRI techniques such as delayed gadolinium-enhanced MRI of cartilage (dGEMRIC), T1 rho, and T2 mapping.
- Loss of the highly negatively charged glycosaminoglycans (GAGs) in damaged hyaline cartilage can be visualized using dGEMRIC and T1 rho.
- Degenerative changes in collagen orientation and hydration of cartilage affect T2 mapping.
- Please see Chapter 111 "Imaging of Articular Cartilage" for further discussion.

## Ultrasound

Diagnostic US is not a commonly used clinical diagnostic tool for OA. US is useful for evaluation of synovitis in arthritis,

**Table 44.1.** Overview of Kellgren and Lawrence and Modified Kellgren and Lawrence Grading Systems for Radiographic Assessment of Knee Osteoarthritis

|  | ORIGINAL KELLGREN AND LAWRENCE CLASSIFICATION | MODIFIED KELLGREN AND LAWRENCE CLASSIFICATION[A] | RADIOGRAPHIC OSTEOARTHRITIS |
|---|---|---|---|
| Grade 0 | No feature of osteoarthritis | No feature of osteoarthritis | No |
| Grade 1 | Doubtful joint-space narrowing and possible osteophytic lipping | Equivocal osteophyte | No |
| Grade 2 | Definite osteophytes and possible joint-space narrowing | Unequivocal osteophyte | Yes |
| Grade 3 | Moderate multiple osteophytes, definite joint-space narrowing, and some sclerosis and possible deformity of bone ends | Joint-space narrowing | Yes |
| Grade 4 | Large osteophytes, marked joint-space narrowing, severe sclerosis, and definite deformity of bone ends | Bone-to-bone appearance | Yes |

[a]Adapted from Guermazi A, et al. *J Bone Joint Surg Am.* 2009;91(suppl 1):54–62.

which may also be seen in both inflammatory arthritis and OA. Utility of US in evaluation of arthritides is discussed in detail in Section 10, "Musculoskeletal Ultrasound."

**Computed Tomography**
- CT is excellent for detailed evaluation of OA findings, such as subchondral bone sclerosis, subchondral cystlike changes, and osteophytes.
- 3D CT is of particular help for orthopedic planning of joint arthroplasty.
- Ionizing radiation and limited soft tissue evaluation restrict the routine use of CT in clinical imaging of OA.

- CT arthrography is the most accurate method for evaluating superficial and focal cartilage defects.

**Treatment Options**
- Conservative treatment includes exercise, pharmacology, bracing, and intraarticular steroid injections in the management of OA.
- Surgical treatment includes joint replacement surgery as an effective intervention for late-stage disease.
- Disease-modifying drugs of OA are still investigational.

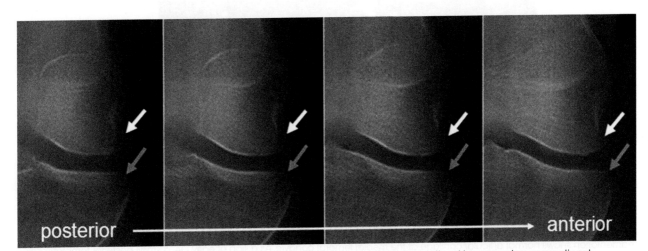

posterior ⟶ anterior

**Figure 44.2.** Tomosynthesis of the knee with OA. Digital tomosynthesis generates cross-sectional images using conventional radiographic image acquisition techniques. Image example shows 4 consecutive sections with 3-mm slice thickness from posterior to anterior with exquisite depiction of femoral (*white arrows*) and small tibial osteophytes (*gray arrows*).

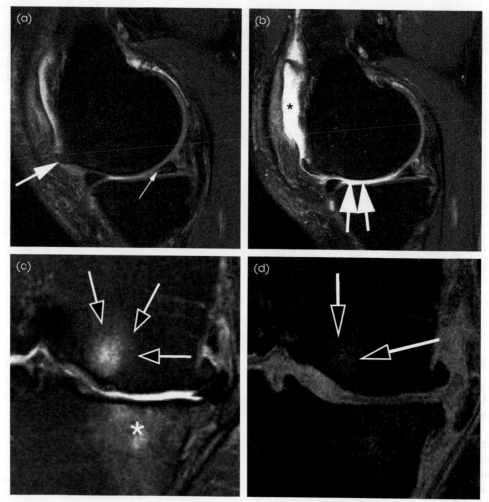

**Figure 44.3.** OA of the knee on MRI. (*A*) Sagittal PD FS MR image at baseline depicts small horizontal tear in the posterior horn of the medial meniscus (*small arrow*). An anterior osteophyte at the medial femoral condyle is shown in addition (*large arrow*). (*B*) At 24-month follow-up there is marked cartilage loss at the medial weight-bearing part of the femur (*arrows*). In addition, there is marked joint effusion (*asterisk*). (*C*) Coronal PD FS MR image shows subchondral bone marrow lesions in the medial femoral condyle (*arrows*) and tibial plateau (*asterisk*). Note in addition marked femoral and tibial cartilage loss, marginal osteophytes and severe meniscal extrusion. (*D*) Corresponding coronal fast low-angle shot (FLASH) MR image, commonly used for cartilage segmentation, barely depicts femoral bone marrow lesion (*arrows*), and shows tibial bone marrow lesion only to minimal extent.

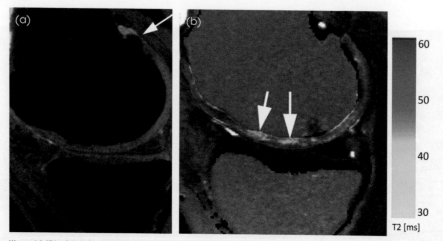

**Figure 44.4.** Compositional MRI of the knee articular cartilage. (*A*) Sagittal FLASH MR image, commonly used for cartilage segmentation shows normal articular cartilage at the medial femoral condyle. As a sign of early OA, a small posterior femoral osteophyte is depicted (*arrow*). (*B*) Corresponding color-coded T2W MR image depicts intracartilaginous T2 values in colors ranging from green to dark blue. There is marked heterogeneity in cartilage T2 with areas of lower T2 values in the weight-bearing parts of the femoral condyle that is not appreciated on morphologic image in (*A*). T2 values show marked interindividual variability and may fluctuate over time. Clinical relevance of early changes in cartilage compositional changes is still being evaluated.

## Key Points

- Radiography is the gold standard in OA imaging, used for grading disease severity.
- MRI enables imaging evaluation of all of the OA-related pathological features including osseous, cartilaginous, and other soft tissue lesions, as well as early findings not detectable by radiography, such as synovitis and BME.

## Recommended Reading

Jacobson JA, Giritsh G, Jian Y, Sabb BJ, radiographic evaluation of arthritis: degenerative joint disease and variations. *Radiology.* 2008;248(3):737–47.

## References

1. Losina E, Weinstein AM, Reichmann WM, et al. Lifetime risk and age at diagnosis of symptomatic knee osteoarthritis in the US. *Arthritis Care Res (Hoboken).* 2013;65:703–11.
2. Kotlarz H, Gunnarsson CL, Fang H, Rizzo JA. Insurer and out-of-pocket costs of osteoarthritis in the US: evidence from national survey data. *Arthritis Rheum.* 2009;60:3546–53.
3. Altman RD, Gold GE. Atlas of individual radiographic features in osteoarthritis, revised. *Osteoarthritis Cartilage.* 2007;15(suppl A):A1–56.
4. Altman R, Asch E, Bloch D, et al. Development of criteria for the classification and reporting of osteoarthritis. Classification of osteoarthritis of the knee. Diagnostic and Therapeutic Criteria Committee of the American Rheumatism Association. *Arthritis Rheum.* 1986;29:1039–49.
5. Kellgren JH, Lawrence JS. Radiological assessment of osteo-arthrosis. *Ann Rheum Dis.* 1957;16:494–502.
6. Hayashi D, Xu L, Roemer FW, et al. Detection of osteophytes and subchondral cysts in the knee with use of tomosynthesis. *Radiology.* 2012;263:206–15.
7. Hayashi D, Guermazi A, Roemer FW. MRI of osteoarthritis: the challenges of definition and quantification. *Semin Musculoskelet Radiol.* 2012;16:419–30.
8. Roemer FW, Guermazi A, Felson DT, et al. Presence of MRI-detected joint effusion and synovitis increases the risk of cartilage loss in knees without osteoarthritis at 30-month follow-up: the MOST study. *Ann Rheum Dis.* 2011;70:1804–809.
9. Zhang Y, Nevitt M, Niu J, et al. Fluctuation of knee pain and changes in bone marrow lesions, effusions, and synovitis on magnetic resonance imaging. *Arthritis Rheum.* 2011;63:691–99.
10. Guermazi A, Roemer FW, Hayashi D, et al. Assessment of synovitis with contrast-enhanced MRI using a whole-joint semiquantitative scoring system in people with, or at high risk of, knee osteoarthritis: the MOST study. *Ann Rheum Dis.* 2011;70:805–11.
11. Guermazi A, Roemer FW, Alizai H, et al. State of the art: MR imaging after knee cartilage repair surgery. *Radiology.* 2015;277:23–43.
12. Guermazi A, Alizai H, Crema MD, Trattnig S, Regatte RR, Roemer FW. Compositional MRI techniques for evaluation of cartilage degeneration in osteoarthritis. *Osteoarthritis Cartilage.* 2015;23:1639–53.
13. Burstein D, Gray M, Mosher T, Dardzinski B. Measures of molecular composition and structure in osteoarthritis. *Radiol Clin North Am.* 2009;47:675–86.
14. Omoumi P, Mercier GA, Lecouvet F, Simoni P, Vande Berg BC. CT arthrography, MR arthrography, PET and scintigraphy in osteoarthritis. *Radiol Clin North Am.* 2009;47:595–615.

# CHAPTER 45

# Imaging of Erosive Osteoarthritis

Daichi Hayashi, Ali Guermazi, and Frank W. Roemer

## Introduction

Erosive osteoarthritis (EOA) has been viewed as a subset of hand OA with joint erosions and is also referred to as an *inflammatory phenotype of OA*. It classically affects the interphalangeal (IP) joints of the hands symmetrically, typically in postmenopausal women with an estimated female-to-male ratio of 12:1. Large joints, such as the shoulder, knee, or hip are rarely involved. There is moderate to severe synovitis superimposed on the typical degenerative changes seen in OA, but the precise etiology is yet to be determined. Radiography is the primary imaging modality used in the diagnosis of EOA.

## Pathophysiology and Clinical Findings

Clinical symptoms of EOA include pain, swelling, and tenderness of the small joints of the hands, as well as throbbing paresthesia of the fingertips and morning stiffness. EOA starts from the DIP joints and later involves the PIP joints. It may also affect the first carpometacarpal (CMC), scaphoid-trapezio-trapezoid, and other carpal joints. The affected articulations are commonly characterized by deformities, which can include subluxations, flexion contractions, Heberden and Bouchard nodes, ankylosis of DIP, and PIP joints and opera-glass deformity. The precise diagnostic criteria of EOA are yet to be determined, including the type, number, and locations of the affected joints.

## Imaging Strategy

Radiography of the hands is the initial diagnostic test. Rarely is additional imaging required. Both US, using gray-scale and power Doppler settings, and MRI, using a small FOV, a dedicated hand or surface coil, intravenous contrast, and fluid-sensitive and T1W sequences, are highly sensitive to the erosions and synovitis that may precede radiographically detectable evidence of disease.

## Imaging Findings

### Radiography

Characteristic radiographic changes of EOA include
- Joint-space narrowing and central joint erosions affecting the IP and first CMC joints of the hand and sometimes the foot.
- Erosion is an essential hallmark for the diagnosis of EOA, and the osteophytosis characteristic of *nonerosive* OA may sometimes be absent or occur later in the disease process.

Disease progression leads to characteristic deformities:

- *Gull-wing* deformity caused by marginal sclerosis and osteophytes of the distal side of the joint (Figure 45.1), although the proximal side is centrally eroded and thinned
- *Saw-tooth* appearance with a jagged joint contour, which may later lead to ankylosis (Figure 45.1)

EOA may resemble psoriatic (PsA) (or reactive arthritis) with the following distinguishing features:

- EOA erosions show *crumbling* of the central bony surface, in contrast to the sharply defined, typically marginal erosions of PsA.
- PsA erosions more typically have a *mouse-ear* configuration, characterized by marginal erosion and periosteal bone proliferation of the distal phalanges of the distal IP joints.
- In PsA, there is frequent involvement of other sites in the body, in particular the SI joints.
- Acroosteolysis, pencil-in-cup deformities, and arthritis mutilans are not observed in EOA.

### Ultrasound
- Gray-scale and power Doppler imaging can detect the characteristic erosions, thickened synovium, effusions, and increased intraarticular power Doppler signal.

### Magnetic Resonance Imaging
- Cortical disruption by erosions, joint effusions, and thickened, enhancing synovium are detected on fluid-sensitive and T1W sequences pre- and postcontrast (Figure 45.2).
- OA changes, including subchondral sclerosis and cystlike changes, and marginal osteophytes are also seen (Figure 45.2).
- In contrast to EOA, PsA more commonly shows the following:
  - Soft tissue swelling and inflammation
  - Periostitis, which is not a feature of erosive OA
  - Marginally located erosions, but central erosions may also be observed

## Key Points
- EOA is a subset of OA with erosions and superimposed synovitis, typically seen in the finger joints.

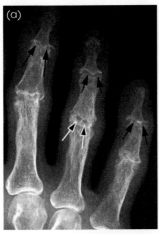
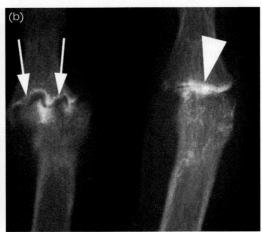

**Figure 45.1.** Articular erosions in erosive OA. (*A*) Gull-wing features are seen in all DIPs (*black arrows*). In addition the PIP joint of digit 4 shows a so-called saw-tooth erosion (*white bordered arrows*). Magnification AP view of another patient (*B*) depicts a classic saw-tooth erosion in the PIP joint (*arrows*), whereas the third PIP joint exhibits a nonerosive appearance of advanced OA with joint-space narrowing and subchondral sclerosis (*arrowhead*).

- Radiography is primarily used for imaging of EOA.
- US and MRI can be useful in detecting erosions, joint effusion, and active synovitis that may precede radiographic changes.
- The most common differential diagnosis of EOA is PsA, which exhibits additional characteristic imaging features such as bony proliferations and periostitis.

## Recommended Reading

Jacobson JA, Girish G, Jian Y, Sabb BJ. Radiographic evaluation of arthritis: degenerative joint disease and variations. *Radiology.* 2008;248(3):737–47.

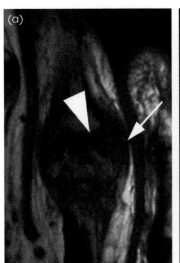
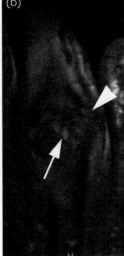

**Figure 45.2.** Erosive OA on MRI. (*A*) Coronal T1W MR image shows subchondral sclerosis (*arrowhead*), capsular thickening reflecting synovitis (*arrow*), and central erosions. (*B*) Corresponding coronal PD FS MR image shows superiorly a subchondral cystlike lesion (*arrow*) and a classic marginal osteophyte (*arrowhead*) along with periarticular soft tissue edema and BME.

## References

1. Kloppenburg M, Kwok WY. Hand osteoarthritis—a heterogeneous disorder. *Nat Rev Rheumatol.* 2011;8:22–31.
2. Belhorn LR, Hess EV. Erosive osteoarthritis. *Semin Arthritis Rheum.* 1993;22:298–306
3. Keats TE, Johnstone WH, O'Brien WM. Large joint destruction in erosive osteoarthritis. *Skeletal Radiol.* 1981;6:267–69.
4. Punzi L, Ramonda R, Sfriso P. Erosive osteoarthritis. *Best Pract Res Clin Rheumatol.* 2004;18:739–58.
5. Greenway G, Resnick D, Weisman M, et al. Carpal involvement in inflammatory (erosive) osteoarthritis. *J Can Assoc Radiol.* 1972;30:95–98.
6. Greenspan A. Erosive osteoarthritis. *Semin Musculoskelet Radiol.* 2003;7:155–59.
7. Yeturi S, Patel P, David G, Rosenthal AK. Lack of uniform diagnostic criteria for erosive OA: a systematic review [abstract]. *Arthritis Rheumatol.* 2015;67(suppl 10). http://acrabstracts.org/abstract/lack-of-uniform-diagnostic-criteria-for-erosive-oa-a-systematic-review/. Accessed December 1, 2015.
8. Vlychou M, Koutroumpas A, Malizos K, Sakkas LI. Ultrasonographic evidence of inflammation is frequent in hands of patients with erosive osteoarthritis. *Osteoarthritis Cartilage.* 2009;17:1283–27.
9. Wittoek R, Jans L, Lambrecht V, Carron P, Verstraete K, Verbruggen G. Reliability and construct validity of ultrasonography of soft tissue and destructive changes in erosive osteoarthritis of the interphalangeal finger joints: a comparison with MRI. *Ann Rheum Dis.* 2011;70:278–83.
10. Kortekaas MC, Kwok WY, Reijnierse M, Stijnen T, Kloppenburg M. Inflammation is associated with erosive development in patients with hand osteoarthritis: a prospective ultrasonography study. *Arthritis Rheumatol.* 2015 Sep 28. doi:10.1002/art.39438. [Epub ahead of print]
11. Mancarella L, Addimanda O, Pelotti P, Pignotti E, Pulsatelli L, Meliconi R. Ultrasound detected inflammation is associated with the development of new bone erosions in hand osteoarthritis: a longitudinal study over 3.9 years. *Osteoarthritis Cartilage.* 2015;23:1925–32.

12. Haugen IK, Bøyesen P, Slatkowsky-Christensen B, et al. Comparison of features by MRI and radiographs of the interphalangeal finger joints in patients with hand osteoarthritis. *Ann Rheum Dis.* 2012;71:345–50.

13. Stomp W, Krabben A, van der Heijde D, et al. Are rheumatoid arthritis patients discernible from other early arthritis patients using 1.5T extremity magnetic resonance imaging? a large cross-sectional study. *J Rheumatol.* 2014;41:1630–37.

14. Tan AL, Grainger AJ, Tanner SF, et al. High-resolution magnetic resonance imaging for the assessment of hand osteoarthritis. *Arthritis Rheum.* 2005;52: 2355–65.

# CHAPTER 46

# Joint Arthroplasties and Prostheses

Kevin B. Hoover and Tim B. Hunter

## Introduction

Joint replacement is the next most common orthopedic procedure after fracture reduction and fixation. Joint replacement is also called an *arthroplasty*, and the terms *prosthesis* or *implant* are sometimes less used to mean joint replacement. Joint replacements in order of decreasing frequency are total knee arthroplasty (TKA), total hip arthroplasty (THA), hip hemiarthroplasty, total shoulder arthroplasty (TSA), and shoulder hemiarthroplasty. Elbow, wrist, hand, and ankle arthroplasties are also performed. Indications include OA-related pain, most commonly, inflammatory arthritis, ON, fracture, and tumor.

## Imaging Strategy

Radiography is routinely acquired pre- and postoperatively in frontal and lateral, orthogonal planes (Table 46.1). Similar acquisition technique before and after surgery is important to compare hardware alignment and balance. CT is frequently used preoperatively for shoulder evaluation after trauma and for evaluating glenoid bone stock. Intraarticular contrast (CT arthrography) is sometimes used to evaluate both bone stock and rotator cuff (RTC) integrity. Knee arthroplasties are evaluated with CT to assess rotational component alignment. Dual-energy CT (DECT) may hold promise for reducing metal-associated artifact. MRI is used preoperatively in the shoulder for evaluating RTC insufficiency. MRI is also used to evaluate painful arthroplasties in the setting of negative radiographs to evaluate for particle disease, including metallosis, using metal artifact reduction software (MARS) and sequences less susceptible to metallic artifact (eg, STIR, FSE, high band width).

Although 3-phase bone scans are used to diagnose arthroplasty infection or aseptic loosening, both may show increased periarticular and articular uptake in all 3 phases, and definitive diagnosis may require surgery and culture. Increased periprosthetic uptake on tagged white blood cell (WBC) scan is more specific for infection. Nuclear studies are most conclusive when they are normal. US and fluoroscopy are useful to guide diagnostic joint aspirations to exclude infection. US can be used for evaluating superficial tendon injury (eg, extensor mechanism, RTC).

Joint replacement is often described as constrained, unconstrained (nonconstrained), or semiconstrained. A fully constrained implant has very limited motion in a given direction, most often in the AP direction or in axial rotation. A semiconstrained implant has an intermediate amount of motion in a given direction, and an unconstrained implant allows full motion in a given direction.

## Knee Arthroplasty

### Indications

- Most commonly primary OA
- Secondary OA caused by trauma, inflammatory arthritis, and ON
- Tumor involving epiphysis
- TKA selection based on degree of muscle, tendon, and ligament support and number of compartments involved
- Contraindicated in unresolved systemic or joint infection
- Joint aspirations performed to exclude joint infection prior to hardware placement or definitive revision

### Imaging Findings

- Three joint compartments (medial, lateral, patellofemoral) are seen.
- TKA replaces all 3 articulating surfaces with cemented components.
  - Unconstrained prosthesis—bicondylar cobalt-chromium femoral component, titanium tibial tray with a polyethylene surface, and a polyethylene patellar component (button)
    - ACL often removed, but PCL commonly preserved in initial TKA (PCL-retaining; Figures 46.1 and 46.2)
  - CT used to assess the rotation of femoral and tibial components
    - Malrotation can be a pain generator.
    - Internal and external rotation of each component in the axial plane is determined relative to bony landmarks and other component.
  - Constrained prosthesis types are as follows:
    - Posterior-stabilized prosthetic replaces the PCL with a central polyethylene post if there is ligamentous laxity and deformity (eg, RA, revision) (Figure 46.3).
    - In coronal plane instability, the varus-valgus is constrained with an unlinked central metallic post (Figure 46.4).
    - A rotating hinge links femoral and tibial components if there is severe damage of soft tissues (eg, revision, tumor) (Figure 46.5).
- Unicompartmental knee arthroplasty is used for isolated compartment OA, most commonly medial (Figure 46.6).

**Table 46.1. Preoperative and Postoperative Radiography**

| JOINT | VIEWS | WHAT TO ASSESS |
|---|---|---|
| Knee | Weight-bearing AP, PA, Lateral, axial | ■ Varus-valgus alignment for correction<br>■ Single versus multicompartment osteoarthritis for arthroplasty selection<br>■ Patellar malalignment for tubercle osteotomy |
|  | Stitched-leg length | ■ Mechanical axis for correction<br>■ Leg length discrepancy for correction |
| Hip | AP, Cross-table lateral | ■ Central positioning of femoral head component within acetabular cup for liner wear<br>■ Acetabular component abduction and anteversion for limited ROM, impingement, dislocation risk<br>■ Straight versus angulated femoral component alignment within the femur for pain, fracture risk |
| Shoulder | AP, scapular Y, and axillary views | ■ Acromiohumeral interval narrowing <7 mm in RTC insufficiency (preoperative)<br>■ Anterior humeral head subluxation suggests subscapularis tendon tear |
| Elbow | True AP and lateral | ■ Humeral component anterior angulation with loosening |
| Wrist and Hand, Foot | AP, oblique, and lateral views | ■ Periprosthetic lucency, subsidence, dislocation, arthrodesis status |
| Ankle | AP, mortise, and lateral views | ■ Periprosthetic lucency, subsidence<br>■ Polyethylene malalignment |

Abbreviations: AP, anterior-posterior; PA, posterior-anterior; ROM, range of motion; RTC, rotator cuff.

■ Cemented metallic femoral and tibial components with polyethylene tray
  ■ Rarely, interpositional hemiarthroplasty, using allograft meniscus, metal or polyethylene

**Complications**
■ Complications occur more often in men versus women.
■ Hematoma and seroma are the most common complications and best seen on cross-sectional imaging or US.
■ Complications include infection and mechanical (aseptic) loosening:
  ■ On serial radiographs, progressive periprosthetic lucency greater than 2 mm and/or subsidence is seen and is often more rapid in infection (Figures 46.2, 46.5 and 46.6C).
  ■ On MRI, a fibrous membrane of intermediate to fluid signal at the bone or cement-prosthesis interface is an early sign of loosening.
  ■ On MRI, infection is suggested by layered or lamellated synovitis, extracapsular soft tissue

edema and collections, sinus tracts, and reactive lymphadenopathy.
  ■ Diagnosis often requires joint aspiration with elevated leukocyte counts (>1700/mm³) and neutrophil percentage (>65%) consistent with infection.
■ Complications include deep venous thrombosis 0.9-1.6% and bleeding 0.4-0.8% over 15 years.
■ Particle disease can be caused by a granulomatous, foreign body reaction to small polyethylene, cement, or metal particles.
■ Periprosthetic fracture, extensor mechanism failure, and stiffness are all complications.

## Hip Arthroplasty

**Indications**
■ Primary and secondary OA (common)
■ Femoral neck fracture
■ Tumor involving joint margins (uncommon)

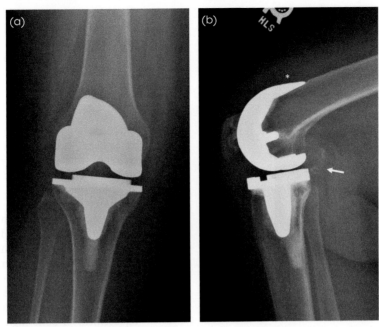

**Figure 46.1.** PCL-retaining cemented TKA. AP (*A*) and lateral (*B*) radiographs show a PCL-retaining cemented TKA with normal orthogonal alignment of the tibial tray to the tibial axis on both views with commonly seen cement posteriorly (*thin arrow*) and suprapatellar effusion (*asterisk*).

- Prosthesis type and use of cement fixation depending on patient activity level, age, and bone stock

**Imaging Findings**
- Hemiarthroplasty replaces only the femoral head and neck.
  - Unipolar, or endoprosthesis—noncemented metallic femoral component used in femoral neck fracture treatment of less mobile patients (Figure 46.7)
  - Bipolar hemiarthroplasty—noncemented prosthetic acetabular cup lined with polyethylene locked

to a cemented or noncemented femoral component (Figure 46.8)
  - Motion within cup and at acetabulum-cup articulation less painful during activity than with unipolar arthroplasty
- THA is typically modular with a metallic stem, often metallic femoral head and a metallic acetabulum and, usually, a polyethylene liner (Figures 46.8 and 46.9).
  - Noncemented components are partially or completely covered with porous coating at bone interface for ingrowth.

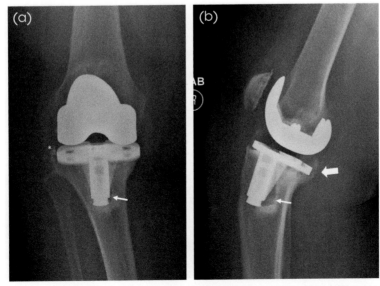

**Figure 46.2.** Failed PCL-retaining cemented TKA. AP (*A*) and lateral (*B*) radiographs show a PCL-retaining cemented TKA with subsidence and angulation (*thick arrow*) of the tibial tray, abnormal widening of the cement-prosthesis interface (*thin arrow*), and cement fracture (*asterisk*).

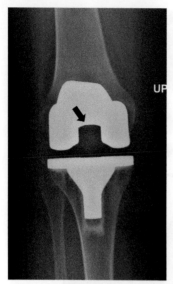

**Figure 46.3.** Posteriorly stabilized TKA. AP radiograph shows a posteriorly stabilized TKA with characteristic square femoral component condylar notch (*thick arrow*).

- Noncemented acetabular components may be fixed with screws.
- Noncemented femoral components common in younger patients (<65 years old) with adequate bone stock.
- Cemented femoral components are more common, especially in hybrid prostheses—noncemented acetabular and cemented femoral components.
  - Cemented acetabular component is used if poor bone stock from tumor or injury.
  - Cement fills the gap between bone and prosthesis, not adhesive.

- Prosthetic head-acetabulum interface may also be metal-on-metal, ceramic-on-metal, or ceramic-on-ceramic.
- Resurfacing arthroplasty replaces articular surface of femoral head alone or with acetabulum (uncommon; Figure 46.10).

**Complications**

- Aseptic loosening, is the most common, suggested by periprosthetic lucency, alignment change, or fibrous membrane formation as seen on MRI.
- Infection, resembling aseptic loosening, may be more rapid or show periostitis.
  - Joint fluid aspirates show elevated leukocyte count (>4200/mm³) and neutrophil percentage (>80%).
  - Infection is generally excluded if serum CRP levels are normal 2 months after arthroplasty, except if the patient is on antibiotics or infected by a low virulence organism (eg, *Propionibacterium acnes*).
  - On MRI with heterogeneous signal intensity synovitis, primarily isointense to skeletal muscle and replacement of bone high T1 fat signal with signal isointense to muscle (Figure 46.11) is seen.
  - Standard treatment is 2-stage revision with hardware removal, antibiotic spacer placement, and 6-12 weeks of intravenous (IV) antibiotics followed by definitive revision.
- Particle disease arising from polyethylene is suggested by the following:
  - Radiographs with off-center femoral head position in the acetabular cup from polyethylene liner wear and periarticular osteolysis by granulomas (Figure 46.9B)
- Adverse local tissue reaction to metal (metallosis), most commonly from metal-on-metal prosthesis, is suggested by the following:
  - Radiographs similar to particle disease, but may be negative

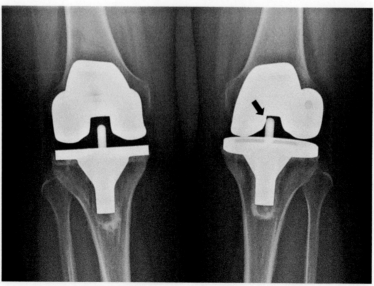

**Figure 46.4.** Constrained bilateral TKA with eccentric left tibial post alignment. AP standing radiograph of the bilateral knees shows varus-valgus constrained bilateral TKA in a patient with Ehlers-Danlos syndrome with eccentric left tibial post alignment (*thick arrow*) caused by component rotation.

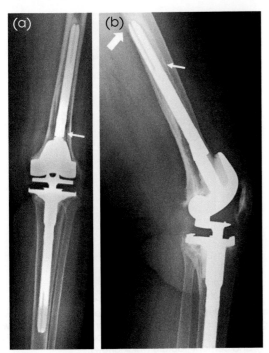

**Figure 46.5.** Failed rotating-hinge linked TKA. AP (*A*) and lateral (*B*) radiographs show a rotating-hinge linked TKA with femoral component loosening with lucency at the bone-cement interface (*thin arrows*), dorsal angulation, and cortical perforation of the proximal femoral component (*thick arrow*) (*B*).

■ Synovitis on MRI containing magnetic susceptibility artifact and replacement of periprosthetic bone fat signal (Figure 46.12)
■ Muscle and tendon destruction by fluid signal masses (pseudotumors); called *aseptic lymphocyte-dominated vasculitis-associated lesions* (ALVAL)

■ Elevated serum and urine ion levels of cobalt and chromium
■ Heterotopic bone formation is common and can limit range of motion and may require surgical resection.
■ Stress shielding with reduction of bone density along femoral stem of prosthesis (Figure 46.13) occurs.
■ Stress loading gives cortical thickening along the femoral stem (Figure 46.14).
■ Dislocations are more common after unipolar prosthesis or revision.
■ Intraoperative or postoperative periprosthetic fracture can occur.

## Shoulder Arthroplasty

**Indications**
■ Primary or secondary OA
■ Comminuted humeral head fracture
■ Tumor involvement of joint
■ Type and fixation of prosthesis dependent on RTC integrity and bone stock

**Imaging Findings**
■ TSA used with a functional RTC (Figure 46.15)
■ Usually noncemented humeral component, cemented polyethylene glenoid component with single (keel) or multiple cemented pegs containing radiopaque wires
■ Reverse total shoulder arthroplasty (RTSA) if RTC insufficiency (Figure 46.16)
■ Prosthetic glenoid ball (glenosphere) attached to glenoid plate (metaglene) fixed with bicortical screws
■ Cupped humeral socket attached to metal diaphyseal stem often noncemented, but cemented if poor bone stock

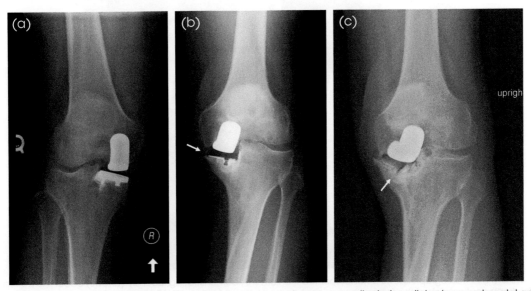

**Figure 46.6.** Unicompartmental knee arthroplasties. (*A*) AP radiograph shows uncomplicated medial unicompartmental arthroplasty with metallic components. (*B, C*) AP radiographs show medial unicompartmental arthroplasty in a knee in varus with cemented metallic femoral and polyethylene tibial (*thin arrow*) components initially with expected prosthetic alignment in the frontal plane (*B*) (*C*) and subsequent cement fracture (*thin arrow*) and polyethylene subsidence 14 years later (*C*).

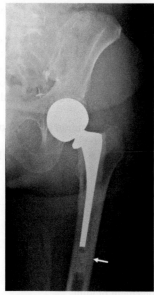

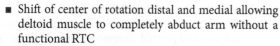

**Figure 46.7.** Unipolar hip hemiarthroplasty. AP radiograph shows an uncomplicated unipolar hemiarthroplasty with a cemented femoral component (*thin arrow*).

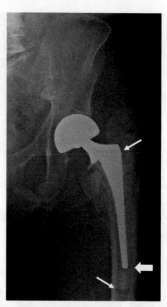

**Figure 46.8.** Failed bipolar hip revision hemiarthroplasty. AP radiograph shows a failed revised bipolar hemiarthroplasty with varus femoral angulation, wide cement-bone lucency (*thin arrows*), and cement fracture (*thick arrow*).

- Shift of center of rotation distal and medial allowing deltoid muscle to completely abduct arm without a functional RTC
- Hemiarthroplasty used if glenoid is well preserved (eg, humeral head fracture, ON, tumor) or poor glenoid bone stock
  - Humeral component often identical to TSA
- Humeral head resurfacing with a curved metal cap fixed with a peg or screw

- Used in ON, large Hill-Sachs fractures, large osteochondral injuries

**Complications**
- Aseptic or septic loosening (Figure 46.17)
- Dislocation, often anterior in RTSA (Figure 46.16)
- Scapular notching in RTSA from contact between humeral cup and inferior glenoid; may loosen glenosphere
- Intraoperative or postoperative periprosthetic fracture

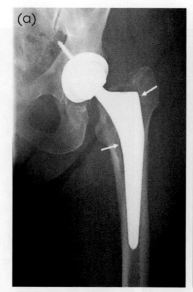

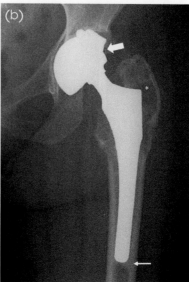

**Figure 46.9.** THAs. (*A*) AP radiograph shows a noncemented titanium THA demonstrating lucency (*arrows*) about the metaphyseal and proximal diaphyseal aspects of the femoral component caused by an infection. (*B*) AP radiograph shows a noncemented left THA with eccentric femoral component positioning in the acetabulum (*thick arrow*) caused by polyethylene liner wear with extensive periarticular osteolysis (*asterisk*) from small particle disease. Endosteal bone formation is also noted at the distal femoral component (pedestal, *thin arrow*) that can be associated with loosening.

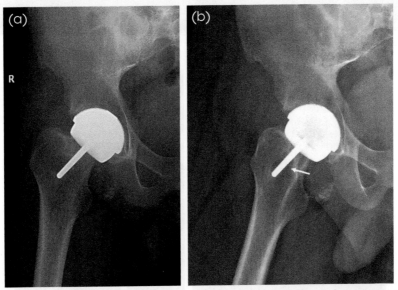

**Figure 46.10.** Resurfacing hip arthroplasty. (*A*) AP radiograph shows a metal-on-metal femoral resurfacing arthroplasty. (*B*) Later AP radiograph shows lucency about the femoral neck stem (*thin arrow*) caused by subsequently developed infection.

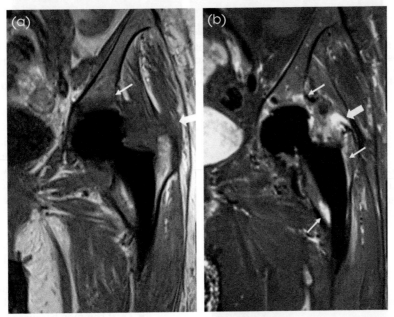

**Figure 46.11.** Infected THA. Using MARS, coronal T1W (*A*) and STIR (*B*) MR images demonstrate replacement of periprosthetic marrow fat with fluid signal infectious material (*thin arrows*) along with tearing of the gluteus tendon attachment on the greater trochanter (*thick arrow*). A draining sinus tract is not shown.

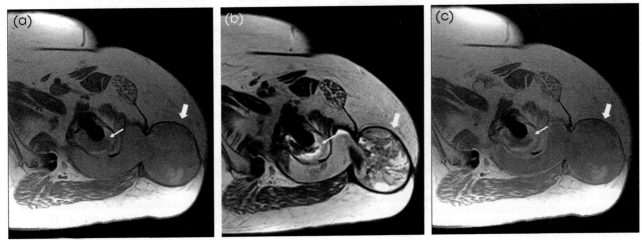

**Figure 46.12.** Adverse local tissue reaction to metal in a 70-year-old-woman with a metal-on-metal THA on MRI. Note a large, soft tissue mass with heterogeneous signal on T1W (*A*) and T2W (*B*) MR images with a low signal capsule (*thick arrows*), herniation through the tensor fascia lata, and replacement of proximal femur bone with peripherally enhancing reactive material (*thin arrows*) on the T1W postcontrast MR image (*C*).

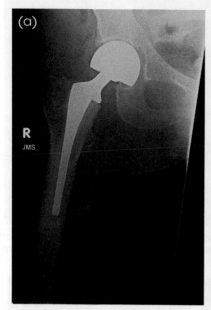
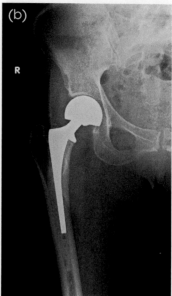

**Figure 46.13.** Stress shielding in a 69-year-old woman with history of femoral neck fracture treated by bipolar hip hemiarthroplasty. (*A*) Initial AP postoperative radiograph of the right hip shows an expected appearance of a bipolar hemiarthroplasty with cemented femoral stem. Note foci of air in the adjacent soft tissues consistent with recent surgery. (*B*) AP radiograph of the same hip obtained 5 months later shows subtle reduction in the femoral cortical thickness along the stem of the implant caused by stress shielding.

## Elbow Arthroplasty

### Indications

- Patient older than 40 years with secondary OA, most often RA or posttraumatic
- Radial head replacement for comminuted, displaced fractures

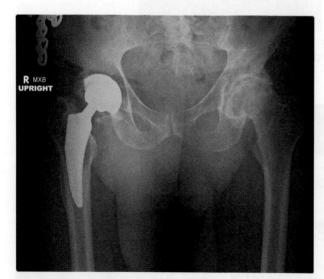

**Figure 46.14.** THA with stress loading. 52-year-old man with right THA 7 years prior. AP radiograph of the pelvis shows the arthroplasty as well as considerable bony proliferation along the lateral aspect of the proximal femoral cortex caused by stress loading from the prosthesis stem.

### Imaging Findings

- Total elbow arthroplasty, hemiarthroplasty, and radial head replacement most common
- Three major types of total elbow arthroplasty
  - Semiconstrained with linked humeral and ulnar components with some varus-valgus movement (Figure 46.18*A, B*)
    - Most common, usually cemented
  - Constrained with rigid, cemented metal-on-metal or metal on polyethylene hinge, linking humerus and ulna
    - Does not allow varus-valgus motion
    - Radial head often resected
    - Least common because of frequency of loosening
  - Unconstrained with unlinked, usually cemented humeral and ulnar components with interposed polyethylene liner
- Hemiarthroplasty with replacement of only the distal humerus in patients with limited function
  - Uncommon, usually from severe trauma
- Radial head replacement common with 1 of 2 types
  - Unipolar stem press-fit or cemented
  - Bipolar with metallic stem articulating via polyethylene liner with prosthetic radial head
- Less common, capitellar arthroplasty alone or with radial head replacement, often metal

### Complications

- Heterotopic ossification reducing mobility
- High revision rates, especially constrained type, because of:
  - Aseptic or septic loosening often with anterior migration of humeral component (Figure 46.18*C, D*)
- Periprosthetic fracture

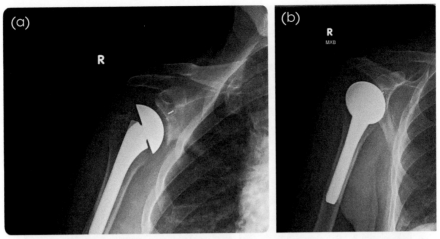

**Figure 46.15.** A 74-year-old woman with TSA. (*A*) Grashey view and (*B*) AP internal rotation view radiographs of the right shoulder show a TSA without evidence of hardware complications.

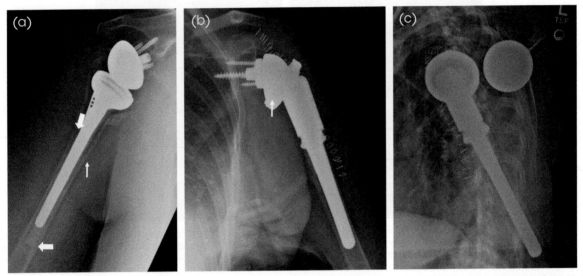

**Figure 46.16.** Infected RTSAs. (*A*) AP radiograph shows an RTSA implant with extensive lucency at the bone-cement interface and irregular cortices (*thick arrows*). Note an attenuated, somewhat moth-eaten humeral cortex with periostitis (*thin arrow*) caused by septic loosening. (*B*) AP and (*C*) scapular Y radiographs of the left shoulder in a different patient show anteriorly dislocated RTSA. AP radiograph (*B*) shows subtle abnormal overlap of the glenosphere and diaphyseal components (*thin arrow*). Anterior dislocation of the humeral prosthesis is better seen on the scapular Y view (*C*).

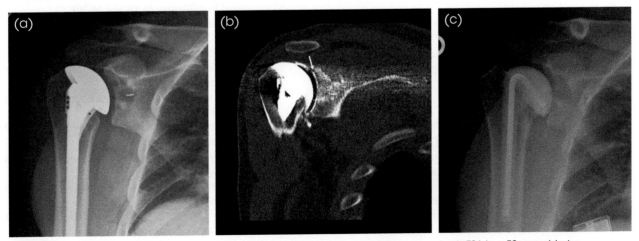

**Figure 46.17.** Shoulder arthroplasty complications. (*A*) AP radiograph demonstrates an anatomic TSA in a 59-year-old who developed an enterococcus infection. (*B*) A coronal reformatted CT arthrogram image demonstrates contrast undercutting the glenoid polyethylene component (*thin arrow*) consistent with loosening. (*C*) Postoperative AP radiograph of the same shoulder shows methyl methacrylate antibiotic spacer placement replacing the humeral component of the prosthesis after explanation of the infected TSA.

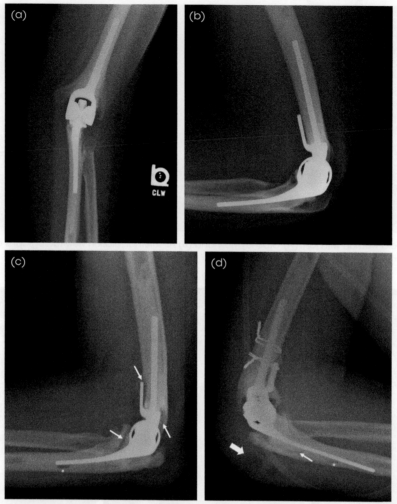

**Figure 46.18.** Semiconstrained elbow arthroplasty (TEA). AP (*A*) and lateral (*B*) radiographs show a normal linked, semiconstrained TEA and radial head resection. (*C*) Lateral elbow radiograph of a different patient shows aseptic loosening with widened prosthesis interfaces (*thin arrows*) and focal lucency at the tip of the ulnar component (*asterisk*) as well as sterile (proven) olecranon bursitis. (*D*) Infected revision arthroplasty of the same patient. Lateral radiograph shows subsequent revision arthroplasty with widened bone-cement interfaces (*thin arrow*) and lucencies about the ulnar component (*asterisk*) as well as periarticular soft tissue emphysema (*thick arrow*) caused by a gas-producing organism.

## Wrist and Hand Arthroplasty

### Indications
- Patient has pain from primary or secondary OA, especially RA.
- Contraindications include previously failed arthroplasty, neuropathy, and weight bearing (eg, cane, walker).

### Imaging Findings
- Wrist arthroplasty less common than surgical fusion (arthrodesis)
  - Requires intact extensor carpi radialis longus and brevis tendons and intact third metacarpal
  - Distal ulna resection to avoid abutment
  - Multiple generations
    - First generation—translucent Silastic, silicone, or elastomer spacer often with metallic grommets at bone interface

- Fourth generation—may be cemented or noncemented and with radial stem, carpal plate, carpal ball (Figures 46.19 and 46.20).
- Less common distal radioulnar joint (DRUJ) arthroplasty
  - Hemiarthroplasty with polymer or metal replacement of the distal ulna that articulates with a native distal radius
  - Prosthesis with a metal distal ulna articulating with a metal radius plate
- Hand and finger arthroplasty primarily of the MCP joints (Figures 46.19 and 46.21)
  - Historically with silicone implants, sometimes with metallic grommets
  - Now uncommon procedure because of long-term failure rates
  - May be associated with surgical PIP joint arthrodesis

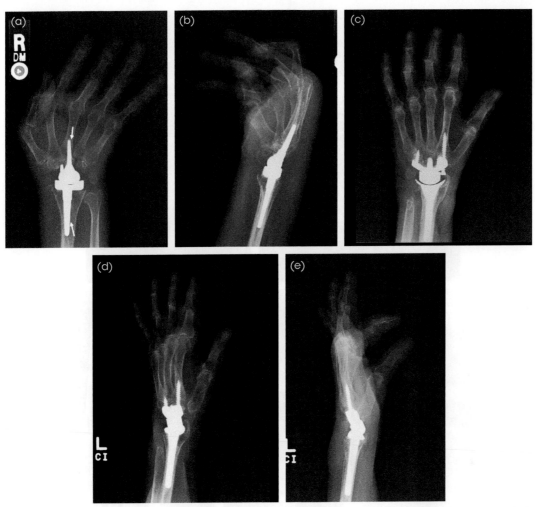

**Figure 46.19.** Total wrist arthroplasty (TWA). PA (*A*) and lateral radiographs (*B*) of a second-generation TWA with cemented radial and noncemented distal components show subtle lucencies about the radial and third metacarpal components (*thin arrows* in *A*) with normal alignment on the frontal and lateral radiographs. PA (*C*), oblique (*D*), and lateral (*E*) radiographs of the left wrist in a 69-year-old woman with RA show a fourth-generation TWA. There are also Silastic implants of the second through fifth PIP joints, which are failing. Figures 46.19*C-E* used with permission from http://medapparatus.com/index.html.

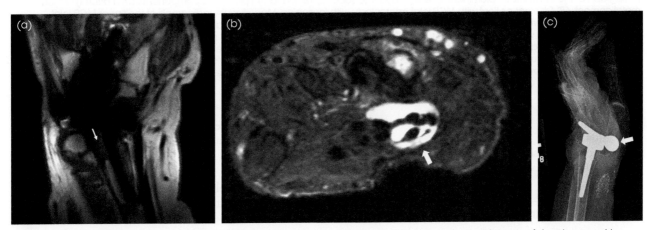

**Figure 46.20.** Failed TWA. (*A*) Coronal T1W MR image of the wrist in a patient with TWA shows abnormal marrow fat replacement in the distal radius (*thin arrow*) caused by particle disease with mild hardware artifact. (*B*) Axial STIR MR image of the same wrist shows tenosynovitis involving the ulnar flexor tendons (*thick arrow*) distal to the wrist with mild hardware artifact. (*C*) Volar TWA dislocation. Lateral radiograph of the wrist in a different patient shows volar dislocation of the distal component of the TWA (*thick arrow*). Note metallic debris in the volar soft tissues of the distal forearm and hand.

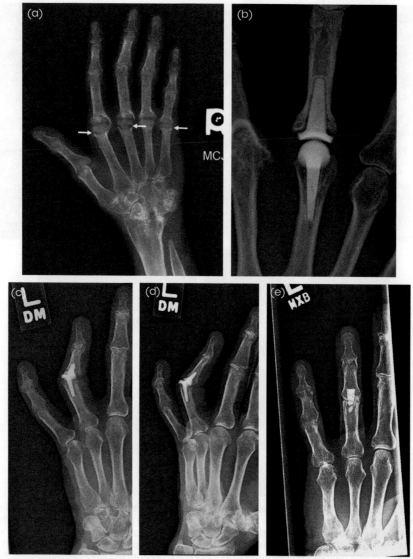

**Figure 46.21.** IP joint arthroplasties. (*A*) Silastic (Swanson) arthroplasties of the second through fifth MCP joints in an RA patient. PA radiograph of the hand shows prominent lucency about the second, third, and fifth prosthetic components (*thin arrows*) without malalignment. (*B*) Different patient with MCP joint arthroplasty with loosening. Magnified PA radiograph of the finger MCP joint shows a prominent periprosthetic lucency involving the phalangeal more than metacarpal components of the pyrocarbon third MCP joint arthroplasty without malalignment. (*C-E*). A 66-year-old woman with infected left ring finger PIP joint arthroplasty. PA (*C*) and (*D*) oblique radiographs show the arthroplasty 1 ½ months after surgery. There is subtle bony erosion at the base of the fourth middle phalanx and subtle lucency around the stem of the prosthesis in the proximal phalanx. (*E*) PA radiograph of the same digit after arthroplasty removal shows placement of an antibiotic cement that is fractured in the proximal phalanx. Note fusion of the interphalangeal joints of the little finger.

**Complications**

- Initially good pain relief, usually with long-term osteolysis, loosening, and dislocation by 10 years (Figure 46.21)

---

## Ankle and Foot Arthroplasty

**Indication**

- Maintain ankle movement in secondary OA patients, most commonly trauma, but also inflammatory arthritis, hemophilia
- Foot arthroplasty, most commonly in RA

- Contraindicated in active local joint or systemic infection, peripheral vascular disease, neuropathic joint

**Imaging Findings**

- Ankle arthroplasty is far less common than arthrodesis.
- The current generation is most commonly nonconstrained with 2 or 3 noncemented components:
  - Replaces articulation of tibia and fibula with the talus
  - Metallic tibial and talar components with unattached (3-component) or attached polyethylene insert (2-component), difficult to distinguish on imaging (Figure 46.22*A–C*)

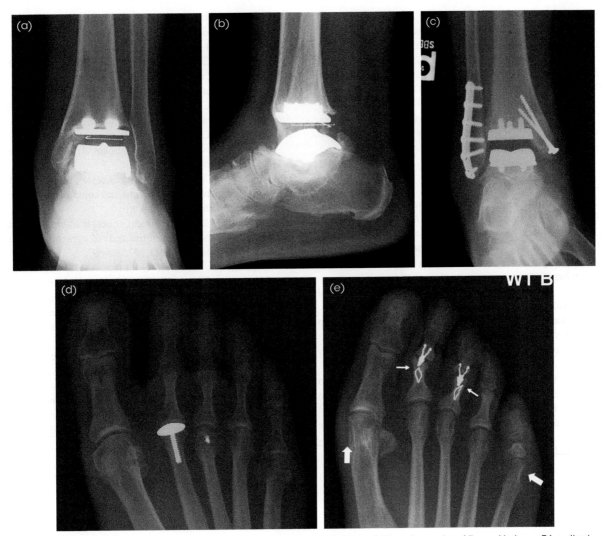

**Figure 46.22.** Ankle and toe joint replacement hardware (TAA). AP (*A*) and lateral (*B*) radiographs of the ankle in an RA patient with subtalar fusion show a normal 3-part TAA. There is an independent free-floating polyethylene liner meniscus that sits between anchored metallic tibial and talar components. (*C*) AP radiograph of a different patient with history of posttraumatic OA shows a 2-part TAA without evidence of hardware complication. This is a second-generation ankle prosthesis with the thick polyethylene weight-bearing surface incorporated either into the tibial or the talar component. Note healed lateral and medial malleolar fractures with intact surgical hardware. (*D*) Second toe MTP joint hemiarthroplasty with early loosening. AP radiograph of the forefoot shows a subtle periprosthetic lucency about the second metatarsal head prosthesis. Note a healed third metatarsal osteotomy site with a surgical anchor in place. (*E*) AP radiograph of the forefoot shows second and third toe Smart Toe implants with proximal fracture (*thin arrows*), third and fourth PIP joint resection arthroplasty, and bunionectomy and bunionettectomy defects (*thick arrows*) of the first and fifth metatarsal heads, respectively.

- Foot arthroplasty has poorer long-term outcomes than arthrodesis or joint resection (resection arthroplasty):
  - Early implants Silastic
  - First metatarsal resurfacing metal hemiarthroplasty less frequent and successful than arthrodesis (Figure 46.22*D*)
  - Interphalangeal joint implants (often Smart Toe) used for arthrodesis (Figure 46.22*E*)

**Complications**
- Aseptic loosening, especially in more active patients
- Early implants with silicone associated with particle disease, fragmentation, synovitis

**Key Points**
- Radiographs are sensitive in detecting findings of loosening, including lucency of more than 2 mm at the bone-cement or bone-prosthesis interface, hardware migration, and reactive bone changes.
- Distinguishing aseptic from infectious loosening often requires correlation with systemic inflammatory markers, joint fluid aspiration, and serial radiographic studies.
- Radiographs can detect particle disease, however, the damage caused by granulomas or pseudotumors are best evaluated with MRI using MARS.

## Recommended Reading

Taljanovic MS, Hunter TB, Miller MD, Sheppard JE. Gallery of medical devices: part 1: orthopedic devices for the extremities and pelvis. *Radiographics*. 2005;25:859–70.

Hunter TB, Taljanovic MS, Wild JR, eds. *Radiologic Guide to Orthopedic Devices*. Cambridge, UK: Cambridge University Press; 2017.

Medical Apparatus: Imaging Guide to Orthopedic Devices. New York, NY: Cambridge University Press; 2013. http://medapparatus.com/index.html.

## References

1. Department of Research & Scientific Affairs, American Academy of Orthopaedic Surgeons. Annual Incidence of Common Musculoskeletal Procedures and Treatment. www.aaos.org/research/stats/CommonProceduresTreatments-March2014.pdf. Published March 2014. Accessed November 2016.

2. Del Pozo JL, Patel R. Clinical practice. Infection associated with prosthetic joints. *N Engl J Med*. 2009;361:787–94.

3. Fritz J, Lurie B, Miller TT, Potter HG. MR imaging of hip arthroplasty implants. *Radiographics*. 2014;34:E106–32.

4. Fritz J, Lurie B, Potter HG. MR imaging of knee arthroplasty implants. *Radiographics*. 2015;35:1483–501.

5. Lin DJ, Wong TT, Kazam JK. Shoulder arthroplasty, from indications to complications: what the radiologist needs to know. *Radiographics*. 2016;36:192–208.

6. Love C, Tomas MB, Marwin SE, Pugliese PV, Palestro CJ. Role of nuclear medicine in diagnosis of the infected joint replacement. *Radiographics*. 2001;21:1229–38.

7. Mulcahy H, Chew FS. Current concepts in total ankle replacement for radiologists: complications. *AJR Am J Roentgenol*. 2015;205:1244–50.

8. Mulcahy H, Chew FS. Current concepts in total ankle replacement for radiologists: features and imaging assessment. *AJR Am J Roentgenol*. 2015;205:1038–47.

9. Mulcahy H, Chew FS. Current concepts in knee replacement: complications. *AJR Am J Roentgenol*. 2014;202:W76–86.

10. Mulcahy H, Chew FS. Current concepts in knee replacement: features and imaging assessment. *AJR Am J Roentgenol*. 2013;201:W828–42.

11. Mulcahy H, Chew FS. Current concepts of hip arthroplasty for radiologists: part 2, revisions and complications. *AJR Am J Roentgenol*. 2012;199:570–80.

12. Mulcahy H, Chew FS. Current concepts of hip arthroplasty for radiologists: part 1, features and radiographic assessment. *AJR Am J Roentgenol*. 2012;199:559–69.

13. Pedersen AB, Mehnert F, Sorensen HT, Emmeluth C, Overgaard S, Johnsen SP. The risk of venous thromboembolism, myocardial infarction, stroke, major bleeding and death in patients undergoing total hip and knee replacement: a 15-year retrospective cohort study of routine clinical practice. *Bone Joint J*. 2014;96-B:479–85.

14. Petscavage JM, Ha AS, Chew FS. Radiologic review of total elbow, radial head, and capitellar resurfacing arthroplasty. *Radiographics*. 2012;32:129–49.

15. Taljanovic MS, Hunter TB, Miller MD, Sheppard JE. Gallery of medical devices: part 1: orthopedic devices for the extremities and pelvis. *Radiographics*. 2005;25:859–70.

16. Nair R. Review article: total wrist arthroplasty. *J Ortho Surg*. 2014;22(3):399–405.

# CHAPTER 47

# Degenerative Spondylosis and Related Conditions

Kevin B. Hoover

## Introduction

Degenerative spondylosis is initiated primarily by intervertebral disc degeneration that results in progressive ligamentous laxity, facet OA, and progressive malalignment. Imaging within the first 6 weeks of back pain is rarely indicated except in instances where there is concern for an aggressive or malignant process, a significant neuromuscular deficit or other concerning *red flags*. Although imaging commonly begins with radiographs, MRI is the most sensitive technique to identify the potential causes of back pain. CT is appropriate in the posttraumatic setting when there is a high fracture risk. Conservative treatment of degenerative back pain is standard with surgery usually limited to patients with red flag signs or symptoms.

## Pathophysiology and Clinical Findings

*Degenerative spondylosis*, or simply *spondylosis*, is a general, loosely used term to describe the spectrum of articular and periarticular findings related to both normal aging and, potentially, pain. The joints and tissues that are involved are the intervertebral disc cartilage, the facet and costovertebral joints, the fibrous supporting ligaments, and the uncovertebral joints in the cervical spine. Intervertebral discs are composed of a central, hydrated nucleus pulposus surrounded by a fibrous envelope attached to adjacent endplates. Displacement of nuclear material (herniated nucleus pulposus) is associated with weakening (eg, bulge, protrusion) and tearing (eg, extrusion, sequestration) of the annulus fibrosus. The most common sites with spondylosis are C5-C7, T11-L1, and L4-S1.

Low back pain (LBP) is the second leading cause of disability worldwide. The lifetime prevalence of LBP is estimated to be 91% and neck pain 67%. In general, pain in spondylosis is associated with activities that increase axial load or stress to the intervertebral disc and facet joints. Referred pain in the extremities is commonly confused with joint-related pain. Clinical history, examination findings, and sometimes diagnostic injections, are essential in identifying, or excluding, the cause(s) of symptoms. Because of the frequency of LBP, imaging is often acquired in its evaluation.

The osseous findings of spondylosis detected on radiographs are not necessarily associated with pain. These degenerative findings increase with age, most precipitously after age 50, even in asymptomatic individuals. More commonly, it is intervertebral disc pathology that is a pain generator. Disc pathology is only indirectly visualized on radiographs and best seen on cross-sectional imaging. The findings of spondylosis on MRI also increase in frequency with age even in asymptomatic individuals. For example, only approximately one-third of asymptomatic patients have normal intervertebral discs on MRI. With aging, there is an increase in prevalence of disc bulges in asymptomatic patients from approximately 30% in 20-year-olds to 84% in 80-year-olds, with similar frequencies of age-related disc height loss. Even the prevalence of malalignment increases in asymptomatic patients from approximately 3% in 20-year-olds to 50% in 80-year-olds. Asymptomatic disc herniations and annular fissures also increase in prevalence with age.

## Imaging Strategy

Most back pain does not require imaging. Spine imaging is most useful in evaluation of concerning, red flag signs or symptoms (Table 47.1), which may require immediate intervention, and in preoperative planning. Radiographs are useful as an initial screen in these patients. CT is useful in evaluating patients with severe or suspected, radiographically occult, fractures. MRI examination is the test of choice in patients with concerning conditions using a spine coil. Standard MRI sequences are sagittal and axial T1W and T2W images, with STIR often added for better marrow evaluation. GRE sequences may be used in the cervical spine to help distinguish endplate osteophytes from disc material. Postcontrast T1W imaging is often obtained in the postsurgical setting to distinguish enhancing, postoperative granulation tissue (epidural fibrosis) from residual or recurrent intervertebral disc material, which rim enhances. Postcontrast imaging is also appropriate if there is concern for infection or malignancy.

## Imaging Findings

### Radiography
- Disc space narrowing (Figure 47.1)
  - Radiolucency, or vacuum phenomenon, is also indicative of disc degeneration.
- Endplate sclerosis (eburnation)
- Endplate osteophytes (Figure 47.1)
  - This is referred to as spondylosis deformans, especially hypertrophic anterior osteophytes.
- Uncovertebral joint osteophytes (cervical spine)

### Table 47.1. Red Flags for Complicated Back Pain

| RED FLAG | POTENTIAL CAUSE OF LBP |
|---|---|
| History of Cancer | Cancer or infection |
| Unexplained weight loss | Cancer or infection |
| Immunosuppression | Cancer or infection |
| Urinary infection | Infection |
| Intravenous drug use | Infection |
| Prolonged use of steroids | Fracture or infection |
| Back pain not improved with conservative management (usually >6 weeks) | |
| History of significant trauma | Fracture |
| Minor fall or heavy lift in the potentially osteoporotic or elderly | Fracture |
| Acute onset of urinary retention or overflow incontinence | Cauda equina syndrome or severe neurologic compromise |
| Loss of anal sphincter tone or fecal incontinence | Cauda equina syndrome or severe neurologic compromise |
| Saddle anesthesia | Cauda equina syndrome or severe neurologic compromise |
| Global or progressive motor weakness in lower extremities | Cauda equina syndrome or severe neurologic compromise |

- Calcification of the ALL
- Facet eburnation with joint narrowing or widening (Figure 47.1)
  - Intraarticular gas (vacuum phenomenon) is also indicative of facet OA.
- Alignment abnormalities
  - Loss or exaggeration of cervical and lumbar lordosis
  - Anterolisthesis (spondylolisthesis) or retrolisthesis (Figure 47.1)
    - This is described for the superior vertebra relative to the next inferior vertebra.
    - Anterolisthesis is commonly graded by percentage malalignment relative to the AP dimension of inferior vertebra:
      - Grade I, 25% or less
      - Grade II, 26-50%
      - Grade III, 51-75%
      - Grade IV, 76-100%
    - Retrolisthesis may be graded by the percentage narrowing of the intervertebral foramina (IVF) by dividing the anterior to posterior dimension into 4 equal units:
      - Grade I is 25% or less.
      - Grade II is 26-50%.
      - Grade III is 51-75%.
      - Grade IV is 76-100%.
      - Alternatively, a measurement (in millimeters) of the amount of displacement can be made.
    - This is related to disc, facet, and ligamentous degeneration (degenerative spondylolisthesis) or to pars interarticularis fracture (spondylolysis and isthmic spondylolisthesis).

- Segmental instability is abnormal motion of a specific vertebral segment:
  - Evaluated on neutral, flexion, and extension lateral radiographs
  - May be associated with degeneration above a fused vertebral segment (junctional syndrome, see Chapter 49, "Spinal Fixation Hardware")
- There is forward or backward displacement of contiguous vertebra relative to another by 4 mm or more.
  - Measurement very dependent on acquisition technique; should be used with caution
  - May be an indication for stabilization surgery
- Pathologic causes can be identified:
  - Fracture with height loss, linear lucencies, retropulsion into canal
    - Discussed in detail in Chapters 1-5 on spine trauma
  - Rapid disc height loss in subacute spondylodiscitis, endplate eburnation and erosion in chronic spondylodiscitis
    - Discussed in detail in Chapter 85, "Pyogenic Spondylodiscitis"
  - Lucent or sclerotic metastasis
    - Discussed in detail in Chapter 63, "Metastatic Disease"

### Computed Tomography

- Traumatic back pain is optimally evaluated to detect fractures.
- Degenerative findings are clearly identified without significant benefit over radiography despite higher radiation dose.
- Sequelae of intervertebral disc degeneration are now routinely evaluated by MRI rather than CT.

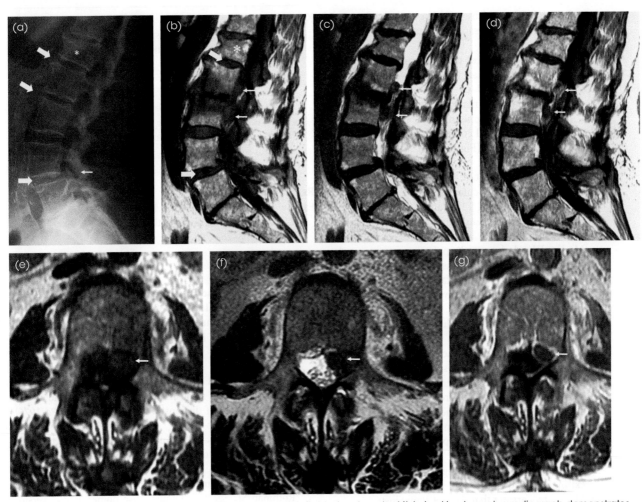

**Figure 47.1.** Severe spondylosis in a 76-year-old woman with left-sided groin pain. (*A*) Lateral lumbar spine radiograph demonstrates spondylosis with moderate compression fracture of the L1 vertebra (*asterisk*); grade I degenerative spondylolisthesis of L4 relative to L5 with facet eburnation and widening (*thin arrow*); severe L5-S1 disc degeneration; multilevel, small anterior endplate osteophytes; and vacuum disc phenomenon at L1-L2, L2-L3, and L4-L5 (*thick arrows*). (*B*) A sagittal T1W MR image demonstrates degenerative spondylolisthesis with areas of very low disc signal associated with vacuum phenomenon (*thick arrows*). Low T1 signal is evident at the L2-L3 disc margins (Modic I) and hyperintense signal at the anterior L4-L5 disc margins (Modic II). Isointense (to muscle) extruded intervertebral disc signal is seen within the spinal canal above and below the L2-L3 disc (*thin arrows*). Relatively normal marrow fat signal is seen within the fractured L1 vertebra consistent with a chronic, healed fracture (*asterisk*). (*C*) A sagittal T2W MR image demonstrates diffuse disc desiccation, severe canal stenosis at L4-L5 at the level of spondylolisthesis, and heterogeneous and hypointense extruded disc material within the spinal canal above and below the L2-L3 disc (*thin arrows*). Low signal at the disc margins at L2-L3 with adjacent high signal is consistent with Modic III and Modic I signal, respectively. Hyperintense signal is seen anteriorly at L4-L5 consistent with Modic II signal. (*D*) A sagittal T1W postcontrast MR image demonstrates rim enhancement of the disc material within the spinal canal above and below L2-L3 (*thin arrows*). (*E, F*) Axial T1W and T2W MR images demonstrate complete effacement of the L3 left lateral recess by low signal extruded disc material (*arrow*). (*G*) An axial T1W postcontrast MR image demonstrates rim enhancement of the extruded disc material (*arrow*). Neoplasm (eg, nerve sheath tumor) would be expected to enhance more diffusely. Greater paravertebral and bone inflammation would be expected with infection.

- CT myelography with intrathecal delivery of contrast is sometimes used:
  - Absence of passage of intrathecal contrast past a point of canal stenosis indicates spinal block.
  - Bony anatomy is optimally visualized for surgical planning.
  - In patients with contraindications to MRI, this is a useful modality.
- CT discography injects contrast into the disc:
  - Increasing injection pressure used to detect if specific symptoms are recreated
  - Now uncommonly used

**Magnetic Resonance Imaging**
- Degenerative disc disease (DDD) is associated with the following:
  - Desiccation or dehydration with loss of nucleus pulposus signal on fluid-sensitive sequences (Figure 47.1C)
  - Linear, fluid signal fissures in the annulus fibrosus
  - Vacuum phenomenon low in signal on all pulse sequences
  - Disc bulge if more than 50% of total circumference or herniation if less than 50% extension beyond vertebral endplate margins on axial images
    - Herniations are subcategorized:

- Protrusions—width of disc material beyond endplate less than the base in any imaging plane
- Extrusions—width of disc material beyond the endplate greater than the base in any imaging plane (Figure 47.1*B*–*G*)
  - Sequestration—herniated fragment that does not contact the originating disc
- Vertebral endplate signal commonly described using the Modic classification (Figure 47.1)
  - Modic I—low signal on T1WI, high signal on fluid-sensitive sequences
    - Represents fibrovascular tissue
  - Modic II—high signal T1WI and T2WI
    - Follows fat signal and represents fatty replacement of marrow
  - Modic III—dark on all pulse sequences and histologically represents dense, woven bone
  - Modic I and III signal associated with LBP
- Canal and IVF stenosis by osteophytes, disc herniations, and facet OA are evaluated:
  - Spinal canal stenosis is best evaluated on sagittal T2W images:
    - Increasing severity from effacement to obliteration of cerebrospinal fluid (CSF) signal
    - Compressive bunching of nerve roots
    - Mass effect on the spinal cord with caliber change and cord signal changes, including syrinx formation.
  - IVF stenosis is best evaluated on sagittal, T1W images in the thoracic and lumbar spines and axial T2W images in the cervical spine:
    - Mild—less than 50% of signal lost around the exiting nerve root
    - Moderate—greater than 50% of signal lost
    - Severe—complete loss of surrounding signal and nerve root compression
- Pathologic causes can also be identified including fracture, infection, and metastasis.

## Treatment Options

- Conservative management guided by physical therapist is the standard of care in acute back pain.
- Surgical decompression is superior to conservative management in patients with spinal stenosis with leg pain and disability.
- Acute disc herniations resulting in muscle weakness are often surgically managed.
- Selective facet and nerve root blocks using fluoroscopic guidance are helpful to establish the diagnosis of radicular or facet pain.
- Medial branch neurotomy using radiofrequency ablation (rhizotomy) may be considered in symptomatic facet degeneration.

## Key Points

- Imaging of degenerative spondylosis is complicated by the overlap of findings in symptomatic and asymptomatic individuals.
- Imaging is most useful in excluding red flag conditions such as fracture, tumor, and infection and routinely starts with radiographs.
- MRI is most useful in surgical candidates to identify the vertebral level of disease and severity of spinal canal and neural foraminal stenosis.

## Recommended Reading

Farshad-Amacker NA, Farshad M, Winklehner A, Andreisek G. MR imaging of degenerative disc disease. *Eur J Radiol.* 2015;84:1768–76.

## References

1. Bogduk N. Degenerative joint disease of the spine. *Radiol Clin North Am.* 2012;50:613–28.
2. Brinjikji W, Luetmer PH, Comstock B, et al. Systematic literature review of imaging features of spinal degeneration in asymptomatic populations. *AJNR Am J Neuroradiol.* 2015;36:811–16.
3. de Schepper EI, Overdevest GM, Suri P, et al. Diagnosis of lumbar spinal stenosis: an updated systematic review of the accuracy of diagnostic tests. *Spine (Phila Pa 1976).* 2013;38:E469–81.
4. Emch TM, Modic MT. Imaging of lumbar degenerative disk disease: history and current state. *Skeletal Radiol.* 2011;40:1175–89.
5. Fardon DF, Williams AL, Dohring EJ, Murtagh FR, Gabriel Rothman SL, Sze GK. Lumbar disc nomenclature: version 2.0: Recommendations of the combined task forces of the North American Spine Society, the American Society of Spine Radiology and the American Society of Neuroradiology. *Spine J.* 2014;14:2525–45.
6. Farshad-Amacker NA, Farshad M, Winklehner A, Andreisek G. MR imaging of degenerative disc disease. *Eur J Radiol.* 2015;84:1768–76.
7. Izzo R, Popolizio T, D'Aprile P, Muto M. Spinal pain. *Eur J Radiol.* 2015;84:746–56.
8. Jacobs WC, Rubinstein SM, Koes B, van Tulder MW, Peul WC. Evidence for surgery in degenerative lumbar spine disorders. *Best Pract Res Clin Rheumatol.* 2013;27:673–84.
9. Leone A, Guglielmi G, Cassar-Pullicino VN, Bonomo L. Lumbar intervertebral instability: a review. *Radiology.* 2007;245:62–77.
10. Patel ND, Broderick DF, Burns J, et al. ACR appropriateness criteria low back pain. *J Am Coll Radiol.* 2016;13:1069–78.

# CHAPTER 48

# Diffuse Idiopathic Skeletal Hyperostosis

Kevin B. Hoover

## Introduction

DISH is a condition characterized by ossification of entheses or the bony attachments of tendons, ligaments, and joint capsules. The diagnosis of DISH is based on spine radiographs that show flowing ossification along the margins of 4 contiguous vertebral bodies and typically with peripheral skeleton enthesopathy. Because the imaging findings of DISH can be confused with the seronegative spondyloarthropathies (SpA), familiarity with its imaging characteristics is useful to preclude unnecessary treatments. Rare cases of symptomatic dysphagia or difficulty breathing, spinal stenosis or fracture, and heterotopic ossification (HO) may require additional imaging evaluation and treatment.

## Pathophysiology and Clinical Findings

The soft tissue ossification of DISH is a condition with a prevalence as high as 42% in men older than age 65. It is preceded by tissue hypervascularity and chronic inflammatory cellular infiltration that is not detectable on imaging. In the spine, there is periosteal new bone formation of the anterior vertebral bodies, focal and diffuse calcification and ossification of the ALL, paraspinal connective tissue, and annulus fibrosus. It is associated with a number of medications and metabolic and constitutional disorders (Box 48.1). Most patients with DISH have no symptoms and are detected incidentally. Symptoms can be related to dysphagia, airway obstruction, and pain and morning stiffness of the thoracic spine. DISH is also associated with hypertrophic osteoarthritis with extensive bone proliferation and periprosthetic ossification after total hip arthroplasty (THA), symptomatic in up to 10% of patients.

## Imaging Strategy

Radiography of the spine is used for diagnosis. In patients with hypertrophic osteoarthritis being evaluated for THA, spine radiographs should be considered to look for DISH. This is because of the association of DISH with potentially debilitating HO after surgery and the availability of prophylactic treatment. In trauma or the rare cases of spinal stenosis, CT and MRI are useful in evaluation because of the propensity for fracture and for operative planning.

## Imaging Findings

### Radiography

- Spine radiographs with flowing ossification along the anterolateral margins of 4 or more contiguous vertebrae is diagnostic of DISH (Figure 48.1).
  - Ossification is limited to the right thoracic spine, likely caused by the inhibitory effect of the pulsating left-sided descending aorta (Figure 48.1B).
- Vertebral body bridging is frequently incomplete.
- Bone production is out of proportion to the minor degree of disc or joint degeneration, unlike spondylosis deformans.
  - Both may result in dysphagia because of esophageal impingement by bone.
- DISH is a rare cause of spinal stenosis because of ossification of the posterior longitudinal ligament (OPLL) and the ligamenta flava.
- Peripheral enthesopathy is common at the calcaneus, olecranon, or patellar entheses and the iliac wings (Figure 48.2).
- SpA, especially AS, also show enthesopathy and spine involvement.
  - SI joint and facet joint inflammation or ankylosis are the most specific findings to distinguish AS from DISH (Table 48.1).
  - Fusion of the costovertebral and facet joints is another distinguishing feature of AS from DISH.
- Spine fracture is an infrequent, important complication of chronic DISH (Figure 48.1D)
  - Less frequent than in AS because of normal bone mineral density
  - Most commonly from hyperextension of the cervical and thoracic spine
  - May result in a pseudoarthrosis at the fracture site
- Hypertrophic osteoarthritis with large marginal osteophytes and ossification of the capsular attachments relative to the severity of disease may be seen.
- HO of periprosthetic soft tissue after hip arthroplasty is also associated with DISH and may be debilitating.

### Magnetic Resonance Imaging

- MRI is not used commonly to diagnose or evaluate DISH, but is used to diagnose SpA (Table 48.1).
- Both DISH and AS may show the following:
  - Edema and ankylosis in the upper SI joints
  - Anterior vertebral corner edema or fat infiltration

**Box 48.1.** Conditions Associated with DISH

Metabolic syndrome and individual conditions: obesity, hypertension, glucose intolerance, hyperuricemia, hypercholesterolemia
Diabetes mellitus
Hypervitaminosis A
Retinoids (eg, isotretinoin, etretinate)

- MRI is optimal in evaluating the degree of spinal canal and cord involvement by fracture or OPLL.
  - GRE pulse sequence can be especially valuable in distinguishing ossification from herniated disc material.

## Computed Tomography
- CT is not routinely used to evaluate DISH.
- CT is superior to radiography to exclude SI joints and facet and costovertebral joint ankyloses seen in SpA.
  - Periarticular bridging heterotopic bone may be seen in DISH.
- OPLL or ligamenta flava ossification is easily detected.

## Treatment Options
- Treatment is rare.
- Surgical removal of anterior cervical spine ossifications may be required in cases of dysphagia.
- NSAID treatment for 2 weeks starting after THA can be used to prevent HO in patients with DISH.

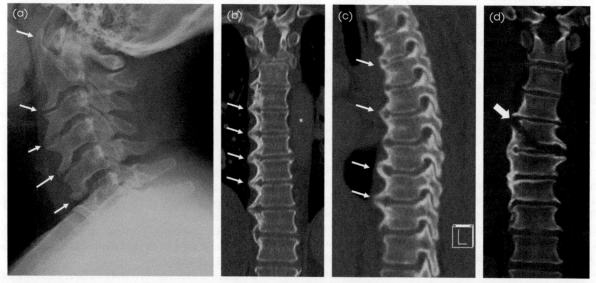

**Figure 48.1.** DISH of the cervical and thoracic spines. (*A*) AP of the cervical spine shows course anterior vertebral ossification (*thin arrows*) extending from the skull base distally with vertebral elongation, incomplete anterior fusion and normal facets. (*B*) Coronal and sagittal CT reformatted images of the thoracic spine show coarse anterior and asymmetric right-sided paraspinal ossifications with relative absence beneath the aorta (*asterisk*) in an obese patient. (*D*) Coronal CT reformatted image of the thoracic spine show an oblique fracture through the vertebral body in a patient with DISH (*thick arrow*).

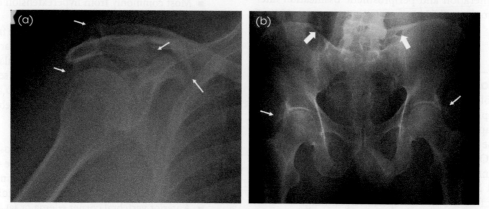

**Figure 48.2.** DISH in a 51-year-old patient chronically treated with retinoids for a skin condition (ichthyosis). (*A*) An internally rotated AP shoulder radiograph demonstrates hypertrophic ossification associated with the AC joint, the AC and coracoclavicular ligaments and subacromial spur. (*B*) AP radiograph of the pelvis demonstrates bilateral ossification of the iliolumbar ligaments (*thick arrows*) and the rectus femoris origins (*thin arrows*).

**Table 48.1. Distinguishing Characteristics of Diffuse Idiopathic Skeletal Hyperostosis and Ankylosing Spondylitis**

| LOCATION | DISH | AS |
|---|---|---|
| SIJ | ■ Anterior, juxtaarticular bridging of syndesmotic joint sometimes with edema (MRI)<br>■ Spares synovial joint | ■ Erosions<br>■ Periarticular sclerosis or edema<br>■ Synovial joint involvement<br>■ Osseous articular fusion |
| Facet joints | ■ Enthesophytes | ■ Erosions, fusion |
| Spine | ■ Course ossifications<br>■ Often incomplete bridging<br>■ Anterolateral, especially right side thoracic spine<br>■ Anterior vertebral body edema or fat (MRI) | ■ Thin syndesmophytes,<br>■ Ankylosis (bamboo spine)<br>■ Circumferential<br>■ Anterior vertebral body edema or fat signal (MRI) |
| Bone | ■ Normal bone mineral density | ■ Osteoporosis |
| Spine fracture | ■ Body (more common than AS) or intervertebral disc | ■ Intervertebral disc |

Abbreviations: AS, ankylosing spondylitis; DISH, diffuse idiopathic skeletal hyperostosis; MRI, magnetic resonance imaging; SIJ, sacroiliac joint.

■ Although conservative treatment is often adequate for spine fractures, surgical stabilization may be required for the rare displaced or unstable fractures.

**Key Points**
■ DISH is common, rarely symptomatic, and usually incidentally detected on radiographs.
■ Flowing osteophytes involving 4 or more vertebral levels in the absence of inflammatory findings are the principle diagnostic findings.
■ Fracture of ankylosed vertebrae, soft tissue impingement, and spinal stenosis caused by ligament ossification are rare.
■ MRI and CT are secondary imaging techniques most helpful in distinguishing DISH from SpA and evaluating spine fractures.

**Recommended Reading**
Taljanovic MS, Hunter TB, Wisneski RJ, et al. Imaging characteristics of diffuse idiopathic skeletal hyperostosis with an emphasis on acute spinal fractures: review. *AJR Am J Roentgenol.* 2009;193:S10–19, quiz S20-4.

**References**
1. Mader R, Novofestovski I, Adawi M, Lavi I. Metabolic syndrome and cardiovascular risk in patients with diffuse idiopathic skeletal hyperostosis. *Semin Arthritis Rheum.* 2009;38:361–65.
2. Mazieres B. Diffuse idiopathic skeletal hyperostosis (Forestier-Rotes-Querol disease): what's new? *Joint Bone Spine.* 2013;80:466–70.
3. Resnick D, Niwayama G. Radiographic and pathologic features of spinal involvement in diffuse idiopathic skeletal hyperostosis (DISH). *Radiology.* 1976;119:559–68.
4. Taljanovic MS, Hunter TB, Wisneski RJ, et al. Imaging characteristics of diffuse idiopathic skeletal hyperostosis with an emphasis on acute spinal fractures: review. *AJR Am J Roentgenol.* 2009;193:S10–19, quiz S20-4.
5. Weiss BG, Bachmann LM, Pfirrmann CW, Kissling RO, Zubler V. Whole body magnetic resonance imaging features in diffuse idiopathic skeletal hyperostosis in conjunction with clinical variables to whole body MRI and clinical variables in ankylosing spondylitis. *J Rheumatol.* 2016;43:335–42.

# CHAPTER 49

# Spinal Fixation Hardware

Kevin B. Hoover and Tim B. Hunter

## Introduction

The spine transmits axial load and facilitates restrained motion during flexion, extension, rotation, and lateral bending. A simplified structural model of the spine divides it into 3 columns: anterior, middle, and posterior (Table 49.1). Stability requires 2 of the 3 columns to be intact. Traumatic, neoplastic, infectious, or degenerative disruption of these columns and pain are indications for surgery. Spinal fusion is used to restore and maintain disc space height, decompress the spinal canal and neural foramina, maintain normal lordosis, and increase the stability of involved segments. Approximately, 1.2 million spine surgeries are performed annually in the United States. The materials commonly used include titanium and Vitallium (an alloy of cobalt, chromium, and molybdenum). Complications include failure of fusion, hardware loosening, injury caused by improper placement, junctional disease (disc degeneration and instability above or below the level of fusion), fracture, and infection.

## Imaging Strategy

Radiographs are routinely used for pre- and postoperative evaluation including AP, lateral, oblique, and flexion and extension lateral views. Bridging bony fusion mass should be detected on radiographs 6-9 months after surgery, and if absent, pseudoarthrosis is diagnosed. In junctional syndrome (disease), exaggerated motion above or below the level of solid fusion, or segmental instability, can be seen between flexion and extension. Evaluation of the cervicothoracic spine junction is limited on radiographs because of overlying structures, and CT may be required for evaluation. Noncontrast enhanced CT imaging with routine multiplanar reformations is optimal for assessing hardware placement and osseous anatomy. CT myelogram can be useful in evaluating intrathecal contents and complications, such as in arachnoiditis, especially if there are contraindications to MRI. MRI is ideal if there is a concern for postoperative complications not directly associated with hardware, such as new radiculopathy, leg pain, sensory changes, and motor weakness or infection. T1W and T2W sagittal and axial MR images without and with gadolinium are useful, especially with metal artifact reduction software (MARS) and sequences less susceptible to artifact (eg, STIR, FSE). Sagittal STIR sequences are optimal for evaluating marrow abnormality. Enhancing postsurgical scar (epidural fibrosis) that impinges on nerve roots can be distinguished from disc material, which does not enhance. Radionuclide bone scan, especially with single photon emission computed tomography (SPECT), with increased tracer uptake at a site of fusion may indicate pseudoarthrosis. Radionuclide white blood cell scans can be also be used for discitis.

## Cervical Spine Instrumentation

### Anterior and Posterior Plate and Screw Fixation

#### Indications

- Anterior plates for multilevel fusion
- Zero-profile device for single-level fusion
- Posterior fusion after trauma and posterior decompression for canal stenosis
- Screw fixation for unstable type II odontoid fractures or anterior displacement greater than 4 mm (Figure 49.1)
- Atlantoaxial instability with neurologic impairment

#### Imaging Findings

- Anterior plates most commonly with disc replacement—anterior cervical discectomy and fusion (ACDF) (Figure 49.2)
  - Anterior approach preferred to posterior primarily because of risk of spinal cord injury and small posterior element size
  - Anchor screws optimally positioned more than 2 mm from endplates and seated in posterior cortex
  - Zero-profile ACDF screws in bodies above and below disc replacement
    - May reduce postoperative dysphagia
- Posterior plates and rods less common than ACDF
  - Limit flexion and extension, including occipital-cervical fusion struts
  - Because of small pedicle size, lateral mass screws used at C3-C6, and pedicle screws used at C2, C7, and T1
- Anterior fixation of displaced odontoid fracture with compression screw and sometimes posterior wiring
- Atlantoaxial subluxation, often treated conservatively; may be posteriorly fused with rods and screws sometimes extending to the occiput (occipital strut)

#### Complications

- Nerve, cord, and dural injury
- Vertebral artery injury
- Postoperative dysphagia
- Fracture nonunion and pseudoarthrosis (Figures 49.1 and 49.2)

**Table 49.1. Anterior, Middle, and Posterior Columns of the Spine**

| COLUMN | COMPONENTS | FUNCTION |
|---|---|---|
| Anterior | ■ Anterior longitudinal ligament (ALL)<br>■ Anterior two-thirds of the vertebral body and annulus fibrosis | ■ Supports majority of the axial load<br>■ Resists extension |
| Middle | ■ Posterior third of the vertebral body and annulus fibrosus<br>■ Nucleus pulposus<br>■ Posterior longitudinal ligament (PLL) | ■ Supports axial load<br>■ Resist flexion |
| Posterior | ■ Pedicles<br>■ Facets<br>■ Ligamenta flava<br>■ Interspinous ligament<br>■ Supraspinous ligament | ■ Resist flexion<br>■ Stability during rotation and lateral bending |

### Interbody Fusion and Disc Replacement
### Indications
- Discectomy for myelopathy or radiculopathy
- Corpectomy for severe fractures and tumor

### Imaging Findings
- Interbody fusions after discectomy use
  - Autograft or allograft bone plug or strut (eg, rib, fibula) (Figure 49.2)
  - Radiolucent polyether ether ketone (PEEK) cage with radiopaque marker
    - May be part of zero-profile ACDF system
    - Without MRI artifact
  - Total disc replacements—metallic plates anchored to endplates with a synthetic core for motion and load absorption (Figure 49.3)

- Used at 1 or 2 cervical or lumbar levels, sometimes with posterior fusion
- Designed to maintain motion and decrease risk of junctional syndrome—disc degeneration and instability above or below the level of fusion
- Vertebral body replacements after corpectomy use
  - Hollow vertebral cages frequently made of titanium and generically called *titanium interbody spacers*
  - Filled with autograft or allograft bone
  - May be expandable to restore vertebral body height (Figure 49.4)

### Complications
- Nonunion
- Migration
- Infection
- Junctional disease
- Particle disease after total disc replacement

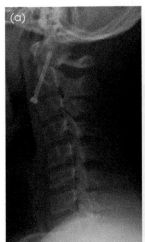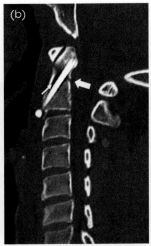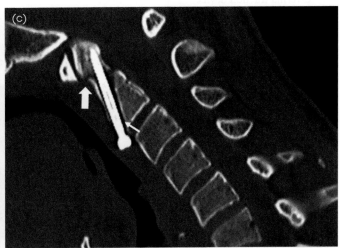

**Figure 49.1.** Odontoid screw placement for type II odontoid fracture. (*A*) Lateral radiograph of the cervical spine shows an odontoid screw transfixing a type II odontoid fracture without evidence for loosening. (*B*) Sagittal reformatted CT image obtained in extension shows a lucency through the well-aligned odontoid fracture (*thick arrow*) and about the screw (*thin arrow*) without bridging bone or callus. (*C*) Sagittal reformatted CT image in flexion shows more obvious lucency about the screw (*thin arrow*) and mild displacement of the fracture site (*thick arrow*) consistent with fracture nonunion and hardware loosening.

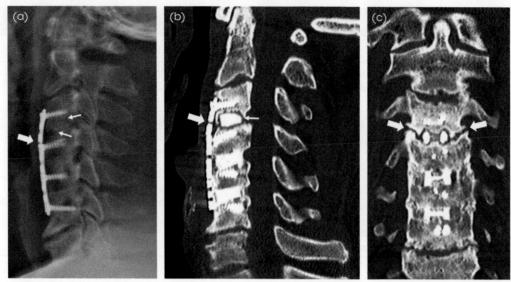

**Figure 49.2.** C3-C6 ACDF with hardware failure. (*A*) Lateral radiograph of the cervical spine demonstrates subtle lucency extending through the anterior plate just inferior to the C3-C4 disc level (*thick arrow*) with additional subtle lucency about the interbody graft (*thin arrows*). (*B*) Sagittal reformatted CT image shows subtle offset of the plate at the site of fracture (*thick arrow*) and lucency around the C3-C4 interbody graft (*thin arrow*). (*C*) Coronal reformatted CT image shows pseudoarthrosis through the C3-C4 level (*thick arrows*).

### External Fixation
### Indications

- Limit motion
- Halos and tongs for upper cervical spine stabilization:
  - Stable C2 fracture, including nondisplaced type II odontoid fracture
  - Occipital condyle fractures
  - Occipitocervical dislocation
- Support instrumented cervical fusion

### Imaging Findings

- Translucent hard (plastic) collars—support chin and occiput and limit motion
- Cranial tongs—pins inserted into skull connected to an external traction device
- Halo vest—metallic ring attached to skull by screws and to translucent thoracic cast by rods to support head

### Complications

- Screw and tong loosening, most common, may be associated with loss of reduction and alignment.
- Infection can occur.

### Thoracic and Lumbar Spine Instrumentation
### Indications

- Stabilizing or treating painful kyphosis or scoliosis
- Trauma
- Congenital or degenerative stenosis
- Developmental, such as dysraphisms
- Multiple column reconstruction, especially posterior lumbar instrumented fusion (PLIF)
- Primary or metastatic neoplastic disease, especially anterior lumbar interbody fusion (ALIF)
- Spinous process distraction and fusion for position dependent spinal claudication

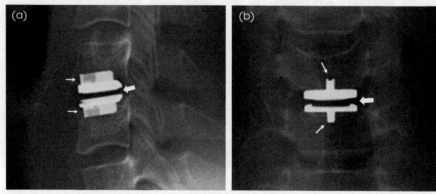

**Figure 49.3.** Cervical disc replacement. Lateral (*A*) and AP (*B*) radiographs of the cervical spine show C5-C6 disc replacement (Synthes Spine ProDisc) with lucent polyethylene ball (*thick arrows*) between endplates fixed to underlying bone with central keels (*thin arrows*).

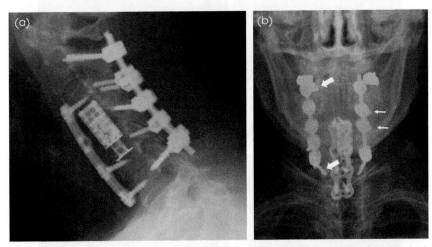

**Figure 49.4.** ACDF, posterior cervical fusion, and titanium cage hardware. (*A*) Lateral radiograph of the cervical spine shows C3-C6 ACDF with an expandable titanium cage extending through the C4 corpectomy site and into the C3 and C5 vertebrae with posterior fusion C2-C6. (*B*) AP radiograph shows medially directed pedicle screws at C2 and C6 (*thick arrows*) with laterally positioned lateral mass screws C3-C5 (*thin arrows*).

- Painful osteoporotic or pathologic vertebral fractures (kyphoplasty, vertebroplasty)

**Imaging Findings**
- Posterior pedicle screws and rods (Figures 49.5-49.9)
  - Screws extend through the pedicles into the vertebral body connected by rods or plates on each side.
  - Bone from the iliac crest(s) are packed around fusion hardware:
    - Solid bone fusion is required for stability or hardware failure will result.
  - Hardware is placed prior to laminectomy or discectomy to stabilize, maximally distract disc space, and decompress the neural foramina.

- This is a simpler and safer approach in thoracic and lumbar spine than an anterior approach.
- Posterior stabilization rod placed for scoliosis with laminar hooks (Figure 49.10). The distraction or compression is used to treat marked adolescent scoliosis, congenital scoliosis, and other severe congenital or developmental deformities.
  - Hooks below lamina distract concave side of curve.
  - Hooks above lamina compress convex side of curve.
- Less common techniques include the following:
  - Anterior approach complete discectomy and interbody fusion— ALIF (Figure 49.7A, B).
    - Over 1-3 levels
    - Less common than in cervical spine
    - Often with zero-profile system and PEEK cages

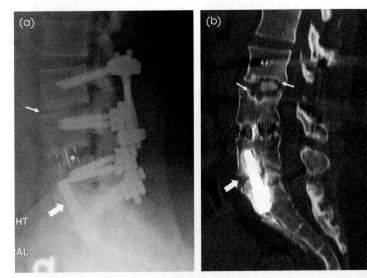

**Figure 49.5.** PLIF and AxiaLIF hardware with intervertebral cage failure at the L3-L4 level. (*A*) Lateral radiograph of the lumbar spine shows L2-S1 posterior fusion with lumbosacral fixation screw (*thick arrow*) and faint cage material seen at the posteriorly subluxated L3-L4 level (*thin arrow*). Note intact PEEK cage at the L4-L5 level (*asterisk*). (*B*) Sagittal reformat CT image shows lucency about the L3-L4 disc graft with eburnation and erosion of the adjacent endplates consistent with pseudoarthrosis (*thin arrows*). Incomplete fusion is noted at the L5-S1 level, as well, with lucency through the disc level (*thick arrow*).

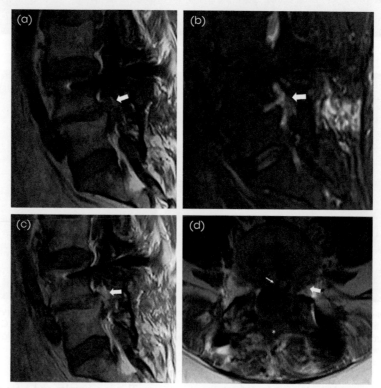

**Figure 49.6.** Subluxated lumbar intervertebral cage and epidural fibrosis causing lateral recess stenosis. (*A-C*) Sagittal T1W (*A*), STIR (*B*), T1W postcontrast (*C*) MR images of the lumbar spine show neural foraminal narrowing by enhancing heterogeneous tissue consistent with epidural fibrosis (*thick arrows*). (*D*) An axial T1WI postcontrast MR image shows narrowing of the spinal canal and left neural foramen by extruded graft material (*thin arrow*) with surrounding enhancing epidural fibrosis tissue (*thick arrow*). A dorsal laminectomy defect is also evident (*asterisk*).

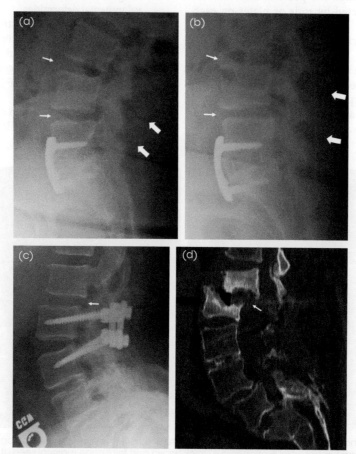

**Figure 49.7.** Early and late changes of junctional disease. (*A*) Extension and (*B*) flexion lateral radiographs in a L5-S1 ALIF patient show relative narrowing of the L4-L5 and L3-L4 disc spaces in flexion above the level of fusion (*thin arrows*) with interspinous distance widening (*thick arrows*) suggestive of exaggerated motion. (*C*) A lateral radiograph of a different patient shows L1-L5 posterior decompression and L2-L3 instrumented fusion with posterior subluxation of L1-L2 (*thin arrow*) and to a lesser extent at L2-L3. (*D*) Sagittal reformatted CT image 3 years later shows severe junctional disease with pseudoarthrosis with vacuum phenomenon, extensive sclerosis, and irregularity of the L1 and L2 vertebral endplates with progressive retrolisthesis (*thin arrow*).

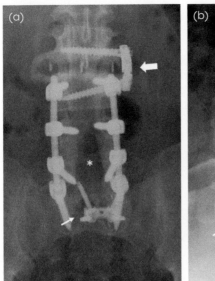
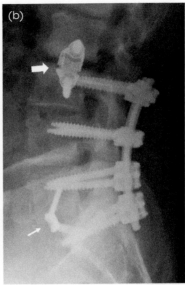

**Figure 49.8.** PLIF, ALIF, and XLIF hardware. (*A*) AP and (*B*) lateral radiographs of the lumbar spine show laminectomy defect consistent with posterior decompression (*asterisk*) and instrumented fusion L3-L5, lateral fusion L2-L3 with a PEEK cage (*thick arrow*), and zero-profile anterior fusion L5-S1 with a PEEK cage (*thin arrow*). There is no radiographic evidence of hardware complications.

- Lateral approach with cage placement and lateral fixation—extreme lateral interbody fusion (XLIF) (Figure 49.8)
  - Retroperitoneal approach through psoas muscle may have less risk of bowel or vascular injury.
- Anterior lumbosacral (L5-S1) fusion with percutaneous discectomy, bone graft placement, and titanium screw (pin) placement—axial lumbar interbody fusion (AxiaLIF)
- Often with posterior pedicle screw stabilization
- Spinous process distraction and fusion
  - Interlaminar lumbar instrumented fusion (ILIF) and interspinous spacers

- ILIF—partial laminectomy (laminotomy), bone graft, and posterior stabilization hardware with or without interbody graft placement
- Interspinous distracting spacers to prevent extension (Figure 49.9).
- Localized lumbar flexion by lumbar spinous process distraction for locally increasing spinal canal diameter and neural foraminal size
- Interbody fusion and disc replacement constructs, as in the cervical spine
- Vertebral augmentation with cement alone (vertebroplasty) or after cavity creation with a balloon (kyphoplasty)
  - Kyphoplasty may increase body height.

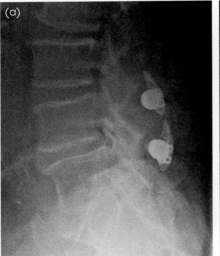
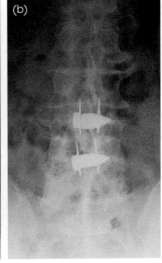

**Figure 49.9.** Interspinous distracting spacers. Lateral (*A*) and AP (*B*) radiographs of the lumbar spine show normal positioning of the interspinous distracting spacers at the L3-L4 and L4-L5 levels without evidence of complications.

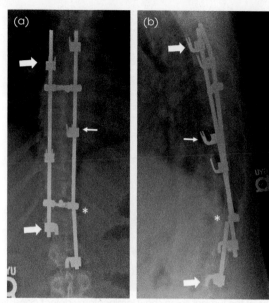

**Figure 49.10.** Distracting stabilization rod failure. (*A*) AP radiograph of the thoracolumbar spine shows paired bilateral posterior thoracolumbar stabilization rods with distracting hooks (*thick arrows*) at T6 and L1 on the right and T5 and L2 on the left with compressive hooks (*thin arrow*) at T10 on the right and T9 on the left. Subtle medial angulation of the left rod is seen at the level of the T12-L1 cross bar (*asterisk*). (*B*) Lateral radiograph shows angulation and displacement of the fractured left sided rod at the thoracolumbar junction (*asterisk*).

- Cylindrical, coiled implants filled with cement have been recently approved.

## Complications

- Intraoperative vascular and bowel injury (ALIF, AxiaLIF, pedicle screw placement)
- Nerve root irritation
- Junctional syndrome (Figure 49.7)
- Infection
- Hematoma
- Neural stretching with paresthesia and radiculopathy, especially XLIF
- Postsurgical scarring and arachnoiditis (Figure 49.6)
- Straightened lumbar lordosis with pain
- Adjacent segment fracture after vertebral augmentation
- Cement extravasation symptoms depending on location (rare)

## Key Points

- Spinal fusion is used to restore and maintain disc space height, decompress the spinal canal and neural foramina, maintain normal lordosis, and increase the stability of involved segments. Failure of fusion results in spinal instability.
- Successful fusion results in added stress to levels above and below fusion that can lead to junctional disease.
- Although postsurgical patients are routinely imaged by radiographs, cross-sectional imaging is important for identified hardware (CT) and soft tissue complications (MRI).

## Recommended Reading

Ha AS, Petscavage-Thomas JM. Imaging of current spinal hardware: lumbar spine. *AJR Am J Roentgenol.* 2014;203:573–81.

Petscavage-Thomas JM, Ha AS. Imaging current spine hardware: part 1, cervical spine and fracture fixation. *AJR Am J Roentgenol.* 2014;203:394–405.

Hunter TB, Taljanovic MS, Wild JR, eds. *Radiologic Guide to Orthopedic Devices.* Cambridge, UK: Cambridge University Press; 2017.

Medical Apparatus: Imaging guide to orthopedic devices. New York, NY: Cambridge University Press; 2013. http://medapparatus.com/index.html.

## References

1. Ha AS, Petscavage-Thomas JM. Imaging of current spinal hardware: lumbar spine. *AJR Am J Roentgenol.* 2014;203:573–81.
2. Hayashi D, Roemer FW, Mian A, Gharaibeh M, Muller B, Guermazi A. Imaging features of postoperative complications after spinal surgery and instrumentation. *AJR Am J Roentgenol.* 2012;199:W123–29.
3. Murtagh RD, Quencer RM, Castellvi AE, Yue JJ. New techniques in lumbar spinal instrumentation: what the radiologist needs to know. *Radiology.* 2011;260:317–30.
4. Petscavage-Thomas JM, Ha AS. Imaging current spine hardware: part 1, cervical spine and fracture fixation. *AJR Am J Roentgenol.* 2014;203:394–405.
5. Young PM, Berquist TH, Bancroft LW, Peterson JJ. Complications of spinal instrumentation. *Radiographics.* 2007;27:775–89.

# 5

Miscellaneous

# CHAPTER 50

# Sarcoidosis

Kevin B. Hoover

## Introduction

Sarcoidosis is a disease of noncaseating granuloma infiltration into a wide variety of tissues, including the musculoskeletal system. Hand radiographs can demonstrate a nearly pathognomonic lacelike appearance of one or multiple phalanges. Both CT and MRI can detect bone and soft tissue involvement that has a nonspecific appearance resembling metastatic disease. Correlation with imaging of the chest is valuable, because musculoskeletal sarcoidosis usually follows pulmonary disease.

## Pathophysiology and Clinical Findings

The organ systems most commonly involved in sarcoid are the lungs, lymph nodes, skin, and eyes. The musculoskeletal system is less commonly involved with a reported bone lesion incidence of 5% based on radiographs. Of those patients with bone involvement, 80-90% also have pulmonary sarcoid. Symptomatic muscle involvement is reported in an estimated 1.4% of sarcoid patients, however, muscle biopsy identifies noncaseating granulomas in 50-80% of patients. Cutaneous involvement is detected in approximately 25% of patients. Joint and tendon involvement is seen in Lofgren syndrome, which is a self-limiting condition consisting of fever, arthralgias (most commonly of the ankles), hilar lymph node enlargement, and erythema nodosum (tender nodules along the anterior lower extremity). Lofgren syndrome is associated with elevated inflammatory cytokine levels. However, there are no specific serologic markers for sarcoidosis. Nonspecific serologic findings include elevated vitamin D levels from production by granulomas, elevated parathyroid hormone from renal failure (secondary hyperparathyroidism), rheumatoid factor in up to half of patients, and elevated creatine kinase and aldolase levels in sarcoid myopathy patients. Tissue biopsy is often required to identify noncaseating granulomas, which are diagnostic.

## Imaging Strategy

Radiographs are the standard first study used to evaluate symptomatic hand or foot involvement. Uncommon, palpable soft tissue lesions are best evaluated by MRI. Although long or large bone osseous involvement may be detected on CT, it is often an incidental finding on studies performed for other reasons. Further characterization of musculoskeletal sarcoidosis by MRI may be useful to identify benign findings such as intralesional fat or fibrosis. Image-guided biopsy, however, is often necessary for diagnosis.

## Imaging Findings

### Radiography

- Hand radiographs detect involvement of the phalanges, which is the most common site of bone involvement (Figure 50.1):
  - Lacelike, lytic involvement of the phalanges of the hands and feet is nearly pathognomonic.
  - Phalanges may become more tubular and suffer from pathologic fractures.
  - If the distal phalanges are involved, acroosteolysis may be mimicked.
- Long bone lesions are less common:
  - Lesions may be occult, lytic, sclerotic, or mixed in appearance.
- Joint and soft tissue involvement is often radiographically occult:
  - Soft tissue swelling, such as dactylitis, may be demonstrated, and subchondral cystlike lesions or erosions are better seen by MRI.
- Osteoporosis and ON may be present secondary to chronic steroid treatment.
- Radiographic skeletal surveys are not useful for detecting diffuse bone involvement.

### Computed Tomography

- CT findings are similar to radiographs.
- Bone lesions may not be visible, and may be lytic, sclerotic, or mixed in appearance.
  - May be detected incidentally on CT scans acquired for unrelated indications
- CT is often used for image-guided bone biopsy.

### Magnetic Resonance Imaging

- MRI is the most sensitive modality to detect musculoskeletal sarcoid.
- Often multiple bone lesions have nonspecific imaging characteristics resembling metastatic disease or multiple myeloma (Figure 50.2):
  - Bone lesions are commonly homogeneously hypointense to muscle on T1W images, hyperintense on fluid-sensitive sequences with postcontrast enhancement.
  - Chronic lesions may be replaced by fat or fibrosis with areas of T1 hyperintensity or hypointensity, respectively.
  - Margins may be poorly defined, sharp, or irregular and brushlike.

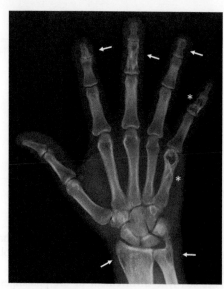

**Figure 50.1.** Sarcoidosis. A 42-year-old man with sarcoid involvement of the hand. PA radiograph of the hand demonstrates lucencies within the distal radius and ulna, metacarpals, and distal phalanges with a sclerotic, remodeled appearance (*thin arrows*). Fifth metacarpal and fifth middle phalanx deformities also suggest healed pathologic fractures (*asterisks*). Soft tissue swelling about the distal second through fifth digits is consistent with soft tissue sarcoid infiltration.

- Cortical involvement is uncommon with large bone lesions.
- In the phalanges, granulomas may extend beyond the cortices with soft tissue involvement that can present as dactylitis.
- Tendon involvement may result in thickening and intermediate to hyperintense signal on fluid-sensitive sequences.

- Tenosynovitis with fluid signal within tendon sheaths may be present.
- Bursitis and joint synovitis may be detected.
- Muscle involvement is common with a variable, nonspecific appearance:
  - Muscle involvement more commonly involves the proximal lower extremities.
  - Multiple muscle nodules may be present and often oriented longitudinally along the myotendinous junction.
    - Central fibrotic area with low signal on all pulse sequences without enhancement is characteristic
    - Surrounded by T2 hyperintense, enhancing granulomatous material
    - Possible negative MRI because of small granuloma size
  - More diffuse involvement may be occult on MRI and resemble polymyositis or steroid myopathy (Figure 50.3):
    - Acutely may show nonspecific, diffuse fluid signal and enhancement.
    - Chronic myositis may show diffuse fatty atrophy.
      - Muscle biopsy may be required to distinguish this from steroid myopathy.
- Subcutaneous, skin and soft tissue masses with lymphadenopathy may be detected.
  - Lesions may be discrete and nodular or indistinct.
  - Signal characteristics are nonspecific—low on T1W images, high on fluid-sensitive sequences with enhancement on the postcontrast sequences.

**Nuclear Medicine**
- Nuclear medicine is not commonly used for evaluation of musculoskeletal sarcoid.
  - Gallium scintigraphy shows uptake along muscle fibers in nodular type, similar to myositis, tuberculous granulomas and lymphoma.

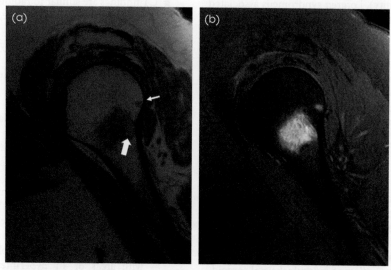

**Figure 50.2.** Osseous sarcoid. A 67-year-old woman with sarcoidosis and right arm pain with a site of osseous sarcoid involvement. (*A*) Sagittal T1W MR image demonstrates a well-circumscribed low signal metaphyseal lesions with areas of hyperintense signal (relative to muscle) consistent with intralesional fat (*thick arrow*). Note an additional small sarcoid lesion with similar signal characteristics at the posterior aspect of the humeral head (*thin arrow*). (*B*) Sagittal STIR MR image demonstrates hyperintense, nonspecific fluid signal in the same lesions. The lesions were occult on radiographs and CT (*not shown*).

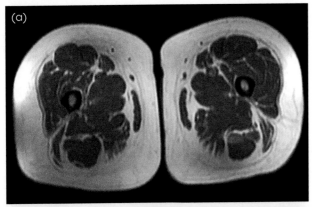

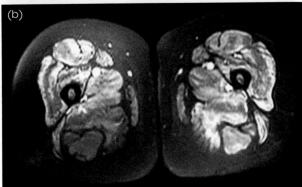

**Figure 50.3.** Sarcoid myopathy. A 51-year-old man with chronic sarcoidosis, on steroids with diffuse myopathy. (*A*) Axial T1W MR image of the bilateral thighs demonstrates normal signal characteristics and absence of fatty muscle atrophy. (*B*) Axial T2W FS MR image of the same region demonstrates diffuse, symmetric muscle edema. The signal abnormality is nonspecific and biopsy identified the noncaseating granulomas of sarcoid.

- Chronic myopathy may have diffuse uptake proportional to degree of active inflammation.
- In positron emission tomography (PET) acquired for other reasons, multifocal skeletal sarcoidosis may be false positive for metastasis on PET.

## Treatment Options

- Systemic corticosteroids are the primary treatment of active sarcoidosis.
- Methotrexate is also effective in acute arthritis or myositis.

## Key Points

- Musculoskeletal sarcoid occurs most commonly in the setting of pulmonary sarcoid.
- The lacelike radiographic appearance of phalangeal sarcoid is nearly pathognomonic.
- Sarcoid of the large and long bones and muscle has a nonspecific appearance that frequently requires biopsy to diagnose.
- Osteoporosis and ON may be detected and caused by chronic steroid use.

### Recommended Reading

Moore SL, Teirstein AE. Musculoskeletal sarcoidosis: spectrum of appearances at MR imaging. *Radiographics*. 2003;23:1389–99.

### References

1. Chatham W. Rheumatic manifestations of systemic disease: sarcoidosis. *Curr Opin Rheumatol*. 2010;22:85–90.
2. Guidry C, Fricke RG, Ram R, Pandey T, Jambhekar K. Imaging of sarcoidosis: a contemporary review. *Radiol Clin North Am*. 2016;54:519–34.
3. Moore SL, Kransdorf MJ, Schweitzer ME, Murphey MD, Babb JS. Can sarcoidosis and metastatic bone lesions be reliably differentiated on routine MRI? *AJR Am J Roentgenol*. 2012;198:1387–93.
4. Moore SL, Teirstein AE. Musculoskeletal sarcoidosis: spectrum of appearances at MR imaging. *Radiographics*. 2003;23:1389–99.
5. Otake S, Ishigaki T. Muscular sarcoidosis. *Semin Musculoskelet Radiol*. 2001;5:167–70.
6. Vardhanabhuti V, Venkatanarasimha N, Bhatnagar G, et al. Extra-pulmonary manifestations of sarcoidosis. *Clin Radiol*. 2012;67:263–76.

# CHAPTER 51

# Amyloidosis

Kevin B. Hoover

## Introduction

Amyloidosis is a group of rare, systemic diseases resulting in osseous, articular and other soft tissue protein deposition. These diseases are categorized as hereditary, reactive, dialysis-related, and immunoglobulin light chain and may show localized or systemic involvement. Imaging is often acquired because of the primary medical condition and symptoms (eg, RA). Although the imaging findings are often nonspecific, the most characteristic finding is abnormal tissue that is dark on all pulse sequences on MRI (Figure 51.1).

## Pathophysiology and Clinical Findings

Amyloidosis is rare with a prevalence estimated at 3-10 cases per million people. The most common type of amyloidosis in developed countries is amyloid light chain amyloidosis (AL), which is seen predominantly in male patients and associated with malignancies, such as multiple myeloma and B-cell lymphoma. Rheumatologic symptoms are the dominant feature in only approximately 9% of AL cases and mimic RA. The *shoulder pad* sign with soft tissue enlargement of the shoulder is characteristic. The most common cause in developing countries is amyloid A (AA) or reactive amyloidosis, secondary to chronic inflammatory conditions of which 70% are rheumatologic, such as RA, AS, psoriatic arthritis, and juvenile idiopathic arthritis. AA amyloidosis less commonly involves the musculoskeletal system. A less common type, dialysis-related amyloidosis (A beta-2 microglobulin [A$\beta$2M]), preferentially involves the musculoskeletal system. Carpal tunnel syndrome and arthropathy mimicking RA are common manifestations of A$\beta$2M. There are a large number of hereditary, autosomal dominant genetic causes most commonly associated with mutation of the TTR (transthyretin) gene. These are associated with neuropathic arthropathy of the lower extremity.

Cardiac involvement is the most common cause of morbidity and mortality in amyloidosis. Carpal tunnel syndrome is the most common indication for surgery. Intramuscular amyloid is rare, except in AL cases, where macroglossia may develop. There are no specific serologic markers of amyloidosis and tissue diagnosis is routinely required. Typically, the subcutaneous abdominal fat tissue is biopsied. However, fat biopsy is usually negative in A$\beta$2M, and synovial biopsy is required instead (Figure 51.2).

## Imaging Strategy

Imaging of the musculoskeletal system is not a standard part of patient workup for amyloidosis. When performed to evaluate the symptomatic patient, radiographic and CT imaging findings of joint involvement (amyloid arthropathy), localized bone or soft tissue involvement (amyloidoma), and diffuse muscle involvement (amyloid myopathy) are nonspecific. MRI may be used to better evaluate articular involvement and may demonstrate low signal amyloid tissue on all pulse sequences without blooming artifact. US is sometimes used to evaluate the shoulder and guide diagnostic biopsy of abnormal tissue. MRI and US (echocardiography) are commonly used for the imaging of cardiac involvement (not discussed).

## Imaging Findings

### Radiography

- Amyloid arthropathy—periarticular lucencies and erosions of variable size involving multiple joints with thin sclerotic margins, resembling RA, are visualized:
  - Associated with joint subluxations, destruction, and contractures
  - Most commonly involves the hips, wrist, shoulders, knees, and spine
- Bone involvement is often periarticular and resembles multiple myeloma, metastasis, and Brown tumors:
  - Pathologic fracture may result.
- Radiography underestimates the extent of disease, which is more accurately determined by CT or MRI.

### Computed Tomography

- Lucencies and erosions of amyloid arthropathy are detected.
- Spondyloarthropathy with vertebral osteolysis, erosions, and disc space narrowing is identified:
  - Associated with A$\beta$2M amyloid
  - Difficult to distinguish from infection (spondylodiscitis)
  - Better evaluated by CT than radiography
- Amyloidomas in bone or soft tissue are more common in AL amyloidosis.
  - Soft tissue lesions often calcify and rarely occur in the extremities.
  - Bone lesions are often lytic and polyostotic without a calcified matrix.

### Magnetic Resonance Imaging

- Amyloid arthropathy can resemble pigmented villonodular synovitis (PVNS), hemophilia, gout, tuberculosis, RA, and synovial chondromatosis.

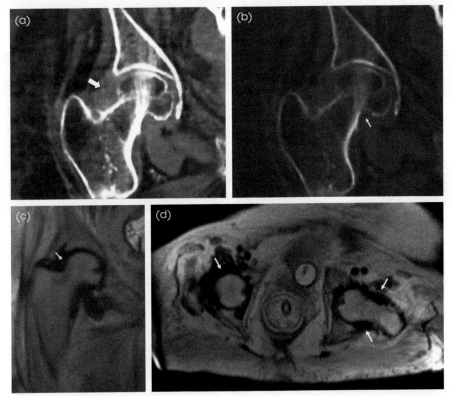

**Figure 51.1.** Amyloidosis. Amyloidosis of the hips. (*A, B*) Coronal reformatted CT images show nonspecific soft tissue density (*thick arrow*) within the right hip joint (*A*) with an eroded (*thin arrow*) and attenuated appearance of the femoral neck (*B*). Coronal (*C*) and axial (*D*) T2W MR images demonstrate low signal tissue within the hip joints, consistent with amyloid (*thin arrows*).

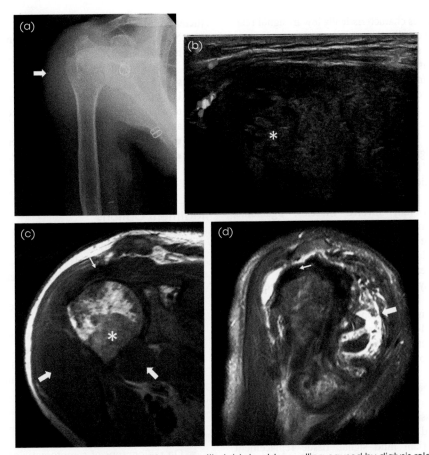

**Figure 51.2.** Dialysis-related amyloidosis. A 76-year-old woman with right shoulder swelling caused by dialysis-related Aβ2M amyloid. (*A*) AP radiograph of the shoulder demonstrates soft tissue swelling overlying the shoulder: shoulder pad sign (*thick arrow*). (*B*) Prebiopsy color Doppler US image demonstrates hypovascular debris with heterogeneous echotexture (*asterisk*). (*C*) Coronal T1W MR image demonstrates hypo- to isointense signal about the shoulder (*thick arrows*) with hypointense signal within the distal rotator cuff (*thin arrow*). Note red marrow reconversion of the metaphysis (*asterisk*) and subarticular epiphysis. (*D*) Sagittal T2W MR image demonstrates low signal within the distal rotator cuff (*thin arrow*) with hypointense debris within a complex fluid collection in the subacromial-subdeltoid bursa overlying the shoulder (*thick arrow*).

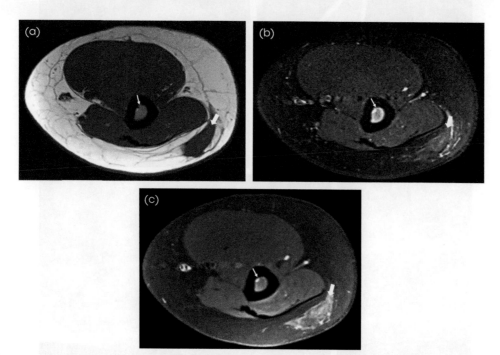

**Figure 51.3.** Idiopathic amyloidosis. A 39-year-old woman with type 1 diabetes with idiopathic amyloidosis. (*A*) Axial T1W, (*B*) T2W FS, and (*C*) postcontrast T1W FS MR images of the arm demonstrates an irregularly contoured mass in the posterolateral subcutaneous tissue (*thick arrow*), which is primarily isointense to muscle (*A, B*) and demonstrates mild enhancement (*C*). Note marrow reconversion (*thin arrows*). Biopsy demonstrated amyloid and the possibility of insulin injection-related deposition was suggested.

- Amyloid tissue is characteristically low in signal relative to muscle on all pulse sequences.
- Appearance is similar to PVNS and hemophilia, however, no hemosiderin or blooming artifact is detected on GRE sequences.
- Amyloid arthropathy is polyarticular.
- Bone amyloidomas are indistinguishable from other polyostotic processes, such as multiple myeloma and metastasis:
  - Shows low signal on T1W sequences, low to high signal on T2W sequences, and moderate enhancement
- Soft tissue amyloid of the musculoskeletal system, which is not articular, is rare:
  - Amyloidomas may involve muscles, ligaments, tendons, fat, and nerves.
  - It is isointense to muscle on T1W images, heterogeneous on fluid-sensitive sequences with heterogeneous enhancement.
  - Myopathy may not be detectable on MRI, requiring biopsy.
  - Fat involvement shows nonspecific reticular signal on T1W and fluid-sensitive sequences.
  - Nerve involvement may result in diffuse enlargement, T2 hyperintensity with variable degrees of enhancement.
- Spondyloarthropathy most often involves the cervical spine.
  - Low signal tissue involves intervertebral discs, facets, synovium, and ligamenta flava.
  - Low, rather than fluid signal, tissue replacement helps distinguish from spondylodiscitis and infection (Figure 51.3).

**Nuclear Medicine**
- Not commonly used in evaluation of amyloid outside highly specialized clinical centers

**Ultrasound**
- US of the shoulder is one of the best characterized techniques to evaluate musculoskeletal involvement of amyloid:
  - Thickening of the rotator cuff tendons
  - Abnormal, echogenic tissue interposed between the tendons, overlying deltoid and between muscle layers

## Treatment Options

- Treatment of amyloid varies by the cause of amyloidosis.
  - AL amyloidosis is treated by chemotherapy with or without steroids or thalidomide, with stem cell transplantation in those patients without cardiac involvement.
  - Primary inflammatory disease is treated in AA amyloidosis.
  - Aβ2M amyloidosis may be stabilized by renal transplantation, but does not regress.
- Localized disease may be treated surgically, which is especially common for carpal tunnel syndrome and is treated by carpal tunnel release.

## Key Points
- On radiographs of symptomatic patients, joint findings are difficult to distinguish from RA.

- Bone amyloidomas cannot be distinguished from metastatic disease or multiple myeloma.
- Low signal material on T1W and fluid-sensitive sequences without blooming artifact on MRI that involves multiple joints is a relatively specific finding.
- Shoulder US can be useful in patients with the shoulder pad sign.
- Biopsy is used for definitive diagnosis.

## Recommended Reading

Takahashi N, Glockner J, Howe BM, Hartman RP, Kawashima A. Taxonomy and imaging manifestations of systemic amyloidosis. *Radiol Clin North Am.* 2016;54:597–612.

## References

1. Beggs SA, Al-Nafussi A, Lambert CM, Porter M, Patton JT. A chronic thigh mass in a 69-year-old man: amyloidoma presenting as a chronic soft tissue mass. *Skeletal Radiol.* 39(12):1237, 1259–61.
2. Hazenberg BP. Amyloidosis: a clinical overview. *Rheum Dis Clin North Am.* 2013;39:323–45.
3. Kay J, Benson CB, Lester S, et al. Utility of high-resolution ultrasound for the diagnosis of dialysis-related amyloidosis. *Arthritis Rheum.* 1992;35:926–32.
4. Kiss E, Keusch G, Zanetti M, et al. Dialysis-related amyloidosis revisited. *AJR Am J Roentgenol.* 2005;185:1460–67.
5. Perfetto F, Moggi-Pignone A, Livi R, Tempestini A, Bergesio F, Matucci-Cerinic M. Systemic amyloidosis: a challenge for the rheumatologist. *Nat Rev Rheumatol.* 2010;6:417–29.
6. Takahashi N, Glockner J, Howe BM, Hartman RP, Kawashima A. Taxonomy and imaging manifestations of systemic amyloidosis. *Radiol Clin North Am.* 2016;54:597–612.
7. Wechalekar AD, Gillmore JD, Hawkins PN. Systemic amyloidosis. *Lancet.* 2016;387:2641–54.

# Section Three

# Tumors and Tumorlike Conditions

Edited by Imran M. Omar

# Osteoid Matrix Bone Tumors

# CHAPTER 52

# Benign Osteoid Matrix Bone Tumors

Abhijit Datir

## Introduction

Osteogenic lesions, or those that form osteoid matrix, are most commonly benign. Enostoses (bone islands) and osteomas are incidentally detected. Osteoid osteomas and osteoblastomas, however, often produce pain and deformity, such as scoliosis. The imaging features and clinical presentation are often characteristic and can help establish a diagnosis without more invasive workups. In many cases, imaging can be helpful to direct definitive therapies, such as radiofrequency ablation.

## Osteoma

### Pathophysiology and Clinical Findings

Osteomas are slow-growing tumors that form dense, mature osteoid matrix. They are found on the surface of bones, usually along the outer table of the calvarium, paranasal sinuses, and mandible. Rarely, they can be seen along long bones. They have been seen in patients from ages 10 to 80, but are most commonly noted in the fourth and fifth decades of life. There is an equal male-to-female ratio, and these lesions are commonly asymptomatic and incidentally noted on imaging studies. Occasionally they can produce symptoms related to mass effect. For example, when they encroach on the paranasal sinuses, they can produce sinus headaches and sinusitis, whereas when they extend into the orbits they can result in diplopia. Osteomas have been associated with Gardner syndrome, which is a familial, autosomal dominant condition consisting of multiple osteomas, numerous intestinal polyps, soft tissue desmoid tumors, and cutaneous masses.

### Imaging Strategy and Findings
- **Radiography**
  - Radiography is usually diagnostic for osteomas. In cases of multiple osteomas, consider Gardner syndrome.
  - Well-marginated, homogenously dense mass of mature osteoid matrix on the surface of bones without continuity with the medullary bone is seen.
  - Osteomas are usually located on the outer table of the calvarium or frontoethmoid sinuses.
  - Osteomas can present along the surfaces of short, tubular bones. In these cases, they are called *periosteal osteomas*.

### Differential Diagnosis
- Parosteal osteosarcoma, sessile osteochondroma, myositis ossificans, focal melorheostosis, calvarial hyperostosis adjacent to meningioma

## Enostosis (Bone Island)

### Pathophysiology and Clinical Findings

An enostosis is a focus of dense, compact bone within the cancellous bone. Although its etiology is not fully known, it is likely developmental, and may either represent hamartomatous proliferation of compact bone or failure of osteoclastic resorption of dense bone. Bone islands are seen throughout the body but tend to occur more commonly at the metaphyses and epiphyses. Most lesions are smaller than 2 cm except in the pelvis. Lesions larger than 2-3 cm are called *giant bone islands* and generally occur within the pelvis. They can continue slowly growing over time. These lesions are usually incidental, and the major diagnostic concern is distinguishing them from more aggressive neoplasms, such as blastic metastases or osteosarcomas.

### Imaging Strategy
- Radiography is diagnostic for 95% of lesions.
- Bone scan can provide helpful supportive evidence of enostosis if it shows either no radiotracer uptake or very mild uptake.
- If lesions are atypical, and demonstrate more pronounced radiotracer uptake or rapid rate of growth, consider biopsy.

### Imaging Findings
#### Radiography
- Round or oval-shaped areas of dense bone within the medullary cavity
- Spiculated margins that blend with surrounding trabeculae (rose-thorn appearance)
- Often oriented along the long axis of the bone

#### Nuclear Imaging
- Bone scintigraphy can exhibit mild increase in radiotracer uptake

### Differential Diagnosis
- Blastic metastases, osteoma, osteoid osteoma, osteosarcoma

## Osteoid Osteoma

### Pathophysiology and Clinical Findings

Osteoid osteomas are small, benign, vascular osteoblastic tumors that account for approximately 10% of all biopsied benign bone tumors. They are classified based on location as *cortical, medullary* (cancellous), or *subperiosteal* (least common). They typically present during first through third decades of life with a male-to-female ratio of 2-3:1. Classically, patients with osteoid osteomas present with characteristic pain that is worst at night and relieved by salicylates.

These lesions are characterized by a central *nidus*, consisting of a vascular connective tissue stroma with varying amounts of calcification and dense reactive bone sclerosis at various stages of maturity. They are most commonly located in the appendicular skeleton, with 50% in the diaphysis or metaphysis of the tibia or femur. Only approximately 13% are intraarticular. When osteoid osteomas occur in the spine, they are most commonly seen within the lumbar spine (60%), and located in the neural arch. However, they can be elusive and are often misdiagnosed clinically as well as on imaging.

### Imaging Strategy
- They are often seen as an incidental finding on conventional radiographs.
- Radiographic features are usually characteristic, and when combined with typical clinical presentation, may even be diagnostic.
- CT is often performed to confirm the diagnosis, and to guide radiofrequency ablation (RFA) of the central nidus.
- MRI is usually not needed, unless there is a diagnostic dilemma. Improved identification of the nidus is possible with high-resolution sequences and dynamic contrast-enhanced gradient-echo techniques.
- Bone scintigraphy now plays little role in the diagnosis or management.

### Imaging Findings
### Radiography
- Typically, intracortical, lucent nidus with surrounding florid reactive sclerosis (Figure 52.1*A*). Nidus usually smaller than 2 cm and round to oval. It may appear lytic, sclerotic, or most commonly of mixed density depending on the degree of mineralization.
- Intramedullary lesions that are intracapsular (such as in the femoral neck) provoke much less reactive sclerosis because of a lower rate of bone production and the

absence of periosteum within the joint capsule, and are therefore difficult to identify. Subperiosteal nidus tends to have more reactive sclerosis than intramedullary or intraarticular lesions.
- A thick rind of reactive sclerosis and solid periosteal reaction may obscure a small nidus. Rarely, the nidus can be multifocal.
- Spinal osteoid osteomas can be difficult to detect initially because of lack of reactive sclerosis. More mature lesions incite reactive sclerosis with a dense (*ivory*) pedicle or lamina (Figure 52.2).

### Computed Tomography
- Classically shows a round or oval soft tissue density nidus with foci of dense mineralization representing mineralized osteoid (Figure 52.1*B*). Associated with perilesional reactive sclerosis.
- *Vascular groove sign*—a recently described finding of thin, serpentine channels in the thickened bone surrounding the nidus (Figure 52.3). This has been shown to be a moderately sensitive (75%) but highly specific (95%) sign for distinguishing osteoid osteoma from other radiolucent bone tumors on CT.

### Magnetic Resonance Imaging
- Nidus seen as heterogeneously hypointense-to-isointense signal on both T1- and T2W sequences, with intense postcontrast enhancement. Perilesional reactive changes involving BME and soft tissue signal are usually present (Figure 52.4).

### Differential Diagnosis
- Infection such as Brodie abscess or intracortical abscess
- Stress fracture

### Treatment Options
- NSAIDs are often used as a first line of treatment in symptomatic patients, given the natural history of spontaneous resolution. However, the current treatment of choice is CT-guided RFA as it is minimally invasive with a reported high success rate.

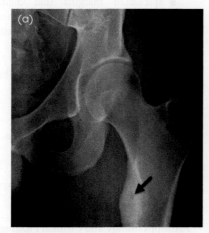 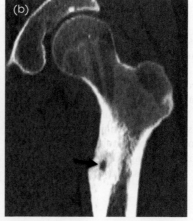

**Figure 52.1.** Osteoid osteoma in a long bone. (*A*) AP radiograph and (*B*) coronal CT reconstruction of the proximal femur show focal intracortical radiolucency (nidus) in the lesser trochanter (*arrows*) with surrounding exuberant sclerosis.

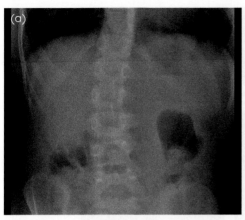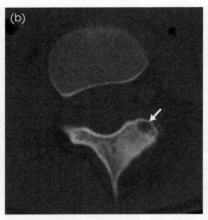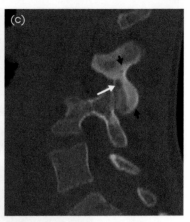

**Figure 52.2.** Spinal osteoid osteoma. (*A*) AP radiograph of the lumbar spine shows mild dextroscoliosis centered at L2, but without focal lesion or abnormality. CT of the lumbar spine with (*B*) axial and (*C*) sagittal reconstructions at the L2 level in the same patient shows a hypodense lesion in the left pedicle (*white arrows*) with surrounding reactive sclerosis (*black arrows*), giving the appearance of an *ivory pedicle*.

■ Findings suggestive of successfully treated nidus after RFA include complete (or almost complete) ossification of treated nidus on CT (Figure 52.5), whereas MRI may continue to show reactive marrow and soft tissue changes despite successful treatment.

## Osteoblastoma

### Pathophysiology and Clinical Findings
Osteoblastoma is a rare tumor that accounts for less than 1% of all primary bone neoplasms. Histologically, it is similar to osteoid osteoma and is differentiated primarily by its size,

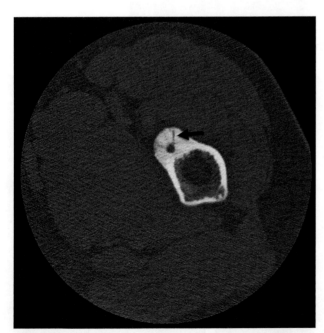

**Figure 52.3.** *Vascular groove sign* in an intracortical osteoid osteoma in the proximal femur. On an axial CT image, there is thin, serpentine hypodensity (*arrow*) coursing through the sclerosis surrounding the central nidus.

being typically greater than 1.5 cm in diameter. Over 80% of patients are younger than age 30 with a male-to-female ratio of 2-3:1. In contrast to osteoid osteoma, osteoblastoma has a predilection for the spine, and is most commonly located in the neural arch. In addition, pain is usually not as acute or severe and rarely relieved by salicylates. Typically, it shows a more aggressive growth pattern with potential for extraosseous involvement and does not resolve spontaneously.

### Imaging Strategy
■ Radiography and CT are usually sufficient to demonstrate the lesion and suggest the diagnosis.
■ MRI may be helpful for evaluation of extraosseous extension.

### Imaging Findings
■ Four distinctive radiologic presentations have been described:
  ■ *Giant osteoid osteoma*—nidus is usually more than 2 cm in diameter; less reactive sclerosis and possibly more prominent periosteal response than osteoid osteoma (Figure 52.6).
  ■ *Blowout expansive lesion*—similar to an aneurysmal bone cyst with small radiopacities in the center; particularly common in spine (Figure 52.7).
  ■ *Aggressive lesion*—simulating a malignant tumor (Figure 52.8). Rare pulmonary metastases have been reported in cases of the aggressive form of osteoblastoma.
  ■ *Periosteal lesion*—exhibits a thin shell of newly formed periosteal bone but without perilesional bone sclerosis.
■ Osteoblastoma may be associated with secondary aneurysmal bone cyst formation.

### Differential Diagnosis
■ Aneurysmal bone cyst
■ Osteosarcoma

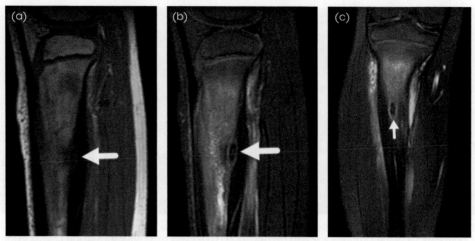

**Figure 52.4.** Osteoid osteoma on MRI. Sagittal (*A*) T1W and (*B*) T2W FS MR images of the proximal tibia show a heterogeneous, hypointense-to-isointense subcortical nidus (*arrows*) with intense marginal enhancement on the coronal postcontrast T1W FS MR image (*C*). Note surrounding intense marrow and soft tissue enhancement consistent with edema.

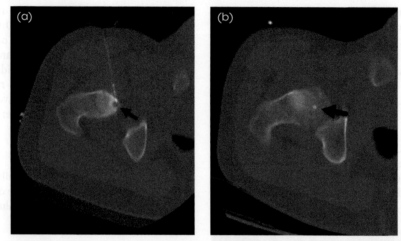

**Figure 52.5.** RFA of osteoid osteoma. (*A*) Pre- and (*B*) post-RFA axial CT images of an intraarticular osteoid osteoma of the femoral neck demonstrate the complete ossification of a radiolucent nidus 3 months following ablation (*arrows*), consistent with successful outcome.

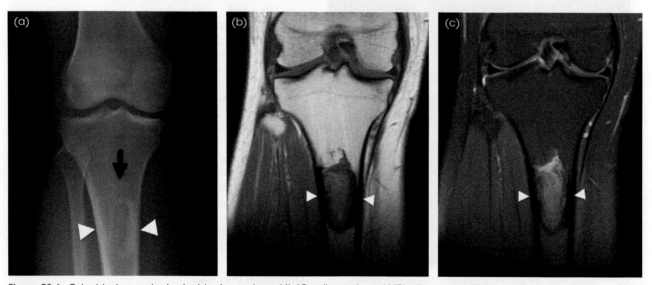

**Figure 52.6.** Osteoblastoma, giant osteoid osteoma type. (*A*) AP radiograph and MRI with coronal (*B*) T1W and (*C*) T2W FS MR images show osteoblastoma in the proximal tibia simulating giant osteoid osteoma (approximately 4 cm in greatest dimension) with more pronounced periosteal response (*arrowheads*) but relatively lesser degree of reactive sclerosis (*arrow*) surrounding the radiolucent nidus.

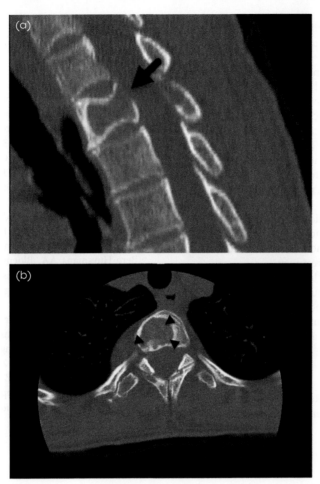

**Figure 52.7.** Osteoblastoma, blowout expansive type. (*A*) Sagittal and (*B*) axial CT images demonstrate an osteoblastoma in a thoracic vertebral body with lytic and expansive appearance causing posterior cortical disruption (*arrow*). In (*A*), there is additional lucency in the spinous process indicating involvement. Note areas of matrix ossification within the tumor (*arrowheads*). On the sagittal reformatted image, there is additional rounded lucency that likely represents additional involvement.

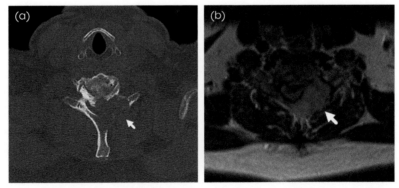

**Figure 52.8.** Osteoblastoma, aggressive type. (*A*) Axial CT image shows aggressive osteoblastoma with cortical destruction in the left neural arch of the cervical vertebra (*arrow*). (*B*) Axial T2W MR image shows associated extraosseous soft tissue component (*arrow*) and intraspinal extension causing mass effect on the spinal cord.

**Treatment Options**

- Options are similar to that for osteoid osteoma for smaller lesions.
- Larger lesions may require en bloc resection with additional bone grafting and internal fixation.

**Key Points**

- Osteoma is a benign, bone-forming tumor seen on the surfaces of bones, usually along the calvarium and frontoethmoid sinuses and incidentally noted on imaging studies.

- Enostosis (bone island) is likely a developmental lesion resulting in a focus of compact bone within the cancellous bone.
- Enostoses (bone islands) can occasionally slowly grow or demonstrate subtly increased radiotracer uptake. However, follow-up imaging or biopsy may be warranted if there is more rapid growth or significant radiotracer uptake.
- Osteoid osteoma has typical findings of intracortical radiolucent nidus and florid perilesional reactive sclerosis, and the pain is commonly relieved by salicylates.
- Most commonly, osteoid osteomas are located within the metadiaphyseal cortex with more than 50% occurring in the femur and tibia.
- Current treatment of choice in symptomatic osteoid osteoma patients is CT-guided RFA, and complete (or almost complete) ossification of treated nidus on CT correlates with successful treatment.
- Osteoblastoma is a benign lesion with histological similarity to osteoid osteoma but with a typically larger size and more variable appearance and clinical presentation.
- The most common location for osteoblastoma is in the spine, especially the neural arch.

### Recommended Reading

Chai JW, Hong SH, Choi JY, et al. Radiologic diagnosis of osteoid osteoma: from simple to challenging findings. *Radiographics* 2010;30:737–49.

Shaikh MI, Saifuddin A, Pringle J, Natali C, Sherzi Z. Spinal osteoblastoma: CT and MR imaging with pathological correlation. *Skeletal Radiol*. 1999;28:33–40.

### References

1. Becce F, Theumann N, Rochette A, et al. Osteoid osteoma and osteoid osteoma-mimicking lesions: biopsy findings, distinctive MDCT features and treatment by radiofrequency ablation. *Eur Radiol*. 2010;20:2439–46.
2. Liu PT, Kujak JL, Roberts CC, de Chadarevian JP. The vascular groove sign: a new CT finding associated with osteoid osteoma. *AJR Am J Roentgenol*. 2011;196:168–73.
3. Sherazi Z, Saifuddin A, Shaikh MI, Natali C, Pringle JAS. Unusual imaging findings in association with spinal osteoblastoma. *Clin Radiol*. 1996;51:644–48.
4. Vanderschueren GM, Taminiau AH, Obermann WR, van den Berg-Huysmans AA, Bloem JL, van Erkel AR. The healing pattern of osteoid osteomas on computed tomography and magnetic resonance imaging after thermocoagulation. *Skeletal Radiol*. 2007;36:813–21.
5. von Kalle T, Langendörfer M, Fernandez FF, Winkler P. Combined dynamic contrast-enhancement and serial 3D-substraction analysis in magnetic resonance imaging of osteoid osteomas. *Eur Radiol*. 2009;19:2508–17.
6. Youssef BA, Haddad MC, Zahrani A, et al. Osteoid osteoma and osteoblastoma: MRI appearances and the significance of ring enhancement. *Eur Radiol*. 1996;6:291–96.

# CHAPTER 53

# Malignant Osteoid Matrix Bone Tumors

Abhijit Datir

## Introduction

Osteosarcoma, or osteogenic sarcoma, is a primary malignant mesenchymal bone tumor in which the malignant tumor cells directly form the osteoid matrix, bone, or both. It is the most common primary bone tumor in children and adolescents, and second most frequent primary malignant bone tumor (following myeloma) if all age groups are considered. It is composed of a number of histologic types that have varying radiologic findings and prognoses, which can affect treatment options. As a result, it is important to recognize differences between the major subtypes when interpreting imaging studies. According to the current World Health Organization (WHO) classification, osteosarcomas are classified into 8 categories (Box 53.1). Approximately 75-85% of all osteosarcomas are the high-grade central or intramedullary type, commonly known as *conventional osteosarcoma*.

## Conventional Osteosarcoma

### Pathophysiology and Clinical Findings

Conventional osteosarcoma is most commonly seen in patients younger than age 25. It is typically seen in the appendicular (peripheral) skeleton, particularly the distal femur, proximal tibia, and proximal humerus (in order of frequency), with 90% in the metaphyseal or metadiaphyseal region and 10% involving the diaphysis. There are 3 histologic subtypes: *osteoblastic* (50%), *chondroblastic* (25%), and *fibroblastic* (25%; may mimic malignant fibrous histiocytoma). This tissue characterization is important because it impacts the selection of neoadjuvant treatment. Less than 5% may show noncontiguous intramedullary lesions within the parent bone or across adjacent joints (so-called skip metastases), which will influence subsequent surgical options. At initial presentation, 5-10% of cases have pulmonary metastases. The 5-year survival rate in patients without distant metastases is between 60 and 80%. In cases of pulmonary metastases at the time of diagnosis, the survival rate decreases to 40%. If metastases are seen in other organs besides the lungs, however, the survival rate is only between 15 and 30%.

### Imaging Strategy

- Diagnosis of bone tumors is generally made on radiography.
- MRI is used for characterizing degree of osseous and soft tissue involvement.
- IV gadolinium-based contrast can be helpful to determine degree of tissue necrosis and to detect areas of soft tissue extension.
- Whole-body bone scintigraphy or, more recently, whole-body MRI can be used for detection of skeletal metastases.

### Imaging Findings

Refer to Figure 53.1.

### Radiography

- Radiographic appearance depends on the degree of malignant osteoid production with a spectrum ranging from purely lytic to densely osteoblastic, although most show a mixed pattern.
- A permeative (or less commonly moth-eaten) type of bone destruction with irregular cortical disruption, wide zone of transition, and associated soft tissue mass is seen.
- Aggressive periosteal reaction, most commonly the *sunburst* pattern (spiculated, divergent periosteal reaction radiating away from an aggressive bone lesion) and a Codman triangle (triangularly shaped periosteal reaction at the edge of an aggressive bone lesion in which the periosteum has been lifted away from the cortex) are seen.

### Magnetic Resonance Imaging

- This is the modality of choice used for staging purposes as well as to assess osseous and soft tissue tumor extension for effective surgical planning.
- Irrespective of precise histology, osseous tumor infiltration shows isointense T1W and heterogeneously hyperintense T2W signal with low signal intensity areas corresponding with matrix mineralization.
- Peritumoral edema is usually less florid when compared to benign counterparts (osteoid osteoma and osteoblastoma), and typically diminishes after adjuvant chemotherapy.

### Computed Tomography

- This modality is the most helpful for detecting metastatic disease, particularly pulmonary metastases.
- Pulmonary metastases can contain osteoid matrix and resemble calcified granulomas.

### Treatment Options

- If limb-salvage surgery is feasible, multidrug chemotherapy is followed by wide resection and endoprosthesis placement.
- Less frequently, amputation is followed by chemotherapy.

**Box 53.1.** WHO Classification of Osteosarcoma

1. Conventional intramedullary/central high-grade
2. Telangiectatic
3. Parosteal
4. Periosteal
5. High-grade surface
6. Low-grade central
7. Secondary
8. Small cell

The following unusual forms of osteosarcoma are viewed as subtypes of conventional osteosarcoma because their biological behavior is similar.

- Osteoblastic osteosarcoma-sclerosing type
- Osteosarcoma resembling osteosarcoma
- Chondromyxoid fibroma-like osteosarcoma
- Chondroblastoma-like osteosarcoma
- Clear cell osteosarcoma
- Malignant fibrous histiocytoma-like (fibrohistiocytic) osteosarcoma
- Giant cell-rich osteosarcoma
- Epithelioid osteosarcoma

## Telangiectatic Osteosarcoma

### Pathophysiology and Clinical Findings
Telangiectatic osteosarcoma is a high-grade tumor, most common in the second decade of life. It most often affects the femur and tibia in the metaphyseal region and accounts for approximately 4% of all osteosarcomas. The male-to-female ratio is 2:1. Histologically, it is composed of multiple hemorrhagic, cystic, or necrotic spaces separated by thin septa, often mimicking an aneurysmal bone cyst (ABC) on histology as well as on imaging. Occasionally, it can also have areas of ABC formation. The prognosis is similar to those patients with conventional osteosarcoma and the 5-year survival rate is approximately 65% for patients who present with local disease only.

### Imaging Findings
Refer to Figure 53.2.

### Radiography
- Advanced cases often show osteolytic destructive lesion with cortical destruction and aggressive periosteal reaction (lamellar, sunburst, or Codman triangle).
- Osteoid matrix mineralization is often subtle or undetectable on radiographs and may be more easily detected on CT. It composes only a small amount of the lesion compared with the volume of cystic spaces.
- It is often associated with soft tissue mass and/or pathologic fracture in larger lesions.

### Magnetic Resonance Imaging
- Hyperintense T1W signal intensity is caused by methemoglobin contents of hemorrhage, and heterogeneous T2W signal intensity with fluid-fluid levels (similar to an ABC) is seen.
- Enhancing thick rim and septae correspond to viable high-grade sarcomatous tissue in hemorrhagic or necrotic spaces.

### Differential Diagnosis
#### Aneurysmal Bone Cyst
- ABC is challenging to differentiate from telangiectatic osteosarcoma because of histologic and radiologic similarities.
- ABC typically shows only an enhancing thin peripheral rim and septae without nodularity or osteoid matrix mineralization.
- ABC is usually less aggressive with associated features such as expansile remodeling and a well-defined margin.

#### Giant Cell Tumor
- Usually located in the subchondral bone with hypointense-to-isointense solid mass on T1W and T2W images
- Often associated with secondary ABC-like changes (14%)

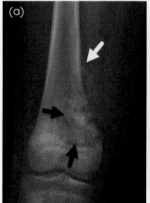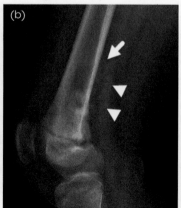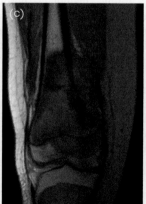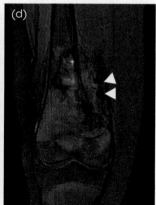

**Figure 53.1.** Conventional central osteosarcoma. (*A*) AP and (*B*) lateral radiographs of the distal femur show aggressive, moth-eaten osseous destruction (*black arrows*) and elevated periosteal reaction (ie, Codman triangle, *white arrows*) in the distal metadiaphysis. It is associated with extraosseous soft tissue mass with osteoid matrix (*arrowheads*). MRI with coronal (*C*) T1W and (*D*) PDW FS sequences confirms the intramedullary lesion with involvement of the distal femoral epiphysis and soft tissue mass. Scattered foci of hypointense signal correspond to osteoid matrix (*arrowheads*).

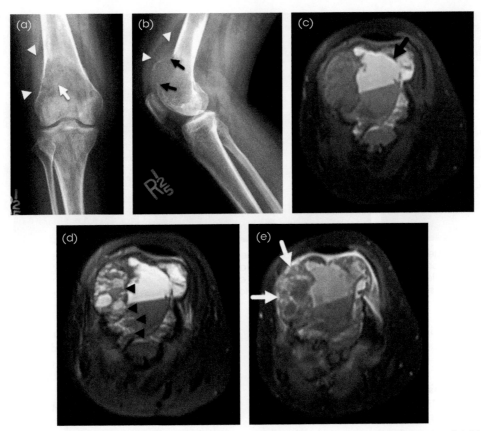

**Figure 53.2.** Telangiectatic osteosarcoma. (*A*) AP and (*B*) lateral radiographs of the knee demonstrate a large distal femoral meta-diaphyseal lytic lesion with cortical destruction, aggressive periosteal reaction (ie, Codman triangle, *black arrows*), thin septa (*white arrow*), and associated extraosseous soft tissue density/mass (*arrowheads*). MRI with axial (*C*) T1W FS, (*D*) T2W FS, and (*E*) contrast-enhanced T1W FS sequences shows multiple fluid-fluid levels (*arrowheads*) with large intratumoral hyperintense T1W signal intensity (*black arrow*) suggestive of hemorrhage in varying stages. Note the relative paucity of the extraosseous soft tissue mass (*white arrows*) with postcontrast enhancement that helps to differentiate this entity from an ABC.

## Surface (or Juxtacortical) Osteosarcoma

- Surface osteosarcoma refers to a group of tumors arising from the bone surface and includes *parosteal, periosteal,* and *high-grade surface* osteosarcomas.
- All 3 types account for less than 10% of all osteosarcomas.

### Parosteal Osteosarcoma
#### Pathophysiology and Clinical Findings

Parosteal osteosarcoma is the most common variety of surface osteosarcoma and arises from the outer fibrous layer of the periosteum. It is a low-grade malignancy seen in the third to fourth decades, with approximately 60% of cases arising from the posterior aspect of the distal femoral metaphysis. Parosteal osteosarcoma accounts for 5% of all osteosarcomas. It has an excellent prognosis with higher than a 90% 5-year survival rate, unless there is dedifferentiation to high-grade osteosarcoma, which occurs in approximately 20% of cases. In some cases, parosteal osteosarcomas may invade the medullary cavity, and some authors have suggested medullary invasion represents higher grade or dedifferentiated tumor. Although medullary invasion has not clearly been associated with a worse prognosis, the presence of medullary invasion necessitates a more aggressive operative resection and is an important imaging finding.

#### Imaging Findings
Refer to Figure 53.3.

- Radiography
  - Characteristic exophytic, lobulated, densely sclerotic mass most frequently arising from, and partially enveloping, the posterior distal femoral metaphysis is seen.
  - The mass is partly adherent to the underlying cortex with the more peripheral component separated from the cortex by a thin radiolucent line (*string sign*) representing interposed periosteum.
- MRI
  - Predominantly hypointense signal on T1W and T2W images corresponding to densely sclerotic radiographic appearance is seen.
  - Areas of unmineralized soft tissue with hyperintense T2W signal likely represent potential dedifferentiation into high-grade tumor, which warrants tissue sampling.
  - Medullary invasion is uncommon and seen in only 15% of cases.

#### Differential Diagnosis
- *Osteochondroma* demonstrates corticomedullary continuity with a T2W hyperintense cartilage cap.

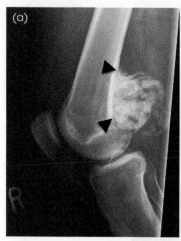 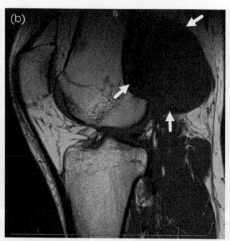 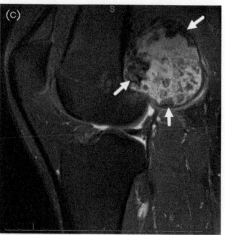

**Figure 53.3.** Parosteal osteosarcoma. (*A*) Lateral radiograph of the knee shows a densely sclerotic extraosseous mass abutting the posterior distal femoral cortex with a thin peripheral intervening radiolucent line (*arrowheads*). MRI with sagittal (*B*) T1W and (*C*) T2W FS sequences demonstrates areas of hypointense signal (*arrows*) consistent with the sclerotic nature of the tumor. The large area of central hyperintense T2W signal raises the suspicion of dedifferentiation into high-grade neoplasm, and needs targeted tissue sampling.

- *Myositis ossificans* is a benign ossified mass within the muscle with gradual ossification from periphery to the center.

### Periosteal Osteosarcoma
#### Pathophysiology and Clinical Findings
Periosteal osteosarcoma is a surface lesion that arises from the outer layer of the periosteum. It most commonly arises from the proximal tibial or distal femoral diaphyses and is usually seen in second to third decades. It accounts for less than 2% of all osteosarcomas.

#### Imaging Findings
Refer to Figure 53.4.

- Radiography
  - Surface lesion with 2 patterns seen
    1. Cortical thickening or erosion (saucerization), and a perpendicular (*hair-on-end*) periosteal reaction
    2. A thin peripheral shell simulating a periosteal chondroma
  - Can wrap around the circumference of the bone
- MRI
  - Spectrum of imaging appearances ranges from features suggestive of periosteal chondroma (caused by chondrogenic elements) with scalloping of the outer cortex to a more aggressive lesion with Codman triangle and a spiculated or sunburst periosteal reaction.

### High-Grade Surface Osteosarcoma
Refer to Figure 53.5.

#### Pathophysiology and Clinical Findings
- Rarest of the surface osteosarcomas, accounting for less than 1% of all osteosarcomas
- Indistinguishable histologically from the intramedullary counterpart (only difference being the surface origin)

### Low-Grade Central Osteosarcoma
#### Pathophysiology and Clinical Findings
- Accounts for less than 1% of all osteosarcomas and occurs in patients older than those presenting with conventional osteosarcoma
- Similar sites of involvement as conventional osteosarcoma (ie, distal femur, proximal tibia and proximal humerus)
- May be indistinguishable from conventional osteosarcoma on imaging, but with slower growth rate and better prognosis

---

### Secondary Osteosarcoma
- Secondary osteosarcoma represents approximately 5-7% of all osteosarcomas.
- It is considered secondary because of malignant transformation in a preexisting bone lesion, such as Paget disease and following radiotherapy.
- Less common examples of preexisting lesion include chronic osteomyelitis, fibrous dysplasia, and medullary infarction.

### Paget Sarcoma
#### Pathophysiology and Clinical Findings
Sarcomatous degeneration is one of the most feared complications of Paget disease. It occurs in 1-3% of patients with Paget disease, and is seen more commonly with increasing osseous involvement of Paget disease. Approximately 50% of Paget sarcomas are osteosarcomas, whereas the remainder are spindle cell and pleomorphic sarcomas or chondrosarcomas. Paget sarcoma is most often seen in the pelvis, femur, and humerus, whereas the spine is typically spared. Paget sarcomas have poor prognosis with survival of less than a year from diagnosis.

#### Imaging Findings
Refer to Figure 53.6.

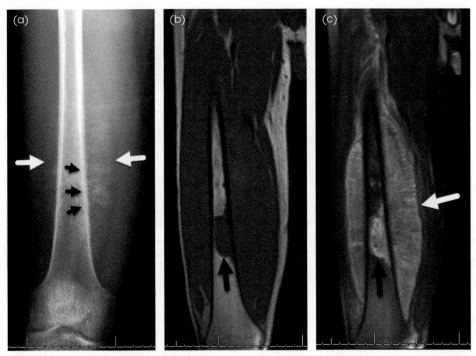

**Figure 53.4.** Periosteal osteosarcoma. (*A*) AP radiograph of the femur demonstrates a large surface lesion arising from the diaphysis with associated periosteal scalloping (*black arrows*) and classic spiculated/sunburst pattern of periosteal reaction (hair-on-end, *white arrows*). MRI with coronal (*B*) T1W and (*C*) T2W FS MR images confirm predominantly extraosseous surface lesion (*white arrow*) with a small intramedullary component (*black arrows*) suggestive of dedifferentiation into high-grade osteosarcoma.

- Radiography and CT
  - CT shows permeative bone lesion with cortical destruction and a soft tissue mass. New bone formation is seen in approximately 20% cases.
- MRI
  - MRI shows isointense-to-hypointense T1W and corresponding hyperintense T2W signal.
  - Loss of T1W marrow signal on MRI may suggest tumor infiltration, although other complications, such as fracture or pseudofracture with hemorrhage and edema should also be considered.
- Definitive diagnosis is based on tissue sampling to differentiate from other etiologies such as metastasis, myeloma, and lymphoma.

**Postradiation Sarcoma**
**Pathophysiology and Clinical Findings**
Approximately 90% of postradiation sarcomas are osteosarcomas or spindle cell sarcomas (fibrosarcoma, undifferentiated high-grade pleomorphic sarcoma). They account for 0.5-5% of all sarcomas, and there is a higher risk in the pediatric population because of increased susceptibility of the immature skeleton to irradiation and longer life span compared to adults.

- Criteria for diagnosis include
  - History of prior radiation therapy
  - Lesion located within the radiation field
  - Latent period of at least 3-4 years
  - Histological evidence of sarcoma, differing significantly from the originally treated tumor

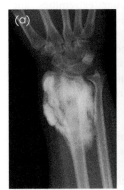
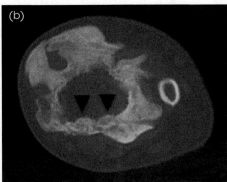
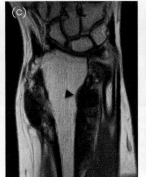
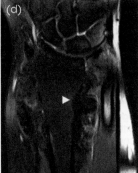

**Figure 53.5.** High-grade surface osteosarcoma. (*A*) PA radiograph, (*B*) axial CT, coronal (*C*), T1W, and (*D*) coronal T2W FS MR images of the wrist show a large lobulated osseous lesion arising from the distal radius cortical surface with minimal scalloping and intramedullary extension (*arrowheads*).

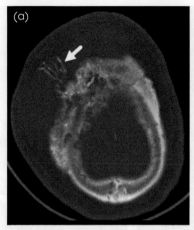
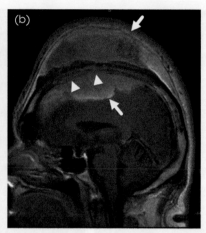

**Figure 53.6.** Paget sarcoma. (*A*) Noncontrast axial CT image shows permeative osseous destruction of the calvarium with new bone formation (*arrow*) on a background of typical mixed lytic-sclerotic changes and diploic widening of Paget disease. (*B*) Noncontrast midline sagittal T1W MR image demonstrates thinning and destruction (*arrowheads*) of the calvarium with a large soft tissue mass extending into the extracalvarial and extraaxial compartments (*arrows*).

### Imaging Findings
Refer to Figure 53.7.

- Radiographic features include permeative bone destruction (>80%), soft tissue mass (>90%) with varying degree of periosteal reaction, and matrix mineralization.
- Cross-sectional imaging shows findings of aggressive neoplasm with osseous destruction and soft tissue involvement.

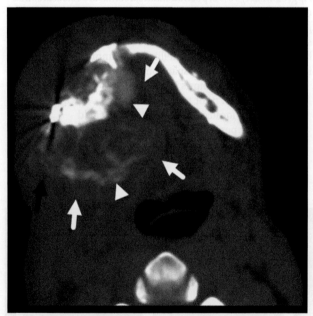

**Figure 53.7.** Postradiation osteosarcoma. A 55-year-old man with history of parotid gland mucoepidermoid carcinoma and treatment including radiation therapy 15 years prior. Noncontrast axial CT image of the mandible shows an aggressive lesion with osseous destruction of the right mandibular ramus (*black arrow*) and large extraosseous mass (*white arrows*) with osteoid matrix (*arrowheads*). This is a biopsy-proven postradiation osteosarcoma.

### Small Cell Osteosarcoma
- Small cell osteosarcoma mimics round cell tumor (such as Ewing sarcoma).
- Radiographically, it is seen as a lucent lesion with permeative margins and large soft tissue mass.
- Histological diagnosis is based on the presence of spindled tumor cells and focal osteoid production.

### Other Types of Osteosarcoma

**Multicentric (Multifocal) Osteosarcoma**
- Simultaneous development of multiple foci of osteosarcoma in multiple bones
- Categorized as *synchronous* (lesions that develop at the same time) or *metachronous* (lesions that develop at different times)
- Must be differentiated from osteosarcoma metastasized to other bones

**Soft Tissue (Extraskeletal) Osteosarcoma**
- This is an uncommon malignant tumor of mesenchymal origin with potential to form neoplastic osteoid, bone, and cartilage.
- It preferentially affects the lower extremities and buttocks.
- Radiographically, it is seen as a soft tissue mass with scattered areas of calcifications and ossifications.
- On cross-sectional imaging, the lesion shows central ossification (referred to as *reverse zoning phenomenon*). This helps to differentiate these lesions from myositis ossificans.

**Giant Cell-Rich Osteosarcoma**
- Aggressive lesion with minimal or absent periosteal reaction, and small soft tissue mass compared with other types of osteosarcomas
- Striking resemblance to giant cell tumor on histology caused by an abundance of giant cells (osteoclasts) and scant tumor osteoid

### Fibrohistiocytic Osteosarcoma

- Recently described entity with resemblance to pleomorphic sarcoma (previously known as malignant fibrous histiocytoma or MFH)
- Tends to involve articular ends of long bones with less periosteal reaction
- Usually exhibits areas of bone formation resembling cotton balls that help to differentiate from pleomorphic sarcoma

### Intracortical Osteosarcoma

- One of the rarest forms of osteosarcoma
- Tumor limited to the cortex without intramedullary or extraosseous soft tissue involvement
- Radiographically seen as a radiolucent lesion with surrounding cortical sclerosis, ranging from 1.0 to 4.2 cm in size

### Gnathic Osteosarcoma

- Arising in the maxilla or mandible, and seen in older patients (fourth to sixth decades)
- A well-differentiated tumor with low mitotic rate and better prognosis

### Syndromic Associations

- Werner syndrome is an autosomal recessive condition characterized by the appearance of premature aging.
- Li-Fraumeni syndrome is an autosomal dominant condition that predisposes patients to various malignancies from an early age.
- Bloom syndrome is an autosomal recessive condition characterized by short stature, development of neoplasms at an early age, and genomic instability.

## Key Points

- Osteosarcoma is the second most common primary malignant bone tumor and forms neoplastic osteoid.
- Seventy-five percent of osteosarcomas occur in patients younger than age 25.

- Osteosarcoma is classified as central (most common), surface (parosteal, periosteal and high-grade), telangiectatic, multicentric, low-grade central, secondary, and other less common types.
- Three histologic subtypes of primary osteosarcoma are based on dominant tissue pattern—osteoblastic (50%), chondroblastic (25%), and fibroblastic (25%).
- Conventional radiographs show aggressive lesion with permeative bone destruction, extraosseous soft tissue mass, and cortical disruption with periosteal reaction (sunburst type or Codman triangle).
- MRI is useful for assessing tumor extent and skip lesions.
- Treatment includes surgery (amputation or limb-salvage, if feasible) and chemotherapy.

### Recommended Reading

Yarmish G, Klein MJ, Landa J, Lefkowitz RA, Hwang S. Imaging characteristics of primary osteosarcoma: nonconventional types. *Radiographics*. 2010;30:1653–72.

### References

1. Discepola F, Powell TI, Nahal A. Telangiectatic osteosarcoma: radiologic and pathologic findings. *Radiographics*. 2009;29:380–83.
2. Dönmez FY, Tüzün U, Başaran C, Tunaci M, Bilgic B, Acunas G. MRI findings in parosteal osteosarcoma: correlation with histopathology. *Diagn Interv Radiol*. 2008;14(3):142–52.
3. Lopez C, Thomas DV, Davies AM. Neoplastic transformation in Paget's disease of bone: pictorial review. *Eur Radiol*. 2003;13:151–63.
4. Murphey MD, Jelinek JS, Temple HT, Flemming DJ, Gannon FH. Imaging of periosteal osteosarcoma: radiologic-pathologic correlation. *Radiology*. 2004;233:129–38.
5. Murphey MD, Robbin MR, McRae GA, Flemming DJ, Temple HT, Kransdorf MJ. The many faces of osteosarcoma. *Radiographics*. 1997;17:1205–31.
6. Sheppard DG, Libshitz HI. Post-radiation sarcomas: a review of the clinical and imaging features in 63 cases. *Clin Radiol*. 2001;56:22–29.

# Chondroid Matrix Bone Tumors

# CHAPTER 54

# Benign Chondroid Matrix Bone Tumors

Benjamin D. Levine and Leanne L. Seeger

## Introduction

The most common benign primary bone tumors are those of cartilage origin. Cartilaginous tumors comprise approximately 24% of all primary bone tumors. Some of these tumors are common, asymptomatic, and often discovered incidentally, whereas others are uncommon and can present with pain. Most cartilage bone tumors have distinguishing imaging characteristics, which together with the clinical findings and anatomic location lead to an accurate diagnosis and guide patient management.

## Osteochondroma

### Pathophysiology and Clinical Findings

Osteochondromas are bony exostoses that are the most common benign bone tumor in all ages, and the most common bone tumor overall in children. Osteochondromas make up 10-15% of all bone neoplasms and 20-50% of all benign bone neoplasms. Most commonly, these tumors are solitary. However, they can be multiple, which is diagnostic of *multiple hereditary exostoses*. Osteochondromas often grow until skeletal maturity, and can develop following surgery and physeal injuries in the setting of Salter-Harris fractures. They are the most common benign tumor caused by radiation and are reported to develop in 6-24% of irradiated patients. Development of osteochondromas has also been associated with stem cell transplantation, representing a cumulative risk of 6.1% of osteochondroma development at 15 years posttransplant. However, other studies have suggested that younger age at transplant plus radiation rather than transplant alone increases risk of osteochondroma development. Most solitary osteochondromas are asymptomatic, and this lesion is more common in males. The symptomatic lesions tend to occur in patients younger than age 20. Approximately half of all osteochondromas arise in the lower extremities, with most around the knee (Figure 54.1). The femur is the most commonly involved bone (30%), followed by the humerus (10-20%). Osteochondromas less commonly occur in the small bones of the feet and hands, scapula, and pelvis.

Complications of osteochondromas include fracture; adventitial bursa formation; impingement on adjacent soft tissue structures, such as nerves and vessels, and malignant transformation (Figure 54.2). The most feared complication is malignant transformation, occurring in approximately 1% of solitary osteochondromas. These transformations occur within the cartilage cap resulting in formation of a secondary chondrosarcoma, or rarely an osteosarcoma.

Although unusual, fractures of osteochondromas can occur following trauma, most commonly around the knee with pedunculated lesions. These may require surgical resection. Adventitial bursa formation around the cartilage cap of an osteochondroma has a reported incidence of 1.5%, occurring most commonly in scapular lesions and lesions about the lesser trochanter of the proximal femur. Vascular compromise from osteochondromas can result in stenosis, occlusion, or pseudoaneurysm. Popliteal artery entrapment syndrome can occur from osteochondromas situated about the knee. Nerve compression is a complication that has been described to involve the radial, sciatic and common peroneal nerves.

### Multiple Hereditary Exostoses

Multiple hereditary exostoses (MHE) is an autosomal-dominant condition in which there are several osteochondromas that are most commonly seen around the knees and ankles in the lower extremity, and the shoulder in the upper extremity. This has a 2:1 male-to-female predominance. The imaging features and complications of exostoses seen in MHE are indistinguishable from solitary osteochondromas although malignant degeneration may occur in up to 15% of patients. More central lesions, such as those around the pelvis and shoulders, have a higher risk of malignant degeneration than more distal ones.

### Subungual Exostosis

Subungual exostoses are osseous excrescences that arise along the dorsal or dorsomedial aspects of the distal phalanges, deep to or around the nail bed. There is a predilection for the toes, especially the great toe. They most commonly occur in younger patients, in the third and fourth decades of life, and present equally in men and women. They are histologically distinct from osteochondromas because there is no cortical or medullary contiguity. They may arise after trauma to the periosteum, which is more loosely adherent to the bone in this region, with subsequent chondromatous metaplasia. Unlike true osteochondromas, the cartilage cap consists of fibrocartilage rather than hyaline cartilage.

### Dysplasia Epiphysealis Hemimelica (Trevor Disease)

Dysplasia epiphysealis hemimelica (DEH) is an unusual developmental condition in which osteochondromas form along the epiphysis. It demonstrates a male-to-female ratio of 3:1 and can lead to limb shortening, gait abnormalities, or

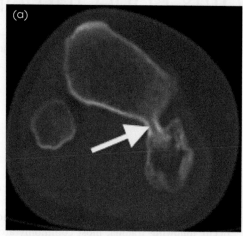
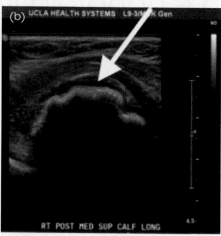

**Figure 54.1.** Pedunculated osteochondroma. A 25-year-old woman with a pedunculated osteochondroma arising from the proximal tibial metaphysis. (*A*) Axial CT image shows the osteochondroma is continuous with the medullary cavity of the bone of origin (*arrow*). (*B*) Transverse US image shows the smooth thin hypoechoic cartilage cap (*arrow*) of the osteochondroma.

palpable masses. It usually presents in a single lower extremity, especially around the knee or ankle. On radiography, the epiphysis may initially appear overgrown and irregular. Later during the disease, stippled calcifications may appear, which become progressively coarsened. As the lesion matures, it may undergo ossification. MRI can help to confirm the epiphyseal origin of this lesion, which will suggest the diagnosis. The unmineralized cartilage components demonstrate typical features on MRI, with high signal on fluid-sensitive sequences and intermediate signal on T1W imaging. The mineralized components are dark in signal on all pulse sequences.

### Turret Exostosis

Turret exostoses are extraosseous excrescences that arise from the dorsal surfaces of the proximal and middle phalanges in the hands. They are likely related to cutaneous laceration with disruption of the underlying dorsal periosteum and subsequent

ossification of a periosteal hematoma. Patients may present with a painful lump that develops after trauma.

### Bizarre Parosteal Osteochondromatous Proliferation (Nora Lesion) and Florid Reactive Periostitis

Bizarre parosteal osteochondromatous proliferation (BPOP) is an unusual lesion that most commonly arises along the metacarpal bones in the hands more than the metatarsal bones in the feet. It usually occurs in patients in the second and third decades of life and is seen equally in men and women. It may be related to prior trauma. In the early phases, there may be ill-defined periosteal proliferation. As the lesion matures, it may become progressively ossified. However, it generally is separate from the underlying bone. Imaging demonstrates broad-based ossification that is applied to the surface of the bone without medullary continuity. No cartilage cap is seen. The imaging features of BPOP overlap with florid reactive periostitis (FRP), which is an uncommon, benign osteochondromatous periosteal reaction that also most commonly occurs around the phalanges in the hands and feet. In some instances, only histologic examination may be able to make the distinction between BPOP and FRP, because BPOP has a thin periosteal layer that covers the osteochondromatous reaction, whereas FRP does not.

### Imaging Strategy and Findings
#### Radiography

- Continuity of medullary cavity and cortex with that of the bone of origin is pathognomonic.
- There are 2 types of osteochondromas:
  - *Pedunculated* lesions have a narrow base and expanded apex.
  - *Sessile* lesions are broadest at the base and smaller at the apex.
- Typically, osteochondromas arise from a metaphyseal/metadiaphyseal location and project away from the adjacent joint.

#### Computed Tomography

- CT is an excellent imaging technique to identify the lesion continuity with the native medullary cavity,

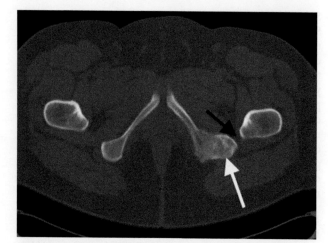

**Figure 54.2.** Sessile osteochondroma. A 21-year-old man with a sessile osteochondroma arising from the ischial tuberosity (*white arrow*). The osteochondroma narrows the ischiofemoral space (*black arrow*) and may be associated with ischiofemoral impingement syndrome in the appropriate clinical setting.

particularly in flat bones or where there is complex anatomy, such as the pelvis or shoulder.

■ CT accurately delineates cartilage calcifications when present.

## Ultrasound
■ Can also be used to evaluate the cartilage cap, which appears hypoechoic

## Magnetic Resonance Imaging
■ MRI is an ideal technique to evaluate complications of osteochondromas, including malignant transformation, fracture, vascular compromise, and nerve impingement with denervation edema.
■ The base of an osteochondroma has the typical MRI signal intensity of normal bone although there may be red marrow-like signal within the stalk.
■ The cartilage cap has typical MRI features of hyaline cartilage (low-intermediate signal on T1W, and hyperintense on T2W images).
■ The cartilage cap in young patients may appear heterogeneous in signal because of active endochondral ossification.
■ The apex of an osteochondroma is covered by a cartilage cap. When measured perpendicular to the surface of the bone at the cartilage cap to bone interface, this cap thickness usually measures less than 2 cm.
  ■ Cartilage cap thickness of 1 cm or less is considered of very low risk for malignant degeneration.
  ■ Cap thickness between 1 and 2 cm may be considered borderline and require closer follow-up imaging.
  ■ Cap thickness of greater than 2 cm in adults strongly indicates malignant transformation to chondrosarcoma.

## Differential Diagnosis
■ Occasionally can resemble myositis ossificans or heterotopic ossification, intraarticular bodies or rarely bone-forming neoplasms

## Treatment Options
■ Surgical resection of benign chondroid lesions is reserved for painful lesions, or those impinging on adjacent structures, such as neurovascular bundles.

---

# Enchondroma

## Pathophysiology and Clinical Presentation
Enchondromas are benign tumors of hyaline cartilage origin and represent the second most common benign cartilage tumor. It was previously thought that enchondromas arise from displaced cartilage rests from the physis into the metaphysis; however, more recent studies have suggested enchondromas are in fact neoplasms. Their estimated prevalence is 2.9%, and these lesions present in the third or fourth decades of life, usually as incidental findings on imaging. Most enchondromas arise in the small bones of the hand, of which 40-50% are in the proximal phalanges, 15-30% in the metacarpals, and 20-30% in the middle phalanges. The carpal bones are a rare site. The most common long bone to be involved is the femur, followed by the humerus and tibia. Approximately 7% of all cases involve the small bones of the feet. Most commonly, enchondromas arise in the long bone metaphyses, but epiphyseal, cortical, and juxtacortical (periosteal) lesions have been described.

## Enchondromatosis (Ollier Disease and Maffucci Syndrome)
Multiple enchondromas, particularly in a unilateral distribution, is called *Ollier disease*. This often results in osseous expansion, deformity, and growth disturbance. If enchondromatosis is seen in association with soft tissue hemangiomas, the condition is called *Maffucci syndrome*. No hereditary predisposition in either condition has been seen. The individual lesions are histologically similar to solitary enchondromas and radiographically appear as expansile lucent lesions with endosteal scalloping and often areas of chondroid matrix mineralization. In patients with Maffucci syndrome, calcified soft tissue phleboliths can indicate the presence of hemangiomas, and hemangiomas often occur near the enchondromas. Although these conditions can result in growth arrest and pathologic fractures, the most worrisome complication is malignant degeneration to chondrosarcoma. The reported risk of malignant degeneration in patients with Maffucci syndrome is at least 20% and is higher than the reported risk for those with Ollier disease.

## Imaging Strategy
■ Differentiation of benign from low-grade malignant chondroid tumors should be made with an approach that combines the clinical, imaging, and histologic findings to arrive at the diagnosis and management.
■ Despite the challenge of differentiating enchondroma from low-grade chondrosarcoma, there are imaging features that have been described:
  ■ Peripheral (appendicular) location favors a benign lesion (enchondroma), whereas a central location (pelvis) favors malignancy (chondrosarcoma).
  ■ Although both lesions commonly arise in the femur; enchondroma is more common distally and chondrosarcoma more common proximally.
  ■ Chondrosarcoma is usually greater in size than enchondroma (>5 cm), and the depth of endosteal scalloping is greater for chondrosarcoma.
  ■ Other features that favor chondrosarcoma rather than enchondroma include male gender, older age at presentation, and the presence of pain. In fact, localized pain that is not attributable to any other cause is a more valuable indicator of chondrosarcoma than any imaging finding.

## Imaging Strategy
Radiography is the initial imaging modality of choice and shows the typical features (Figure 54.3). Enchondromas seen on MRI are most commonly incidental. However, MRI can be used to characterize lesions with atypical radiographic or clinical features, such as those presenting with pathologic fracture and callus formation. It is often difficult to differentiate

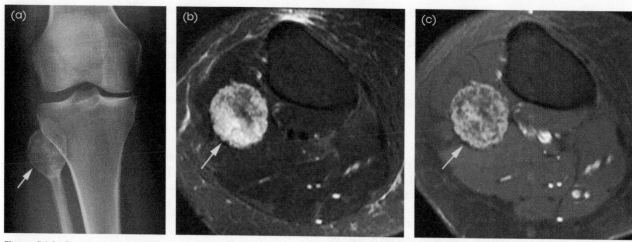

**Figure 54.3.** Enchondroma. A 48-year-old woman with palpable lateral right knee lesion. (*A*) AP radiograph of the knee demonstrates a lobular, expansile, largely sclerotic lesion with endosteal scalloping, cortical thinning, and ring-and-arc matrix mineralization (*arrow*), consistent with an enchondroma. (*B*) Axial STIR MR image shows the typical hyperintense cartilage signal with lobulated margins, consistent with an enchondroma (*arrow*). (*C*) Axial T1 FS postcontrast MR image demonstrates ring-and-arc enhancement (*arrow*) typical of low-grade chondroid lesions.

enchondroma and low-grade chondrosarcoma with imaging alone (Figure 54.4).

### Imaging Findings
### Radiography and Computed Tomography
- Typically, lobular lesions may show endosteal scalloping and variable bone expansion especially in small tubular bones.
- Cortical disruption and periostitis usually do not occur in the absence of a pathologic fracture.
- Curvilinear calcifications with a *ring-and-arc* morphology is typical of chondroid matrix lesions.
- In the long bones, enchondromas may be located either centrally or eccentrically and do not typically show a sclerotic margin.

### Magnetic Resonance Imaging
- Signal characteristics similar to hyaline cartilage, intermediate on T1W and hyperintense on T2W images,

often with thin hypointense septa between the lobules of cartilage on T2W images
- May have curvilinear dark foci corresponding to areas of matrix calcification
- Usually enhance peripherally following gadolinium-based contrast injection and may demonstrate central ring-and-arc enhancement as well

### Treatment Options
- For benign enchondromas in which surgery is warranted, curettage followed by placement of bone graft material is usually curative.

---

## Periosteal Chondroma

### Pathophysiology and Clinical Presentation
Periosteal chondroma is a rare benign cartilage tumor that is located on the surface of the cortex, beneath the periosteum.

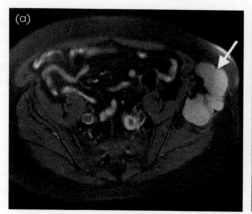
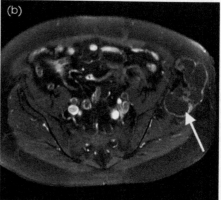

**Figure 54.4.** Grade 1 chondrosarcoma. A 52-year-old man with grade 1 chondrosarcoma. (*A*) Axial T2W FS MR image of the pelvis shows a hyperintense, lobular expansile lesion (*arrow*) arising in the left iliac wing from the cartilage cap of a sessile osteochondroma. (*B*) Axial T1W FS postcontrast MR image demonstrates peripheral and septal enhancement typical of cartilage (*arrow*).

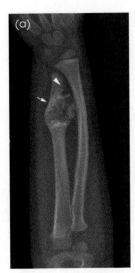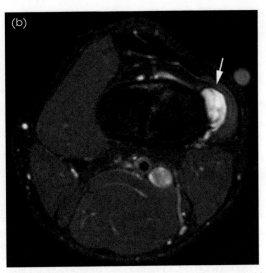

**Figure 54.5.** Periosteal chondromas in separate patients. (*A*) AP radiograph of the forearm in a 3-year-old girl shows a partially mineralized lesion arising along the distal ulnar diaphysis (*arrow*). The lesion is associated with saucerization of the underlying bone (*arrowhead*), which indicates that it is a surface lesion. (*B*) Axial T2W FS MR image in an 18-year-old man demonstrates a lobulated lesion along the surface of the distal lateral femoral metaphysis that is nearly as bright as fluid (*arrow*). This is appearance is typical of a chondroid lesion.

It usually grows slowly and presents with localized pain and swelling. No age or gender predilection is seen.

### Imaging Findings
**Radiography and Computed Tomography**

- Cortical pressure erosion (saucerization), a thin periosteal shell of bone, cartilage matrix mineralization, and mild elevation of the bone cortex at the margin of the lesion

**Magnetic Resonance Imaging**

- Typical signal characteristics of chondroid tissue already described (Figure 54.5) are seen.
- Periosteal chondromas are usually smaller than periosteal chondrosarcomas, a feature that can be used to differentiate them. Most lesions of periosteal chondromas measure less than 2.5 cm maximally, whereas most periosteal chondrosarcomas measure more than 5 cm. Some authors have suggested a 3-cm cutoff may be helpful to distinguish between periosteal chondroma and chondrosarcoma.

## Chondroblastoma

### Pathophysiology and Clinical Findings
Chondroblastoma is a rare benign cartilage tumor that is usually epiphyseal or apophyseal. The lesion may extend into the metaphysis, but isolated diaphyseal or metaphyseal lesions are rare. Approximately 75-80% of all cases involve the long bones. The foot is the second most common location, and lesions are most often seen in the talus and calcaneus. Other described sites include the scapula, acromion, ribs, sacrum, patella, and small bones of hands and feet. It is more common in males, and the mean age at presentation has been found to be 19.9 years. Although rare, chondroblastoma metastases, especially to the bones and lungs, have been reported.

### Imaging Findings
**Radiography and Computed Tomography**

- Demonstrates a lytic lesion with a thin, sclerotic, geographic margin, lobular contour, and chondroid matrix mineralization (30%)

**Magnetic Resonance Imaging**

- Lesions most commonly demonstrate intermediate signal on T1W imaging and intermediate to low signal on fluid-sensitive sequences. Postcontrast T1W imaging shows peripheral or septal enhancement.
- The lesion typically demonstrates periostitis, BME, and surrounding soft tissue edema (Figure 54.6).
- Reactive joint effusion and synovitis are seen.
- Fluid-fluid levels may indicate secondary ABC development, reported in approximately 15% of cases.
- MRI is particularly useful to evaluate for recurrence where histologically proven recurrent lesions demonstrate marrow edema. Conversely, resolution of reactive marrow edema suggests no recurrence.

### Treatment Options

- Although typically treated with curettage and bone grafting, CT-guided RFA has also been described.

## Chondromyxoid Fibroma

### Pathophysiology and Clinical Presentation
Chondromyxoid fibroma (CMF) is a rare, benign bone lesion. Histologic evaluation of these tumors is difficult, as they cannot be classified as solely cartilaginous or fibrous lesions; however, these tumors may resemble chondroblastoma. The mean age at presentation of CMF is approximately 25 years with an age range of 3-70 years. CMF is most common in an eccentric, intramedullary, and

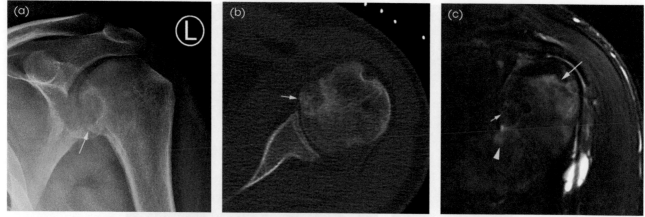

**Figure 54.6.** Chondroblastoma. A 30-year-old man with chronic left shoulder pain. (*A*) AP radiograph of the shoulder shows a well-defined lytic lesion with sclerotic margins in the proximal humeral epiphysis (*arrow*). (*B*) Axial CT image shows the epiphyseal lytic lesion along the anterior proximal humeral epiphysis with internal mineralization (*arrow*). (*C*) Coronal T2W FS MR image shows heterogeneous but lower signal within the lesion (*short arrow*) surrounded by pronounced BME (*long arrow*) and reactive soft tissue edema (*arrowhead*). There is an additional, probably reactive biceps tendon sheath effusion.

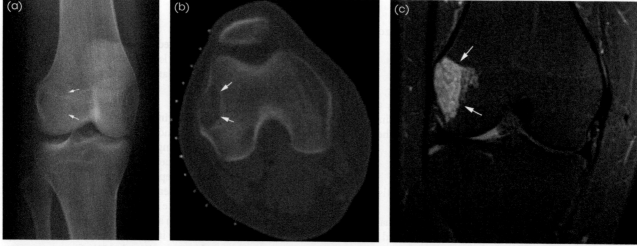

**Figure 54.7.** Chondromyxoid fibroma in a 16-year-old girl with knee pain. (*A*) AP radiograph of the pelvis demonstrates a subtle geographic, lytic lesion in the lateral femoral condyle (*arrows*). (*B*) Axial CT through the distal femur shows the lytic lesion (*arrows*) has a faint sclerotic rim and focal cortical osteolysis along its lateral surface. (*C*) Coronal T2W FS MR image of the lesion shows lobulated hyperintense signal (*arrows*). The lesion was diagnosed as a chondromyxoid fibroma on CT-guided biopsy.

metaphyseal location. In the lower extremity, epiphyseal and cortical locations are rare.

### Imaging Findings
### Radiography and Computed Tomography

- Imaging is classically described as a geographic, well-defined, expansile lytic tumor with a sclerotic rim (Figure 54.7).
- Although internal trabeculation is common within the lesion, radiographically evident matrix mineralization is uncommon (2-15% of lesions).

### Magnetic Resonance Imaging

- Features are nonspecific and not well reported because of the rarity of the tumor.

### Treatment Options

- Curettage with allograft bone or polymethylmethacrylate is the preferred treatment with a low rate of reported recurrence.

### Key Points

- Benign chondroid matrix bone tumors are the most common benign primary bone tumor overall, although they represent a broad spectrum of differing neoplasms.
- Imaging plays an important role in their diagnosis and management, with radiography being the mainstay modality of choice for their initial workup.
- MRI and CT can provide increased diagnostic confidence and accuracy and have become essential tools that guide clinical management of the benign cartilage bone tumors.

## Recommended Reading

Robbin MR, Murphey MD. Benign chondroid neoplasms of bone. *Semin Musculoskelet Radiol.* 2000;4(1):45–58.

## References

1. Bernard SA, Murphey MD, Flemming DJ, Kransdorf MJ. Improved differentiation of benign osteochondromas from secondary chondrosarcomas with standardized measurement of cartilage cap at CT and MR imaging. *Radiology.* 2010;255:857–65.

2. Bloem JL, Mulder JD. Chondroblastoma: a clinical and radiological study of 104 cases. *Skeletal Radiol.* 1985;14:1–9.

3. Douis H., Saifuddin A. The imaging of cartilaginous bone tumours. I. Benign lesions. *Skeletal Radiol.* 2012;41:1195–212.

4. Flemming DJ, Murphey MD. Enchondroma and chondrosarcoma. *Semin Musculoskelet Radiol.* 2000;4:59–71.

5. Lee KC, Davies AM, Cassar-Pullicino VN. Imaging the complications of osteochondromas. *Clin Radiol.* 2002;57:18–28.

6. Lersundi A, Mankin HJ, Mourikis A, Hornicek FJ. Chondromyxoid fibroma: a rarely encountered and puzzling tumor. *Clin Orthop Relat Res.* 2005;439:171–75.

7. Murphey MD, Choi JJ, Kransdorf MJ, Flemming DJ, Gannon FH. Imaging of osteochondroma: variants and complications with radiologic–pathologic correlation. *Radiographics.* 2000;20:1407–34.

8. Murphey MD, Flemming DJ, Boyea SR, Bojescul JA, Sweet DE, Temple HT. Enchondroma versus chondrosarcoma in the appendicular skeleton: differentiating features. *Radiographics.* 1998;18:1213–37.

9. Robinson P, White LM, Sundaram M, et al. Periosteal chondroid tumors: radiologic evaluation with pathologic correlation. *Am J Roentgenol.* 2001;177:1183–88.

10. Ryzewicz M, Manaster BJ, Naar E, Lindeque B. Low-grade cartilage tumors: diagnosis and treatment. *Orthopedics.* 2007;30:35–46.

# Malignant Chondroid Matrix Bone Tumors

Benjamin D. Levine and Leanne L. Seeger

## Introduction

Chondrosarcoma refers to a malignant tumor that produces cartilage matrix. It represents approximately 3.5% of all biopsied primary bone tumors and 20-27% of all primary sarcomas, and is overall the third most common primary malignant bone tumor. A variety of histological subtypes of chondrosarcoma exist, including intramedullary, clear cell, mesenchymal, and dedifferentiated chondrosarcoma. An additional subtype is the extraskeletal myxoid chondrosarcoma. As this is not a bone tumor, it will not be discussed.

There is further classification into primary (lesions arising de novo) and secondary (tumors arising in preexisting lesions, such as enchondroma or osteochondroma) lesions. Finally, chondrosarcoma can be further characterized by location and may be central, peripheral, or juxtacortical. Central chondrosarcomas arise in the medullary cavity; peripheral chondrosarcomas arise in the cartilage cap of an osteochondroma; and juxtacortical lesions arise on the surface of bone.

## Conventional Intramedullary Chondrosarcoma

### Pathophysiology and Clinical Findings

Intramedullary (central) chondrosarcoma is the most common subtype and is classified histologically into 3 grades: grade 1 (low grade), grade 2 (intermediate), and grade 3 (high grade). Grade 1 chondrosarcoma is the most common and also the most difficult to differentiate from enchondroma on both imaging and histologically. Therefore, any differentiation between enchondroma and low-grade chondrosarcoma should be made only in a multidisciplinary team setting where clinical, imaging, and histologic findings specific to each case can be accounted. These tumors usually present in the fourth and fifth decades of life, and are twice as common in men. Patients present with pain in 95% of cases, although intramedullary chondrosarcoma can present with pathologic fracture in 3-17% of cases. The most common site of intramedullary chondrosarcoma is the long bones, with the femur and humerus being the most commonly involved bones. Axial skeleton involvement is also relatively common, with 25% of tumors involving the pelvis and 8% the ribs. Scapular lesions are commonly seen as well, and occur in approximately 5% of cases. Metaphyseal locations (50%) are more common than diaphyseal (36%), epiphyseal (16%), or subarticular sites. Central pelvic chondrosarcoma most often involves the ilium,

particularly in the region of triradiate cartilage. Solitary sternal chondroid lesions are more likely to be chondrosarcomas rather than enchondromas. Chondrosarcoma of the rib most commonly is located anteriorly at the costochondral junction. The overall 5-year survival rate of central chondrosarcoma is reported at 76%. Outcome also appears to be influenced by the site of the lesion with overall survival highest for chest wall lesions and lowest for pelvic lesions.

### Imaging Strategy and Findings

- Preoperative imaging workup of chondrosarcoma includes MRI for local staging and CT of the chest to assess pulmonary metastases. PET/CT may be helpful to evaluate for metastatic disease. Bone scintigraphy may provide little added benefit.

### Radiography

- Imaging shows a mixed lytic and sclerotic lesion with ring-and-arc type calcifications typical of chondroid matrix mineralization.
- Chondroid matrix is evident in 60-78% of cases.
  - Higher-grade tumors are often associated with less mineralized matrix.
- Moth-eaten or permeative bone destruction suggests higher-grade lesion or dedifferentiation.
- Lobular areas of endosteal scalloping, expansion, cortical destruction, and soft tissue mass formation may also be seen. Deep endosteal scalloping (greater than two-thirds cortical depth) and lesion size greater than 5 cm are signs concerning for central chondrosarcoma rather than enchondroma. In fact, central chondrosarcoma is nearly always greater than 4 cm in size.

### Computed Tomography

- CT is helpful to further characterize matrix mineralization, the presence and depth of endosteal scalloping, and soft tissue mass formation (Figure 55.1).
- Chondrosarcoma usually enhances more uniformly than enchondroma following contrast administration because of increased cellularity.

### Magnetic Resonance Imaging

- Lobular margins with punctate areas of signal void caused by matrix mineralization are seen.
- High T2W signal intensity in the noncalcified areas of tumor is visualized.
- Septal and peripheral lobular enhancement occurs after intravenous contrast administration.

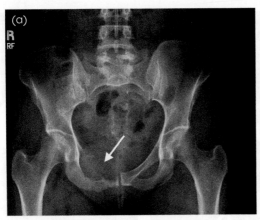
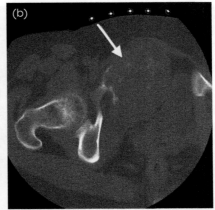

**Figure 55.1.** Grade 2 chondrosarcoma. A 43-year-old woman with destructive pelvic osseous lesion. (*A*) AP radiograph of the pelvis shows an expansile lytic lesion in the right superior pubic ramus with areas of cortical disruption (*arrow*). (*B*) Axial CT image during biopsy planning of the lesion shows ring-and-arc calcifications consistent with cartilage matrix (*arrow*).

- Perilesional BME is uncommon, but may suggest chondrosarcoma rather than enchondroma.
- Entrapped fat within chondrosarcoma suggests low-grade lesion on MRI, whereas soft tissue extension is concerning for high-grade chondrosarcoma.

### Treatment Options
- Histological grade of central chondrosarcoma usually dictates surgical management:
  - Grade 1 is usually treated successfully with intralesional curettage.
  - Grades 2 and 3 are usually treated with wide surgical excision and limb salvage. As with other sarcomas, outcome of chondrosarcoma depends on histological grade, surgical margins, and staging. Grade 1 chondrosarcoma is rarely metastatic at presentation.

## Clear Cell Chondrosarcoma

### Pathophysiology and Clinical Findings
Clear cell chondrosarcoma is a low-grade, epiphyseal-located tumor of the long bones. Histologically, the tumor cells show abundant cytoplasm. Patients usually present in the third to fifth decades of life, and the tumor is more common in men. The long bones are involved in 85-90% of cases of clear cell chondrosarcoma, with the proximal femur being the most common location (68%). The flat bones are uncommonly involved.

### Imaging Findings
#### Radiography and Computed Tomography
- Imaging shows a predominantly lytic, epiphyseal lesion with a variable zone of transition (Figure 55.2).
- Matrix mineralization is seen in 30% of cases, and a sclerotic rim in approximately 20% of cases.

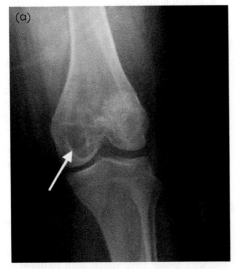
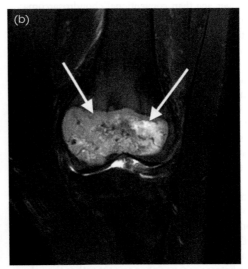

**Figure 55.2.** Clear cell chondrosarcoma. A 13-year-old girl with a distal femoral lytic lesion. (*A*) AP radiograph of the knee shows a lytic lesion in the distal femoral epiphysis with a partially sclerotic rim (*arrow*). (*B*) Coronal T2W FS MR image shows hyperintense signal in the same lesion, suggestive of cartilage (*arrows*).

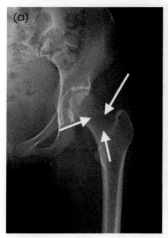
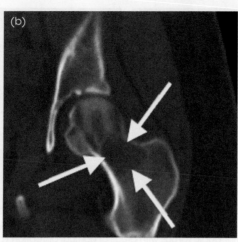
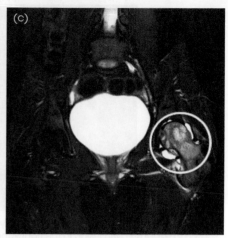

**Figure 55.3.** Mesenchymal chondrosarcoma. A 30-year-old patient with a permeative lytic lesion in the femoral neck. (*A*) AP radiograph of the left hip shows a permeative lytic lesion in the left femoral neck (*arrows*). (*B*) Coronal CT image of the left hip confirms the lytic lesion in the left femoral neck. (*C*) Coronal STIR MR image of the pelvis shows that the lesion also involves the femoral head in addition to the neck (*circle*), with surrounding BME and a hip joint effusion.

- Mild bone expansion may occur, and the proximal humerus has been shown to exhibit a more aggressive growth pattern.

**Magnetic Resonance Imaging**
- Lesions are heterogeneous because of hemorrhage, mineralization, and possible cystic degeneration.
- Perilesional BME is uncommon, which is a finding that aids in its differentiation from the benign epiphyseal lesion, chondroblastoma.

## Mesenchymal Chondrosarcoma

**Pathophysiology and Clinical Findings**
Mesenchymal chondrosarcoma comprises only 2-13% of all bone chondrosarcoma and represents a high-grade variant of chondrosarcoma. Mesenchymal chondrosarcoma usually presents at a younger age than conventional chondrosarcoma, with a mean age of approximately 25 years. The femur is the most commonly affected bone, followed by the ribs, pelvis, humerus, tibia, and fibula. A 5-year survival rate of 52% has been reported.

**Imaging Findings**
**Radiography and Computed Tomography**
- Aggressive, permeative or moth-eaten bone destruction often with periosteal reaction (Figure 55.3) is seen.
- Two-thirds of cases demonstrate chondroid matrix mineralization.
- Large soft tissue mass formation is common.

**Magnetic Resonance Imaging**
- Features of mesenchymal chondrosarcoma differ from conventional chondrosarcoma in that there is heterogeneous T2W signal that is intermediate rather than hyperintense.
- Uniform or heterogeneous enhancement rather than the typical septal or peripheral enhancement of low grade conventional chondrosarcoma is seen.

## Dedifferentiated Chondrosarcoma

**Pathophysiology and Clinical Findings**
Dedifferentiated chondrosarcoma comprises approximately 11% of central chondrosarcomas and is characterized by a high-grade, noncartilaginous sarcoma associated with a preexisting low- to intermediate-grade chondrosarcoma. The noncartilaginous component is usually a conventional high-grade osteosarcoma. There is an equal frequency in men and women with the mean age at diagnosis of 59-66 years. The femur, followed by the pelvis, and then humerus are the most common locations for dedifferentiated chondrosarcoma with most arising in the central medullary cavity. Nearly one-third of dedifferentiated chondrosarcomas present with pathologic fracture and one-fifth with metastatic disease.

**Imaging Findings**
- Imaging appearance is predominantly that of a high-grade chondrosarcoma.

**Radiography**
- Cortical thickening, endosteal scalloping, and periostitis are often present with cortical destruction being commonly seen on approximately 60% of radiographs and 90% of CT and MRI studies (Figure 55.4).
- The key to diagnosis of dedifferentiated chondrosarcoma is the identification of chondroid and nonchondroid components, with areas of aggressive osseous tumor matrix adjacent to areas of chondroid tumor matrix.

**Magnetic Resonance Imaging**
- T2W imaging shows typical well-differentiated chondroid tumor including high signal and peripheral and septal enhancement, and an adjacent component with lower T2W signal with uniform enhancement on T1W postcontrast sequences representing the high-grade sarcoma.

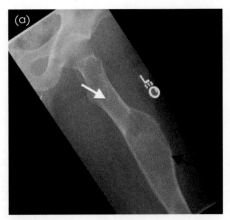 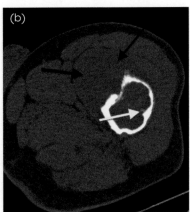 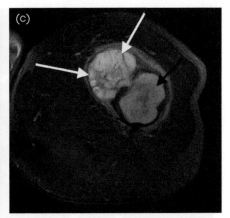

**Figure 55.4.** Dedifferentiated chondrosarcoma. A 59-year-old man with an expansile lytic lesion in the femur. (*A*) Lateral radiograph of the femur shows an expansile lytic lesion with aggressive periosteal reaction (*black arrow*). Note the satellite cartilage lesion more proximally (*white arrow*). (*B*) Axial CT image shows the expansile lesion with cartilage matrix (*white arrow*) and large soft tissue mass (*black arrows*). (*C*) Axial T2W FS MR image shows the hyperintense intramedullary mass (*black arrow*) with associated large soft tissue component (*white arrows*). MRI signal characteristics are that of cartilage.

- Such a *bimorphic* pattern on MRI has been identified in 75% of dedifferentiated chondrosarcomas and is useful for image-guided biopsy targeting of the high-grade component.

## Periosteal Chondrosarcoma

### Pathophysiology and Clinical Findings
Periosteal chondrosarcoma originates from the surface of the bone. It is an uncommon tumor, comprising only approximately 4% of all chondrosarcomas. These lesions most commonly present in the third and fourth decades of life, and are located in the femur, followed by the humerus and tibia, and rarely the ilium, fibula, and ribs. The lesion is located on the surface of the bone with associated thinning or thickening of

the underlying cortex and chondroid matrix mineralization. Cortical destruction is uncommon.

### Imaging Findings
#### Radiography and Computed Tomography
- Thin peripheral shell of calcification is common.

#### Magnetic Resonance Imaging
- Lobular pattern of typical chondroid tumors is seen (Figure 55.5).
- Surrounding BME is uncommon.
- It is difficult to differentiate periosteal chondrosarcoma from periosteal chondroma. The main differentiating feature is tumor size; chondromas have a mean size of 2.2 cm, whereas chondrosarcomas have a mean size of 5.3 cm.

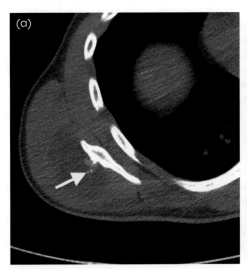 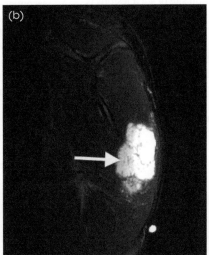 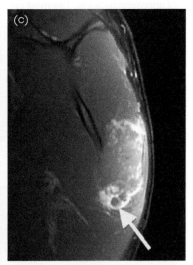

**Figure 55.5.** Periosteal chondrosarcoma. A 32-year-old man with a periosteal lesion. (*A*) Axial CT image shows a periosteal lesion along the inferior scapular body with cartilage calcifications (*arrow*) and periosteal reaction. (*B*) Sagittal T2W FS MR image shows typical hyperintense cartilage signal of the mass (*arrow*). (*C*) Sagittal T1W FS post contrast MR image shows typical peripheral and lobular enhancement pattern of a cartilage tumor (*arrow*). Note that the large size of the lesion favors periosteal chondrosarcoma rather than periosteal chondroma.

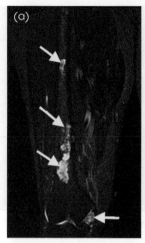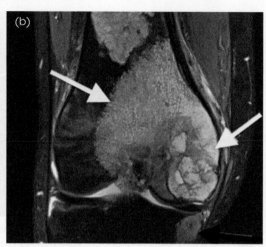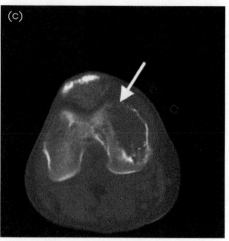

**Figure 55.6.** Ollier disease and secondary chondrosarcoma. A 52-year-old man with multiple enchondromatosis (Ollier disease) and secondary chondrosarcoma. (*A*) Coronal T2- weighted FS MR image of the femur demonstrates multiple cartilage lesions, most consistent with multiple enchondromas (*arrows*). (*B*) Three years later, T2W FS MR image shows marked interval enlargement of the medial femoral condyle cartilage lesion (*white arrows*) and development of a new lesion in the medial tibial plateau (*black arrow*). (*C*) Axial CT image during biopsy planning of the medial femoral condyle lesion shows marked expansion with areas of cortical disruption (*arrow*). Biopsy showed secondary chondrosarcoma.

Periosteal chondroma also tends to be seen in younger patients than periosteal chondrosarcoma.

> Knowledge of these imaging features can improve diagnostic accuracy and help guide clinical management.

## Secondary Chondrosarcoma

### Pathophysiology and Clinical Findings

Chondrosarcoma that arises in association with a benign chondroid lesion, such as an enchondroma or osteochondroma, is termed *secondary chondrosarcoma*. Secondary chondrosarcoma occurring within an underlying enchondroma has a similar imaging appearance as conventional central chondrosarcoma (Figure 55.6), which has been previously discussed. Secondary chondrosarcoma arising from a solitary osteochondroma is estimated to occur at a rate of approximately 1%. The most common site of such lesions is the pelvis, hip, or shoulder.

### Imaging Strategy and Findings

- Diagnosis of malignant transformation in an osteochondroma depends on identification of the cartilage cap thickness which can be assessed with ultrasound, CT, or MRI.
- Cartilage cap thickness of 2 cm or greater is strongly indicative of malignant transformation.

### Key Points

- Chondrosarcoma is the third most common primary malignant bone tumor.
- Conventional intramedullary chondrosarcoma is its most common subtype, although other less common forms such as clear cell, mesenchymal, dedifferentiated, and periosteal subtypes do exist.
- There are specific imaging features that can aid in the diagnosis of chondrosarcoma and these distinct subtypes.

### Recommended Reading

Logie CI, Walker EA, Forsberg JA, Potter BK, Murphey MD. Chondrosarcoma: a diagnostic imager's guide to decision making and patient management. *Semin Musculoskelet Radiol.* 2013;17(2):101–15.

### References

1. Bernard SA, Murphey MD, Flemming DJ, Kransdorf MJ. Improved differentiation of benign osteochondromas from secondary chondrosarcomas with standardized measurement of cartilage cap at CT and MR imaging. *Radiology.* 2010;255:857–65.
2. Collins MS, Koyama T, Swee RG, Inwards CY. Clear cell chondrosarcoma: radiographic, computed tomographic, and magnetic resonance findings in 34 patients with pathologic correlation. *Skeletal Radiol.* 2003;32:687–94.
3. Douis H, Saifuddin A. The imaging of cartilaginous bone tumours. II. Chondrosarcoma. *Skeletal Radiol.* 2013; 42:611–26.
4. Eefting D, Schrage YM, Geirnaerdt MJ, et al. Assessment of interobserver variability and histologic parameters to improve reliability in classification and grading of central cartilaginous tumors. *Am J Surg Pathol.* 2009;33:50–57.
5. Kaim AH, Hugli R, Bonel HM, Jundt G. Chondroblastoma and clear cell chondrosarcoma: radiological and MRI characteristics with histopathological correlation. *Skeletal Radiol.* 2002;31:88–95.
6. Littrell LA, Wenger DE, Wold LE, et al. Radiographic, CT, and MR imaging features of dedifferentiated chondrosarcomas: a retrospective review of 174 de novo cases. *Radiographics.* 2004;24:1397–409.

7. MacSweeney F, Darby A, Saifuddin A. Dedifferentiated chondrosarcoma of the appendicular skeleton: MRI-pathological correlation. *Skeletal Radiol.* 2003;32:671–78.

8. Murphey MD, Choi JJ, Kransdorf MJ, Flemming DJ, Gannon FH. Imaging of osteochondroma: variants and complications with radiologic– pathologic correlation. *Radiographics.* 2000;20:1407–34.

9. Murphey MD, Walker EA, Wilson AJ, Kransdorf MJ, Temple HT, Gannon FH. From the archives of the AFIP: imaging of primary chondrosarcoma: radiologic–pathologic correlation. *Radiographics.* 2003;23:1245–78.

10. Robinson P, White LM, Sundaram M, et al. Periosteal chondroid tumors: radiologic evaluation with pathologic correlation. *AJR Am J Roentgenol.* 2001;177:1183–88.

11. Skeletal Lesions Interobserver Correlation among Expert Diagnosticians (SLICED) Study Group. Reliability of histopathologic and radiologic grading of cartilaginous neoplasms in long bones. *J Bone Joint Surg Am.* 2007;89:2113–23.

12. Yoo HJ, Hong SH, Choi JY, et al. Differentiating high-grade from low-grade chondrosarcoma with MR imaging. *Eur Radiol.* 2009;19:3008–3014.

# Fibrous Matrix Bone Tumors

# CHAPTER 56

# Benign Fibrous Matrix Bone Tumors

Albert Song

## Introduction

Fibrous lesions of the bone are part of a broad category, encompassing developmental, reactive, and neoplastic entities. Neoplastic lesions can be fibroblastic/myofibroblastic and fibrohistiocytic in cell origin, and include benign fibrous histiocytoma and nonossifying fibroma. Nonossifying fibroma and benign fibrous histiocytoma are histologically indistinguishable from one another. The WHO classifies these lesions into a single entity and differentiates the two by clinical presentation and appearance on imaging. Fibrous dysplasia is a fibroosseous developmental lesion associated with GNAS1 gene mutations. These lesions represent bone replaced by fibrous tissue and irregular trabecula made of woven bone. Finally, desmoplastic fibromas are the intraosseous equivalent of soft tissue fibromatosis.

## Nonossifying Fibroma and Benign Fibrous Histiocytoma

### Pathophysiology and Clinical Findings

Nonossifying fibromas (NOFs) are one of the most common benign lesions of bone and are discovered incidentally in patients younger than age 15. Lesions are asymptomatic but can present with pain in the presence of pathologic fracture. The term *nonossifying fibroma* has been used synonymously with fibrous cortical defect, benign cortical defect, metaphyseal cortical defect, and fibroxanthoma. Some authors distinguish NOF from a fibrous cortical defect when lesions are larger than 3 cm. Although malignant degeneration has been reported, its true occurrence remains controversial.

NOFs occur in long bones, particularly the tibia and femur. Polyostotic NOF is associated with Jaffe-Campanacci syndrome and neurofibromatosis type 1. NOFs are usually metaphyseal and tend to be eccentrically intramedullary or intracortical.

Benign fibrous histiocytoma (BFH) is a rare lesion that typically occurs in patients who are older than age 20, although a range from 6 to 74 years has been reported. Although 15% of BFH lesions present incidentally, most patients experience pain. BFH most commonly occurs in the long bones but may also occur in the pelvis. BFH can be metaphyseal, diaphyseal, or epiphyseal, and it also tends to be eccentrically intramedullary or intracortical.

## Fibrous Dysplasia

### Pathophysiology and Clinical Findings

Fibrous dysplasia (FD) can be either monostotic or polyostotic. Polyostotic FD is associated with multiple syndromes including McCune-Albright syndrome (café-au-lait spots, precocious puberty, diabetes, and endocrine dysfunction), Mazabraud syndrome (soft tissue myxomas), diabetes mellitus, Cushing disease, and others. Most cases occur in adolescence or young adulthood without gender predilection. Although some cases are asymptomatic, these lesions can be locally aggressive, and patients often present with pain, deformity, or palpable abnormality. Additionally, some patients may present with pathologic fracture. FD is an intramedullary and often central lesion, usually found in the diaphysis and metaphysis. It may appear elongated if the lesion grows longitudinally along with long bone growth. Monostotic disease most commonly affects the craniofacial bones, proximal femora, and ribs. Polyostotic disease most commonly occurs in the femur, tibia, and pelvis. When the craniofacial bones are involved, patients may present with nerve compression. Up to 4% of lesions may degenerate into malignancy, most commonly osteosarcoma.

## Imaging of Nonossifying Fibroma, Benign Fibrous Histiocytoma, and Fibrous Dysplasia

### Imaging Strategy
- NOF, BFH, and FD have similar imaging features; however, skeletal location (including whether the lesion is centrally or eccentrically positioned within the medullary cavity, and whether it is metaphyseal or diaphyseal), and pattern of attenuation may be helpful in distinguishing these conditions from one another.
- Radiography is the primary choice of imaging because the vast majority of cases of benign fibrous lesions of the bone will be either confidently diagnosed or recognized as nonaggressive on radiography.
- Lesions that are indeterminate or demonstrate aggressive features, such as a wide zone of transition, cortical breach or soft tissue mass should be evaluated with MRI.
- CT is useful to better evaluate subtle cortical breakthrough, identify matrix mineralization, or for surgical planning.
- Bone scintigraphy is of varying sensitivity and often not specific but may be useful in the detection of polyostotic disease.

### Imaging Findings
### Radiography
- Benign fibrous lesions of bone have similar appearances on radiography.

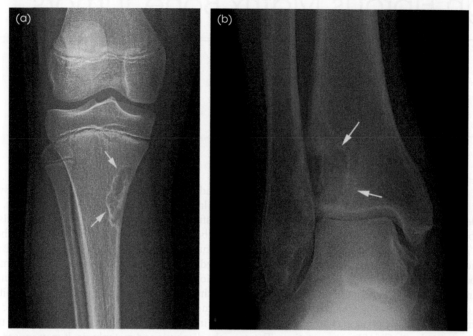

**Figure 56.1.** Comparison of NOF and BFH. On radiography both NOF (*A*) and BFH (*B*) are lucent lesions with sclerotic, well-defined margins (*arrows*). They can both have septations but no matrix mineralization. NOFs occur in children and resolve by adulthood, whereas BFH lesions are found in adults and can be painful. NOFs are metaphyseal or metadiaphyseal, whereas BFH can also occur in the epiphysis. Both NOF and BFH are eccentrically located.

- Lesions are lucent with narrow zones of transition, thin sclerotic margins, and internal septations (Figure 56.1).
  - Lesions may have a bubbly appearance because of internal septations.
- With the exception of FD, they lack matrix mineralization.
- When large or eccentric and intracortical, lesions tend to expand and thin the cortex.
  - In extreme cases, deformities may occur.

- Presence of nonaggressive periosteal bone formation suggests development of a stress riser or pathologic fracture.
- Aggressive radiographic features include wide zones of transition, cortical destruction, and aggressive periosteal bone formation (Figure 56.2).
- Rapid growth, increased bone destruction, and soft tissue mass are other features indicative of malignancy.

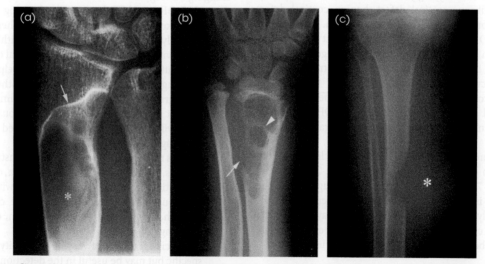

**Figure 56.2.** Three fibrous lesions of bone from least to greatest degree of aggressiveness, 2 of which are benign and 1 of which is malignant. FD of the distal radius in a 34-year-old man (*A*) shows sclerotic margination (*arrow*). Notice the elongated morphology, as this developmental lesion grows longitudinally with the long bone. Ground-glass attenuation (*asterisk*) is caused by intralesional irregular trabeculae. In comparison, this example of desmoplastic fibroma of the distal radius in an 11-year-old boy who presented with swelling after a football game (*B*) is locally aggressive. The cortex is severely expanded and thinned (*arrow*). Internal septations (*arrowhead*) create a soap bubble appearance. The third lesion is an undifferentiated high-grade pleomorphic sarcoma (previously known as MFH, which is further discussed in Chapter 57, "Malignant Fibrous Lesions of the Bone") of the tibia in an 82-year-old woman (*C*). Although still geographic, the margins are very ill defined. There is cortical destruction with a large soft tissue mass (*asterisk*).

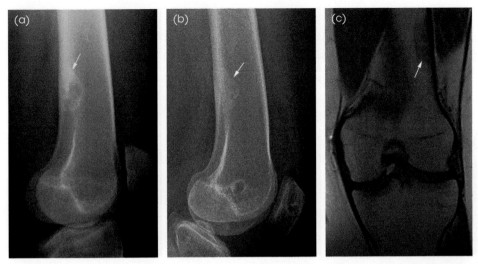

**Figure 56.3.** Healing NOF. NOF of the tibia on these 2 serial lateral radiographs (*A* and *B*) demonstrates the typical pattern of regression as ossification of the lesion begins at the diaphyseal side of the lesion and progresses to the epiphyseal aspect of the lesion (arrows). Eventually, the lesion will completely ossify and become indistinguishable to the surrounding bone. The internal signal of this ossifying NOF on this coronal T1W MR image (*C*) shows fatty marrow replacement of the lesion (arrow), consistent with healing.

- As the patient reaches osseous maturity, NOFs will ossify from the diaphysis to the epiphysis, usually completely resolving without a trace (Figure 56.3).
- FD appears as a lucent lesion with ground-glass attenuation that represents fibrous tissue, and increased opacity represents increased intralesional woven bone (Figures 56.2*A* and 56.4).

### Magnetic Resonance Imaging
- Lesions tend to have regions void of signal on all sequences, representing collagen-rich areas.
- Fibrous stroma is intermediate to hyperintense on T2W images, hypointense on T1W images with variable enhancement (Figure 56.5).
- MRI is more sensitive for occult fracture detection than both CT and radiography.
- MRI is useful for the detection of marrow invasion or extraosseous soft tissue extension, indicating aggressive behavior.

### Treatment Options
- Most lesions do not require intervention.
- Larger BFHs and NOFs can be treated with curettage and bone graft.
- Reconstructive surgery may be performed for deformity correction.

## Osteofibrous Dysplasia

### Pathophysiology and Clinical Findings
Osteofibrous dysplasia, or ossifying fibroma, is similar to FD histologically but has a cortical location. It almost always occurs in the anterior mid tibial diaphysis, and is usually seen in patients younger than age 10 with a male predominance. Patients may present with painless swelling, mild tenderness, or anterior tibial bowing deformity. The lesion usually spontaneously regresses but may slowly enlarge. Complications include pathologic fracture and pseudoarthrosis. This lesion has been associated with adamantinoma, which is a malignant lesion that occurs in the same location and can exist concurrently. As a result, some authors have suggested both lesions represent a spectrum of histologic findings.

### Imaging Findings
#### Radiography
- Expansile, ground-glass appearance centered in the anterior mid tibial diaphyseal cortex
- May have a lobulated sclerotic rim

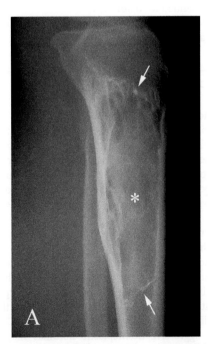

**Figure 56.4.** FD. Lateral radiograph of the proximal tibia in a 34-year-old patient who presented with leg pain shows a centrally occurring intramedullary lucent lesion. The margins are sclerotic and well-defined (*arrows*). Again, notice the elongated shape of the lesion in this. Attenuation here is ground glass (*asterisk*), but can vary depending on extent of internal trabeculation.

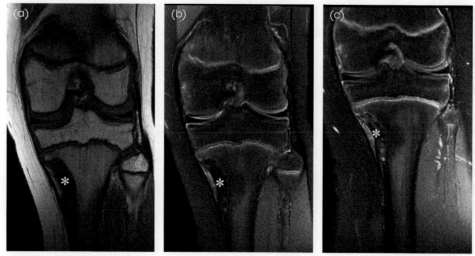

**Figure 56.5.** Benign fibrous bone lesions tend to have similar signal characteristics on MRI. In this example of a proximal tibial NOF, the lesion (*asterisk*) is hypointense on coronal T1W (*A*) and heterogeneous on T2W (*B*) MR images. Areas devoid of signal represent fibrous matrix. The lesion demonstrates variable enhancement on the coronal T1W FS MR image (*C*).

- Lack of aggressive osteolysis or periosteal reaction

### Magnetic Resonance Imaging
- Nonspecific appearance
- Useful to detect aggressive features such as soft tissue extension or bone destruction, which favor adamantinoma or other aggressive process

### Treatment Options
- Conservative management is recommended. Lesions frequently recur after resection.
- If the patient is skeletally immature, bracing is recommended for deformity.
- Surgical correction of deformity can be considered after skeletal maturity.

## Desmoplastic Fibroma

### Pathophysiology and Clinical Findings
Desmoplastic fibroma is a rare, locally aggressive intraosseous lesion usually occurring in patients younger than age 40 with a slight male predominance. It most commonly presents in the pelvis and long bones, such as the femur, humerus, and radius. The lesion generally arises in the diaphysis but often extends into the metaphysis. Patients present with localized pain and swelling.

### Imaging Findings
### Radiography
- Desmoplastic fibroma does not have a specific imaging appearance. The bone looks expanded with cortical thinning or thickening and may have a sharp zone of transition. Occasionally, the lesion may have a thickened pseudotrabeculated appearance (Figure 56.2A).
- More aggressive desmoplastic fibromas may demonstrate osteolysis and soft tissue extension and can mimic malignant lesions.

### Magnetic Resonance Imaging
- Lesions are isointense or hypointense to skeletal muscle on T1W and fluid-sensitive imaging.
- T2W signal is often heterogeneous, and the areas of lower signal may be related to collagen deposition.
- Following IV gadolinium administration, heterogeneous enhancement is seen.

### Treatment Options
- Wide excision is treatment of choice for desmoplastic fibromas; however, local recurrence is common.
- Curettage of desmoplastic fibromas is not recommended because of its locally aggressive behavior and up to 72% recurrence rate. Even with en bloc resection, up to 17% of lesions recur locally.

### Key Points
- Benign fibrous lesions of bone are clinically and radiologically nonaggressive and often do not require intervention.
- NOF and BFH are radiologically and histologically identical. NOFs tend to be asymptomatic, present in younger patients, and are located in the metaphysis. Conversely, patients with BFH tend to be older and present with pain. In addition, these lesions may occur in the epiphysis, metaphysis, or diaphysis.
- Large or complicated benign fibrous lesions may require intervention, usually curettage and bone grafting.

### Recommended Reading
Miller TT. Bone tumors and tumorlike conditions: analysis with conventional radiography. *Radiology.* 2008;246(3): 662–74.
Kumar R, Madewell JE, Lindell MM, Swischuk LE. Fibrous lesions of bones. *Radiographics.* 1990;10(2):237–56.

## References

1. Asnes RS, Berdon WE, Bassett CA. Hypophosphatemic rickets in an adolescent cured by excision of a non-ossifying fibroma. *Clin Pediatr (Phila)*. 1981;20(10):646–48.

2. Fletcher CD, Hogendoorn P, Mertens F, Bridge J, eds. *WHO Classification of Tumours of Soft Tissue and Bone*. 4th ed. Lyon, France: IARC Press; 2013.

3. Gebhardt MC, Campbell CJ, Schiller AL, et al. Desmoplastic fibroma of bone. A report of eight cases and a review of the literature. *J Bone Joint Surg Am*. 1985;67(5):732–47.

4. Graudal N. Desmoplastic fibroma of bone. Case report and literature review. *Acta Orthop Scand*. 1984;55(2):215–19.

5. Kumar R, Madewell JE, Lindell MM, Swischuk LE. Fibrous lesions of bones. *Radiographics*. 1990;10(2):237–56.

6. Leehey DJ, Ing TS, Daugirdas JT. Fanconi syndrome associated with a non-ossifying fibroma of bone. *Am J Med*. 1985;78(4):708–10.

7. Miller TT. Bone tumors and tumorlike conditions: analysis with conventional radiography. *Radiology*. 2008;246(3):662–74.

8. Peterson HA, Fitzgerald EM. Fractures through non-ossifying fibromas in children. *Minn Med*. 1980;63(2):139–44.

# CHAPTER 57

# Malignant Fibrous Lesions of the Bone

Albert Song

## Introduction

Malignant fibrous matrix lesions of bone include undifferentiated high-grade pleomorphic sarcoma and fibrosarcoma. Acknowledging its complex and poorly defined nature, WHO reclassified MFH as undifferentiated high-grade pleomorphic sarcoma. The constant evolution of classification and terminology of malignant fibrous lesions of bone is a source of much confusion, complicating the diagnosis and epidemiologic study of these lesions. The true incidence of undifferentiated high-grade pleomorphic sarcoma and fibrosarcoma are probably understated.

## Pathophysiology and Clinical Findings

Both undifferentiated high-grade pleomorphic sarcoma and fibrosarcoma consist of spindle cells, which are characteristically organized in a herringbone configuration in fibrosarcoma. These cells are highly disorganized and heterogeneous in undifferentiated high-grade pleomorphic sarcoma, and thus also referred to as *pleomorphic fibrosarcoma*. Histiocytic infiltration and epithelioid cells are also found in undifferentiated high-grade pleomorphic sarcoma. Both lesions are diagnoses of exclusion, and therefore require extensive tissue sampling to exclude a specific line of cellular differentiation. Presence of osteoid or chondroid matrix would indicate osteosarcoma or chondrosarcoma respectively.

Patients with malignant fibrous lesions of bone typically present with pain, limited range of motion, swelling, and pathologic fracture. Most cases present in patients older than age 40, with only 10-15% presenting in those younger than age 20. Up to one-third of lesions are secondary, arising from other bone conditions such as Paget disease of bone, bone infarct, chronic osteomyelitis, previous radiation treatment, or dedifferentiation of a low-grade sarcoma (Figure 57.1). Half of cases metastasize, most commonly to the lungs. With localized disease, a greater than 50% 5-year survival rate can be achieved with wide excision and negative margins.

## Imaging Strategy for Malignant Fibrous Lesions

### Radiography
- This is the initial examination of choice.
- Often, these lesions will appear aggressive on radiography and warrant biopsy.
  - The lesion location relative to the joint is useful information for surgical planning.

### Computed Tomography
- CT can be performed to exclude matrix mineralization, evaluate presence or degree of cortical destruction, and detect pathologic fracture.
- CT of the chest is routinely obtained to survey for metastatic disease.

### Magnetic Resonance Imaging
- MRI allows for better assessment of marrow and soft tissue mass extension. It is essential to describe the tumor's spatial relationship to any adjacent neurovascular bundles for presurgical planning.
- Regional lymph nodes may be within the FOV and should be evaluated for tumor involvement.

### Nuclear Imaging
- In bone scintigraphy, although nonspecific, lesions show avid uptake of radiotracer and may be used to detect synchronous or distal metastatic osseous lesions.

### Ultrasound and Image-Guided Biopsy
- Although US can be used for image-guided percutaneous biopsy when a significant soft tissue component exists, it cannot penetrate cortical bone and cannot be used to guide biopsy of intraosseous lesions in which there is an intact cortex.
  - CT is superior for image-guided percutaneous needle biopsy of intraosseous lesions.
  - Historically, the needle tract for percutaneous biopsy has been resected along with the tumor. Therefore, it is important to involve the surgeon when planning approach for biopsy.

## Imaging Findings
Refer to Figure 57.2.

### Radiography and Computed Tomography
- This imaging tends to show large, lucent, eccentric intramedullary lesions most commonly in the metaphysis or metadiaphysis of long bones. The most common bones affected are the femur, tibia, humerus, and the pelvis.
- Aggressive features, including wide zone of transition, cortical destruction, and aggressive periosteal bone formation, are seen.
- Lesions may be moth-eaten or permeative in appearance.
- Rapid growth, increased bone destruction, and soft tissue mass are other features indicative of malignancy.
- Occasionally, aggressive bone destruction may result in formation of a sequestrum, in which a partially destroyed piece of bone becomes separated from the rest of the bone.

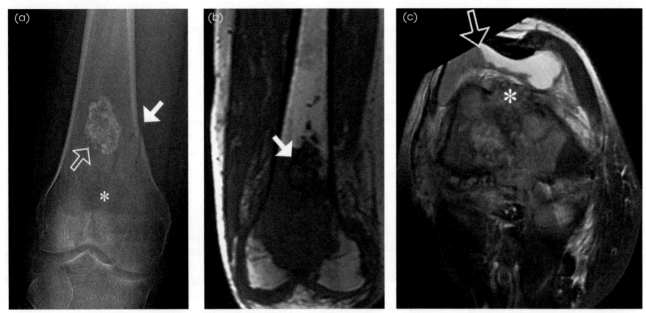

**Figure 57.1.** Undifferentiated high-grade pleomorphic sarcoma dedifferentiating from a chondroid matrix lesion. An ill-defined lesion (*asterisk*) is seen arising from an enchondroma at the distal femoral metaphysis with a medial partial articular pathological fracture (*white arrow*) on the AP view of the distal femur (*A*). There is subtle erosion of the distal lateral margin of the enchondroma (*arrow*). Coronal T1W (*B*) MR image shows a hypointense mass in the distal femoral metaphysis arising from the enchondroma (*arrow*). The mass is heterogeneous on axial T2W FS MR image (*C*) with cortical destruction at the trochlear sulcus of the distal femur and soft tissue extension (*asterisk*) into the knee joint. Notice the fluid-fluid level (*arrow*) within the joint effusion because of hemarthrosis secondary to the intraarticular pathologic fracture.

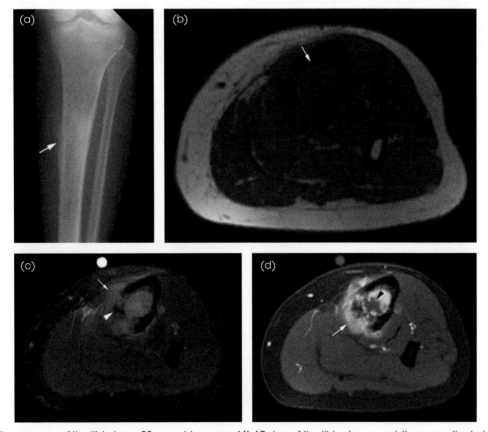

**Figure 57.2.** Fibrosarcoma of the tibia in an 82-year-old woman. (*A*) AP view of the tibia shows a subtle permeative lesion at the proximal tibial metadiaphysis. There is irregular periosteal new bone formation at the medial proximal diaphysis (*arrow*). On MRI, the lesion is hypointense on T1W (*B*) and hyperintense on T2W FS (*C*) axial MR images. There is destruction of the medial cortex with sequestrum formation (*arrowhead*) and soft tissue extension invading the subcutaneous and posterior compartments (*arrow*). (*D*) The lesion shows heterogeneous enhancement (*white arrow*) on T1W FS postcontrast MR image. Central regions of nonenhancement (*black arrowhead*) represent tumor necrosis, which is a poor prognostic indicator.

### Magnetic Resonance Imaging

- Soft tissue components are usually isointense to hypointense to skeletal muscle on T1W imaging and heterogeneously hyperintense on T2W imaging with areas of variable enhancement.
- There are often confluent regions of low signal on MRI, which represent collagen-rich areas, calcification, or hemosiderin deposition caused by intralesional hemorrhage.
- Central nonenhancing soft tissue represents tumor necrosis.
  - Large regions of necrosis are an indicator of poor prognosis.

### Treatment Options

- Wide surgical excision is recommended.
- Chemotherapy has been shown to minimally improve overall and disease-free survival.
- Neoadjuvant, intraoperative, and postoperative radiation therapy has been shown to decrease local recurrence but has not shown improved 5-year survival rate.

## Key Points

- Radiography is the modality of choice for the initial evaluation of malignant fibrous bone tumors.
- Radiographic features, such as wide zone of transition, cortical destruction, aggressive periosteal bone formation, and soft tissue mass, are characteristic of malignant fibrous lesions of bone.
- MRI is often performed to evaluate bone marrow and soft tissue extent of disease. Invasion of the neurovascular bundle and local lymph nodes are best assessed on MRI.
- Malignant fibrous lesions of bone are diagnoses of exclusion. Histologic diagnosis requires extensive soft tissue sampling.

- Image-guided percutaneous soft tissue sampling should be performed in consultation with orthopedic oncology.

### Recommended Reading

Miller TT. Bone tumors and tumorlike conditions: analysis with conventional radiography. *Radiology*. 2008;246(3):662–74.

Kumar R, Madewell JE, Lindell MM, Swischuk LE. Fibrous lesions of bones. *Radiographics*. 1990;10(2):237–56.

### References

1. Dahlin DC, Ivins JC. Fibrosarcoma of bone. A study of 114 cases. *Cancer*. 1969;23(1):35–41.
2. Fletcher CD, Hogendoorn P, Mertens F, Bridge J, eds. *WHO Classification of Tumours of Soft Tissue and Bone*. 4th ed. Lyon, France: IARC Press; 2013.
3. Huvos AG, Higinbotham NL. Primary fibrosarcoma of bone: a clinicopathologic study of 130 patients. *Cancer*. 1975;35(3):837–47.
4. Kumar R, Madewell JE, Lindell MM, Swischuk LE. Fibrous lesions of bones. *Radiographics*. 1990;10(2):237–56.
5. Larsson SE, Lorentzon R, Boquist L. Fibrosarcoma of bone. a demographic, clinical and histopathological study of all cases reported to the Swedish cancer registry from 1958–1968. *J Bone Joint Surg Br*. 1976;58-B(4):412–17.
6. Miller TT. Bone tumors and tumorlike conditions: analysis with conventional radiography. *Radiology*. 2008;246(3):662–74.
7. Papagelopoulos PJ, Galanis E, Frassica FJ, Sim FH, Larson DR, Wold LE. Primary fibrosarcoma of bone. Outcome after primary surgical treatment. *Clin Orthop Relat Res*. 2000 Apr;(373):88–103.
8. Taconis WK, Mulder JD. Fibrosarcoma and malignant fibrous histiocytoma of long bones. Radiographic features and grading. *Skeletal Radiol*. 1984;11(4):237–45.

# Normal Bone Marrow and Bone Marrow Lesions

# CHAPTER 58

# Normal Bone Marrow and Benign Bone Marrow Lesions

Jonathan D. Samet

## Normal Bone Marrow

### Physiology and Distribution

As people age, bone marrow composition progressively converts from hematopoietic (red) marrow to fatty (yellow) marrow. At birth, the bone marrow is entirely cellular (red marrow). Starting from fingers and toes and spreading toward the spine, the red marrow slowly converts to fatty marrow. By skeletal maturity, the extremities have converted mostly to fatty marrow. In a given long bone, the epiphysis becomes fatty first, followed by the diaphysis and then the metaphysis. In infants for example, the epiphyseal ossification centers will be the first to become fatty replaced, within 6 months after radiologic visualization. Residual red marrow is commonly seen in the metaphyses, especially the proximal humerus and femur (Figure 58.1*A, B*; Table 58.1).

### Imaging Findings
#### Magnetic Resonance Imaging
- Fatty marrow
  - Demonstrates high signal intensity on T1W and T2W non-fat-suppressed sequences compared to skeletal muscle, and is similar to subcutaneous adipose tissue
  - Fat saturation routinely used on fluid-sensitive sequences including T2W FS, STIR, and also PD sequences.
    - With fat suppression, the bright signal from fatty marrow decreases, similar to subcutaneous fat, increasing the conspicuity of pathologic signal.
- Red marrow
  - Compared with skeletal muscle on fat-suppressed, fluid-sensitive sequences, red marrow is mildly hyperintense but hypointense to fluid.
  - On T1W imaging red marrow is relatively hypointense.
  - Even in prominent red marrow, foci of T1 hyperintense signal representing areas of interspersed yellow marrow can be seen within the hypointense signal, which is a reassuring sign that it is not a pathologic process.
  - In long bones, the morphology of normal red marrow is ill-defined, referred to as flame-shaped, fanning away from the physis (Figure 58.1*C*).
  - Chemical-shift imaging can help determine if there is malignant marrow replacement.
    - When fat and water are present in a given voxel, the magnitude vectors at their resonant frequency will be at 180 degrees to one another at specific times on 1.5 and 3 T, therefore canceling each other out. This will cause a dependable drop in signal when equal amounts of fat and water are present in the same voxel. Normal red marrow is not entirely cellular (which largely consists of water) and still contains a large percentage of fat (approximately 40% fat and 40% water). Therefore, there is a predictable signal drop (hypointensity) seen on opposed-phase (out-of-phase) sequences for red marrow, typically 15-20%. For comparison, yellow marrow is 80% fat and 15% water, and there is very little drop in signal on opposed-phase sequences.

## Benign Bone Marrow Lesions

### Red Marrow ReconversionPathophysiology and Clinical Findings

The bone marrow is a dynamic organ; when stressed, recovering, or in response to medications, it can become physiologically hyperactive. Previously seen regions of fatty marrow can undergo so-called red marrow reconversion, typically in the reverse direction compared to aging. For the radiologist who may not be aware of the cause of marrow reconversion at the time of interpretation, this can be a troubling finding on MRI, and possibly mistaken for a malignancy. If it appears diffuse, the findings can mimic leukemia, and if spotty, it could be confused for metastatic disease. However, the MRI characteristics of red marrow already discussed will also hold true in cases of red marrow reconversion. For example, in conditions that produce anemia, such as sickle cell anemia, the bone marrow produces more red marrow to counteract the effects of anemia (Figure 58.2). Thalassemia can also induce hyperplasia of the hematopoietic marrow secondary to chronic anemia and is discussed in Chapter 74, "Anemias." Obesity and smoking have also been reported to produce red marrow reconversion. Oncologic patients receiving granulocyte-macrophage colony-stimulating factor (GM-CSF) to intentionally restart the bone marrow after chemotherapy, have a characteristic hypercellular red marrow reconversion pattern on imaging. As with all of radiology, a thorough history is critical in correctly interpreting the imaging findings.

## Table 58.1. Benign and Malignant Bone Marrow Conditions

| BENIGN MARROW CONDITIONS | MALIGNANT MARROW CONDITIONS |
|---|---|
| Red marrow reconversion | Neuroblastoma |
| Edema | Leukemia |
| Infarction | Lymphoma |
| Osteomyelitis | Multiple myeloma |
| Intraosseous fat deposits | Ewing sarcoma |
| Infiltration (Gaucher disease) | |
| Chronic recurrent multifocal osteomyelitis (CRMO) | |

### Bone Marrow Edema
#### Pathophysiology and Clinical Findings

BME is a nonspecific response of the marrow to trauma, infection, neoplasia, and many other insults. In the setting of trauma, this BME, thought to reflect microtrabecular injury, is referred to as *bone contusion*. In cases of overuse, repetitive injury, it is known as an *osseous stress reaction*. The location, MRI signal, and morphology, combined with the history will lead one to the correct diagnosis. In many instances, this appearance does not correspond to true edema histologically, and some authors have preferred terms such as *marrow edema-like signal abnormalities*. However, *bone marrow edema* and *BME* are shorter terms that are familiar to imagers and clinicians, and will be used throughout this book.

### Imaging Findings
- MRI
  - T2 hyperintense compared with skeletal muscle and brighter than red marrow
  - Can be associated with dark signal on T1W imaging
  - Ill-defined morphology and patchy distribution, typically centered at the site of pathology whether it is related to bone contusion or osteomyelitis (Figure 58.3)
  - Should search carefully for subtle fracture lines that may represent stress fractures or incomplete posttraumatic fractures
  - Lines are usually T1 and T2 hypointense, depending on the chronicity; can be T2 hyperintense if fluid-filled

### Osteonecrosis

ON can be secondary to many etiologies, including idiopathic, sickle cell disease, drug related (steroids), and prior infection. Medullary ON is commonly called *bone infarct* and is commonly seen in the metaphysis and diaphysis of long bones (Figure 58.4). ON seen in the epiphyses is commonly referred to as avascular necrosis. The findings of ON are more thoroughly discussed in Chapter 115, "Osteonecroses and Osteochondroses."

### Bone Marrow Infection (Osteomyelitis)

Osteomyelitis produces a spectrum of imaging findings depending on age and type (Figure 58.5). In pediatric patients, osteomyelitis of long bones occurs near sites of active endochondral ossification, the physis. Therefore, it is most commonly seen in the metaphysis adjacent to the physis. The epiphysis and diaphysis are uncommonly affected in isolation. In adults, it is commonly seen as contiguous spread of infection from the soft tissues, for example, in the diabetic foot. Acute infarcts in sickle cell disease may be difficult to distinguish from osteomyelitis (see Chapter 74). The imaging

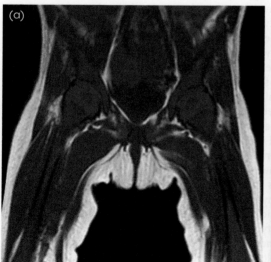
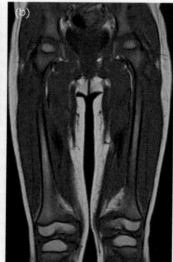
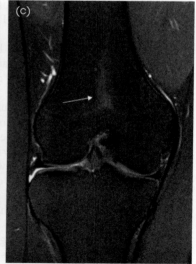

**Figure 58.1.** Normal distribution of hematopoietic marrow at different ages on MRI. (*A*) Coronal T1W image of the pelvis in a 5-month-old patient with normal bone marrow signal. The femoral ossification centers have formed but remain cellular. Red marrow persists in all visualized bones. Image courtesy of Mary Wyers, MD, Chicago, IL. (*B*) Coronal T1W image of both femora in a healthy 2-year-old child. The visualized marrow in the epiphyses and diaphyses are predominantly fatty. Subtle red marrow is seen in the metaphyses. (*C*) Coronal PD FS of the knee shows normal red marrow in the distal metaphysis projecting away from the physis. Note the characteristic flame shaped slightly PD hyperintense appearance (*arrow*).

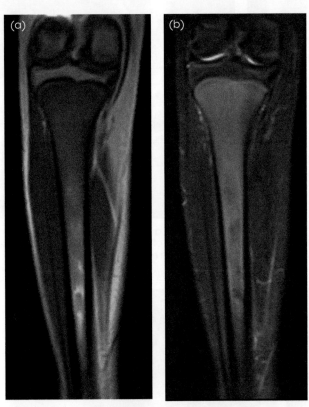

**Figure 58.2.** Hematopoietic marrow in a patient with sickle cell disease. Coronal T1W (*A*) and coronal STIR (*B*) MR images of the tibia in a 13-year-old child with sickle cell disease with prominent red marrow in the metaphysis and diaphysis, greater than would be expected for a healthy child. This is consistent with red marrow reconversion.

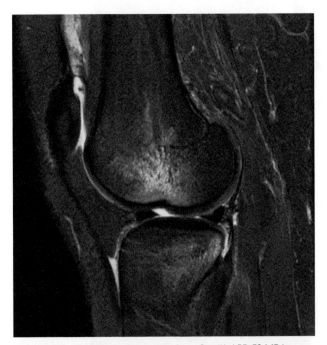

**Figure 58.3.** BME related to contusions. Sagittal PD FS MR image of the knee in a patient with ACL tear showing classic *kissing* contusion BME pattern from a pivot shift mechanism of injury. The BME signal is more hyperintense compared to the grayish red marrow superior to the contusion.

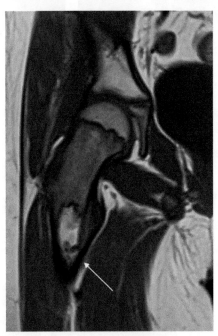

**Figure 58.4.** ON. Coronal T1W image of the femur in an oncologic patient performed because of areas of suspicious hypermetabolic activity on recent PET/CT. MRI showed a fat-containing lesion in the proximal right femur, consistent with a bone infarct (*arrow*).

findings of osteomyelitis are more thoroughly discussed in Chapter 86, "Osteomyelitis of the Long and Flat Bones."

### Intraosseous Fat Deposits
### Pathophysiology and Clinical Findings
In the setting of trauma and infection, the fatty marrow can occasionally liquefy, which is thought to be related to bursting of fat cells. This can produce a fatty globule within the marrow space or in the surrounding soft tissues. On fracture follow-up, these fat globules can be mistaken for primary bone lesions or bone destruction in the setting of osteomyelitis.

### Imaging Findings
- MRI (Figure 58.6)
  - Apparent lesions will follow fat signal on all sequences, confirming the diagnosis of fat globule.
  - A fat-fluid level can be observed in the soft tissues in the setting of acute osteomyelitis, secondary to bone marrow fat leaking out of the intramedullary space.

### Posttherapeutic Conditions
### Pathophysiology and Clinical Findings
Oncology patients receiving chemotherapy, radiation, or bone marrow-altering medications, or who are recovering from therapy can have dramatic alterations in bone marrow composition, which can manifest diffusely or focally depending on the type. Radiation therapy attempts to treat all tumor cells in its path, but also affects soft tissues and bone marrow.

### Imaging Findings
- MRI

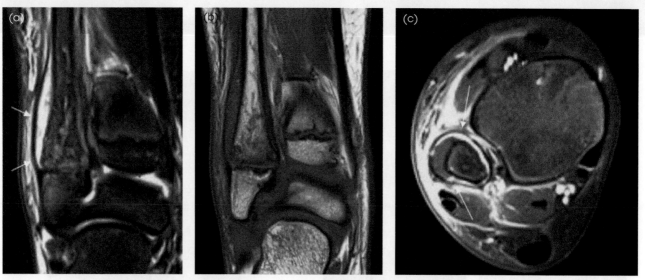

**Figure 58.5.** Osteomyelitis. (*A*) Coronal STIR, (*B*) coronal T1, and axial T1W FS postcontrast images in a patient with osteomyelitis of the fibula, complicated by subperiosteal abscess. The hypointense periosteum (*arrows* in *A*) is elevated off the cortex of the fibula because of the underlying subperiosteal abscess. In (*C*), the subperiosteal abscess is circumferential, with rim enhancement on postcontrast (*arrows*).

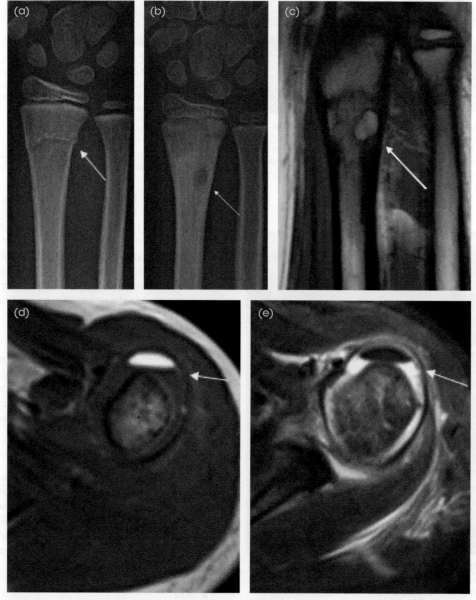

**Figure 58.6.** Intramedullary fat globules. (*A*) Initial and (*B*) follow-up radiographs of the wrist show a buckle type fracture of the radius (*arrow*). A new lucent lesion was detected, which prompted the MRI (*arrow*). (*C*) T1W coronal MRI image shows a fat-containing region corresponding to the radiograph, consistent with a posttraumatic fat globule. (*D*) Axial T1W and (*E*) axial T2W fat-suppressed MRI images in the setting of acute osteomyelitis of the proximal humerus. There is a subperiosteal fluid collection containing a fat-fluid level (*arrow*), which can occur in osteomyelitis.

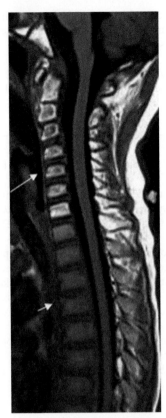

**Figure 58.7.** Postradiation hypoplastic marrow. Sagittal T1W image of the cervical spine demonstrates prominent bone marrow fat in multiple vertebrae (*long arrow*), which is starkly contrasted with normal bone marrow in levels inferior to the radiation portal (*short arrow*). Image courtesy of Maura Ryan, MD, Chicago, IL.

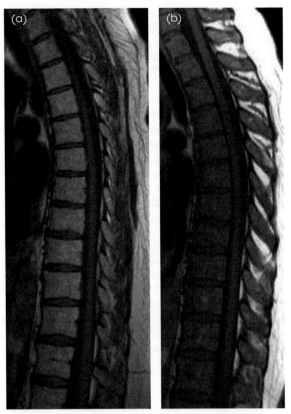

**Figure 58.8.** Red marrow reconversion. (*A*) Sagittal T1W image of the thoracic spine in a woman being treated for breast cancer. (*B*) Sagittal T1W image obtained 2 months after (*A*), demonstrates a dramatic decrease in T1 signal of the bone marrow. This is characteristic of red marrow reconversion.

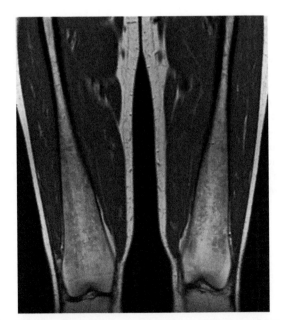

**Figure 58.9.** Marrow replacement. Coronal T1W image of the femora in a 36-year-old patient with Gaucher disease. There is widening of the marrow space typical of the Erlenmeyer flask deformity. There is patchy hypointense T1 signal in the marrow consistent with Gaucher cell infiltration.

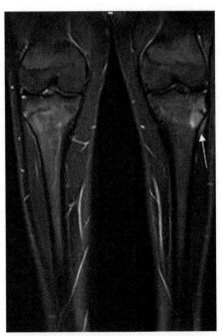

**Figure 58.10.** CRMO. Coronal STIR MR image from a whole-body MRI of the lower extremities demonstrates patchy edema in the proximal tibiae in a periphyseal distribution in this 14-year-old patient with CRMO. The BME is more prominent in the left tibia (*arrow*).

- It affects the bone marrow in a characteristic pattern on MRI, wiping out the red marrow components.
- The bone marrow responds by becoming predominately fatty replaced, producing striking T1 hyperintense signal in the affected areas.
- As radiotherapy portals are very precise, the MRI shows a stark difference between adjacent normal marrow unaffected by the radiation (Figure 58.7).
- Chemotherapy drugs can cause an unwanted but expected bone marrow suppression as a side effect to treatment.
    - When recovering following therapy, the bone marrow can become hypercellular, producing *rebound red marrow reconversion* (Figure 58.8).
    - GM-CSF is a medication that stimulates the bone marrow and helps it to recover.

### Bone Marrow Infiltration
#### Pathophysiology and Clinical Findings
The bone marrow can be infiltrated by benign and malignant cells that will alter the MRI signal appearance. A commonly cited example is Gaucher disease, which is a benign lysosomal storage disorder in which macrophages filled with glucosylceramide (Gaucher cells) deposit in multiple organs including the bone marrow (see Chapter 83, "Lipidoses").

#### Imaging Findings
- Radiography
    - Over time, the shape of the tubular long bones will expand giving a characteristic *Erlenmeyer flask deformity*, caused by widening of the metadiaphysis.
- MRI
    - Depending on the degree of marrow infiltration, the Gaucher accumulation will appear as hypointense on T1W imaging and slightly hyperintense on fluid-sensitive sequences (Figure 58.9).

### Chronic Recurrent Multifocal Osteomyelitis
#### Pathophysiology and Clinical Findings
Chronic recurrent multifocal osteomyelitis (CRMO) is a benign inflammatory noninfectious bone marrow condition seen in the pediatric setting but can also occur in adults. SAPHO (synovitis, acne, pustulosis, hyperostosis, and osteitis) syndrome, is thought by some to be the adult version of CRMO. There are some minor differences, and it is controversial whether this represents the same disease.

#### Imaging Findings
- Radiography
    - Multifocal bone marrow lesions typically in locations similar to where osteomyelitis is found, for example, metaphyses of long bones

- Predilection for the clavicles as well, which is atypical for hematogenous osteomyelitis, unless associated with a septic sternoclavicular joint
- MRI
    - Lesions appear as focal areas of BME on T1W and T2W imaging and can have surrounding periostitis and soft tissue inflammation (Figure 58.10).

### Key Points
- At birth, the bone marrow is entirely hematopoietic (cellular).
- With age, there is a predictable marrow conversion from red to fatty marrow—overall peripheral to central skeleton, and within a long bone (Epiphysis→Diaphysis→Metaphysis).
- Hematopoietic marrow can have overlapping features with pathologic conditions. However, the presence of interspersed fat, T1 signal brighter than skeletal muscle, sparing of the epiphyses, and symmetric distribution are features that can help distinguish red marrow from other entities.
- Trauma and infarction can produce fat-containing bone marrow lesions.
- Osteomyelitis can be infectious or noninfectious (CRMO).

### Recommended Reading
Nouh MR, Eid AF. Magnetic resonance imaging of the spinal marrow: basic understanding of the normal marrow pattern and its variant. *World J Radiol.* 2015;7(12):448–58.
Ollivier L, Gerber S, Vanel D, Brisse H, Leclère J. Improving the interpretation of bone marrow imaging in cancer patients. *Cancer Imaging.* 2006;6:194–98.

### References
1. Ejindu VC, Hine AL, Mashayekhi M, Shorvon PJ, Misra RR. Musculoskeletal manifestations of sickle cell disease. *Radiographics.* 2007;27(4):1005–21.
2. Khanna G, Sato TS, Ferguson P. Imaging of chronic recurrent multifocal osteomyelitis. *Radiographics.* 2009;29(4):1159–77.
3. Laor T, Jaramillo D. MR imaging insights into skeletal maturation: what is normal? *Radiology.* 2009;250(1):28–38.
4. Ricci C, Cova M, Kang YS, et al. Normal age-related patterns of cellular and fatty bone marrow distribution in the axial skeleton: MR imaging study. *Radiology.* 1990;177(1):83–88.

# CHAPTER 59

# Malignant Marrow Bone Tumors

Jonathan D. Samet

## Diffuse Malignant Bone Marrow Diseases

### Pathophysiology and Clinical Findings

Diffuse malignant bone marrow diseases will all have a similar appearance on MRI, characterized by hypointense signal on T1W imaging and hyperintense signal on T2W imaging. The difficulty is deciding how dark is too dark on T1W pulse sequences and how bright is too bright on T2W sequences. As discussed in Chapter 58, "Normal Bone Marrow and Benign Bone Marrow Lesions," bone marrow changes composition throughout life. The fattier, less cellular the marrow is, the easier it becomes to identify a diffuse malignant process that is hypercellular by definition. This is because hypercellular malignant marrow conditions produce significant hyperintensity on fluid-sensitive sequences and hypointensity on T1W sequences, which differs greatly from the expected fatty marrow signal. Conversely, in younger pediatric patients, diffuse malignant processes and normal red marrow may have overlapping features. Therefore, experience with the normal marrow appearance at each age range is a necessary foundation. Certain guidelines can be used to distinguish red marrow from marrow infiltration and/or replacement.

### Imaging Findings

- On T1W imaging, malignant marrow is generally hypointense to adjacent skeletal muscle.
- On fluid-sensitive sequences, malignant marrow signal is significantly hyperintense, having a much brighter signal that the expected grayish red marrow signal.
- In patients younger than age 1, the T1 signal is so dark normally that the STIR signal becomes the only useful factor.
- In the spine, the T1 marrow signal in the vertebral body should be brighter than the adjacent discs.
- Certain portions of bone, such as the epiphyses, are less likely to undergo complete loss in fatty signal. Therefore, a diffuse marrow abnormality that affects the epiphyses suggests malignancy.
  - Conditions causing chronic anemia, such as sickle cell disease, are the exception to this. Thus, the clinical history is vital to proper MRI interpretation.
- The decision to perform a bone marrow aspirate and biopsy will not usually rest solely on the radiologist's interpretation, except in the minority of cases where the complete blood count is normal.
- Hematopoietic marrow has a symmetric distribution, whereas neoplastic lesions tend to have an asymmetric, nodular, or patchy distribution. Imaging the contralateral extremity can be helpful to determine whether the marrow signal is symmetric and in a distribution compatible with red marrow. On occasion, diffuse marrow replacement, such as in leukemia, can also produce a symmetric appearance. However, unlike red marrow, it will not usually spare the epiphyses.
- Chemical shift artifact
  - Most malignant marrow processes replace the normal fat within marrow with malignant cells, thus altering the expected distribution in red marrow.
  - This absence of fat in malignant marrow produces a lack of signal drop when comparing in-phase to opposed-phase imaging (Figures 59.1 and 59.2). Most solid tumor neoplasms, such as metastases, replace the fat within the intramedullary cavity, reducing the degree of signal drop.
  - However, if there is not enough of a malignant cellular infiltrate at the time of scanning, there may still be a drop of signal on the opposed-phase sequence, producing a false-negative result. For example, leukemia and myeloma may infiltrate the marrow without replacing it, leading to a signal drop on the opposed-phase imaging and often producing a false-negative result.
  - Therefore, chemical shift imaging may be more reliable to confirm a malignant process rather than exclude it.

## Diffuse Pediatric Malignant Bone Marrow Processes

### Pathophysiology and Clinical Findings

The main diffuse malignant pediatric bone marrow processes encountered are metastatic neuroblastoma and leukemia. Leukemia will show diffuse or nearly diffuse T1 hypointense and STIR hyperintense signal in the visualized bone marrow (also discussed in Chapter 78, "Lymphoproliferative and Myeloproliferative Disorders"). At first glance, the marrow can look almost normal because of the diffusely symmetric abnormality. However, the degree of T1 hypointensity is significant and darker than adjacent skeletal muscle. Additionally, the STIR signal is very hyperintense. The expected fatty epiphyses will typically be replaced by leukemic cells, a helpful indicator on MRI that one is dealing with a diffuse marrow replacement process (Figure 59.3).

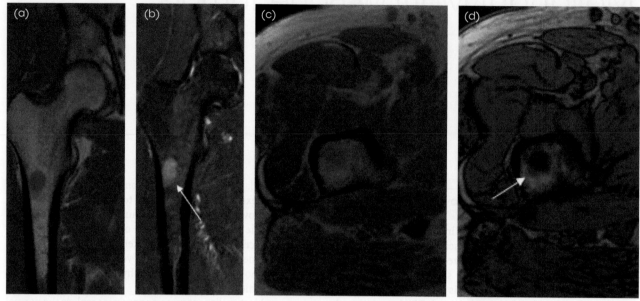

**Figure 59.1.** Chemical shift imaging of marrow neoplasm. (*A*) Coronal T1W, (*B*) Coronal STIR, (*C*) axial in-phase, (*D*) axial opposed-phase MR images of the right femur in a 74-year-old man with prostate cancer and new lesion (*arrow*) found on prostate MRI. There is a significant drop in signal (*arrow*) from in- to opposed-phase consistent with normal red marrow. Follow-up bone scan (*not shown*) was negative.

Osseous involvement in neuroblastoma takes 2 main forms, which are a part of the staging process for the disease. *Bone* involvement refers to a focal lesion and *bone marrow* involvement refers to more diffuse involvement (Figure 59.4). This staging and distinction is made through a combination of imaging and bone marrow aspirate/biopsy.

## Diffuse Adult Malignant Bone Marrow Processes

In adults, the most common diffuse malignant marrow processes include multiple myeloma and leukemia. Intraosseous lymphoma can be focal or multifocal. Myelofibrosis is a myeloproliferative disorder in which the bone marrow is replaced by fibrotic connective tissue (discussed in Chapter 78).

## Multiple Myeloma

### Pathophysiology and Clinical Findings

Plasma cell neoplasms include monoclonal gammopathy of undetermined significance (MGUS), isolated plasmacytoma of bone, extramedullary plasmacytoma, and multiple myeloma (see Chapter 76, "Plasma Cell Dyscrasias"). Patients can be asymptomatic or symptomatic, presenting with pain, fatigue, and pathologic fractures. Multiple myeloma is a plasma cell dyscrasia associated with a monoclonal protein. It is most common in older patients with a median age of diagnosis of 65 years. The 5-year survival rate is 49%. The myeloma cells induce osteoclasts, which leads to osteopenia and fractures, particularly compression fractures of the spine. It often produces multiple osteolytic lesions on radiography and CT.

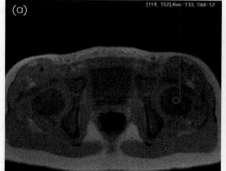
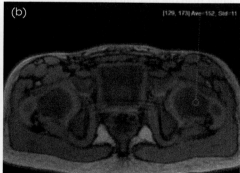

**Figure 59.2.** (*A*) Axial in-phase and (*B*) axial opposed-phase MR images in a 5-year-old patient with acute leukemia show lack of signal drop in the left femoral head from in-phase to opposed-phase consistent with a marrow replacement process.

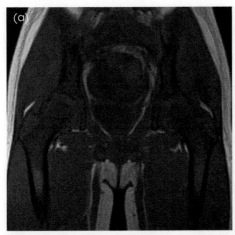
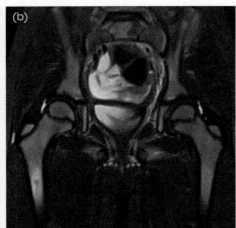

**Figure 59.3.** Marrow neoplastic conditions. (*A*) Coronal T1W and (*B*) STIR MR images of the pelvis in a 5-year-old patient with acute leukemia. There is diffuse T1 hypointense bone marrow signal, including the epiphyses, which are darker than skeletal muscle. On STIR, there is striking diffuse hyperintense signal throughout the marrow.

## Imaging Strategy

Although clinical parameters, including bone marrow plasma cell percentages, high calcium levels, renal insufficiency, and anemia are used for staging, there are imaging criteria that if met can contribute to the diagnosis of active multiple myeloma:

- One or more osteolytic bone lesions on skeletal radiography, CT, or PET/CT
- More than 1 focal lesion on MRI studies larger than 5 mm

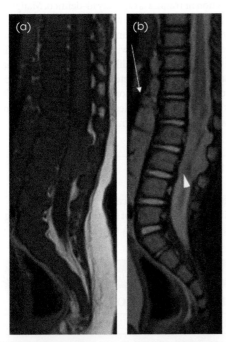

**Figure 59.4.** (*A*) Sagittal T1 and (*B*) STIR MR images of a 9-month-old patient with metastatic neuroblastoma. The bone marrow is diffusely hypointense on T1W imaging and hyperintense on STIR. Note the partially imaged retroperitoneal neuroblastoma (*arrow* in *B*), which invades the spinal canal (*arrowhead* in *B*). (Image courtesy of Maura Ryan, MD, Chicago, IL.)

## Imaging Findings
### Radiography

- Lesions are mainly lytic but can be sclerotic in POEMS (polyneuropathy, organomegaly, endocrinopathies, monoclonal gammopathy, and sclerodactyly) syndrome. Radiography is commonly used for staging, but insensitive for detecting lesions.

### Magnetic Resonance Imaging

- MRI is excellent for evaluating bone marrow; findings will depend on tumor burden.
- Appearance of marrow ranges from normal, focal lesions, diffuse, or focal lesions with diffuse pattern.
- Active myelomatous lesions are T2/STIR hyperintense and demonstrate enhancement on postcontrast imaging (Figure 59.5).
- On follow-up MRI, treated myelomatous lesions may show a decrease in size, and/or postcontrast enhancement. In addition, the internal composition of the lesion may return to more normal fatty marrow, with increased intrinsic T1 signal.

### Nuclear Imaging

- The technetium 99m methylene diphosphonate (MDP) bone scan is insensitive because myeloma lesions are typically lytic. Bone scan uptake relies on osteoblastic activity.
- Fluorine 18-fluorodeoxyglucose ([18]F-FDG)-PET offers high sensitivity and specificity and may have value in prognosis and treatment assessment.

## Lymphoma

### Pathophysiology and Clinical Findings

Lymphoma of bone mostly represents secondary involvement from disseminated lymphoma (also see Chapter 78). Primary lymphoma of the bone is rare, accounting for less than 5% of primary bone tumors. It is typically non-Hodgkin type and can be seen in the long bones, particularly the diaphysis

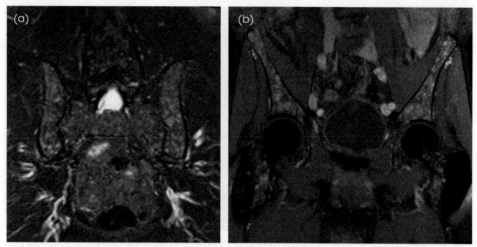

**Figure 59.5.** (A) Coronal STIR and (B) coronal T1W fat-suppressed postcontrast coronal MR images of the pelvis in a 66-year-old patient with active multiple myeloma. Innumerable STIR hyperintense, enhancing lesions are seen in the pelvis and proximal femora.

and metadiaphysis, and the flat bones of the axial skeleton. Conversely, secondary lymphoma has a predilection for the axial skeleton.

### Imaging Strategy
- The goal is to distinguish primary intraosseous lymphoma from secondary osseous involvement of disseminated lymphoma because single primary lymphoma of bone would be stage I non-Hodgkin lymphoma, whereas secondary osseous involvement in disseminated lymphoma is stage IV disease.
- With secondary osseous lymphoma, there will typically be multiple other sites of disease lymphoma (ie, nodal disease plus bone lesions).

### Imaging Findings
**Radiography**
- Permeative lytic, mixed lytic/sclerotic, and less commonly sclerotic lesions are seen.
- Periosteal reaction is not a dominant feature.

**Magnetic Resonance Imaging**
- Focal marrow replacing lesion that is darker than skeletal muscle on T1W imaging and is hyperintense on T2W imaging. It demonstrates enhancement following IV contrast administration.
- Extraosseous soft tissue masses are associated.

- There is a notable disproportionate lack of cortical destruction given the extent of marrow involvement and soft tissue mass.

## Focal Malignant Marrow Lesions
When faced with a focal bone marrow signal abnormality, malignant lesions will have certain worrisome characteristics distinguishing them from their benign counterparts. Morphology, location, and signal intensity are key to making this distinction. In general, the greater degree of BME surrounding a lesion, the higher likelihood it is benign. BME on T1W and T2W sequences from infection or trauma is typically ill-defined. Malignant lesions on MRI, including primary and metastatic lesions, are more often circumscribed and rounded. For primary bone tumors, such as osteosarcoma and Ewing sarcoma, there is often an associated soft tissue mass. Unlike benign marrow signal, the T1 fatty marrow signal is completely replaced, and T1 hyperintense signal from fat within the lesion cannot be detected. Conversely, if fat within a bone marrow lesion is detected, it is a reassuring finding arguing against malignancy (Table 59.1).

## Ewing Sarcoma

### Pathophysiology and Clinical Findings
The Ewing sarcoma family of tumors includes Ewing sarcoma of bone, extraosseous Ewing tumor, and peripheral primitive

### Table 59.1. Comparison of Benign and Malignant Bone Marrow Lesions on Magnetic Resonance Imaging

| BENIGN MARROW LESION | MALIGNANT MARROW LESION |
|---|---|
| Contains fat centrally (ie, bone infarct) | No fat (T1 hypointense) |
| Ill-defined | Rounded, circumscribed |
| No associated soft tissue mass | May have associated soft tissue mass |
| Greater degree of surrounding bone marrow edema | Lesser degree of surrounding bone marrow edema |
| No endosteal scalloping | Endosteal scalloping |

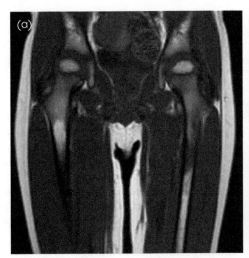
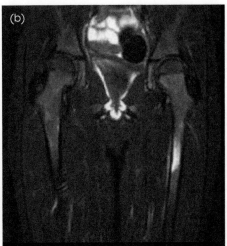

**Figure 59.6.** Adductor insertion avulsive syndrome versus Ewing sarcoma. (*A*) Coronal T1W and (*B*) STIR MR images of the femora in a 10-year-old boy with leg pain. Focal but ill-defined BME is seen in the proximal left femur with associated periosteal reaction. This was initially misdiagnosed as Ewing sarcoma and was biopsied, but pathology was benign. Findings are characteristic of adductor insertion avulsive syndrome.

neuroectodermal tumor (PNET). PNETs of the chest wall are also known as Akins tumors. These tumors are grouped together because of the discovery that in 90% of cases, there is a shared genetic translocation between chromosomes 11 and 22.

Ewing sarcoma of bone is a malignant bone tumor, most common in children and adolescents. It occurs less frequently than osteosarcoma and has a different histologic makeup that is composed of small round blue cells. The reported incidence is 200 cases per year. The most common sites are the bones of the pelvis, extremities, and ribs. Within a long bone, the metadiaphysis followed by diaphysis are the most common sites. This is in contrast to osteosarcoma, which more commonly arises in the metaphysis. There is a better prognosis for younger patients, distal extremity lesions, smaller tumor size, and absence of metastatic disease. The 5-year survival rate is 78% for children younger than age 15, and 60% for ages 15-19. An important benign mimic of Ewing sarcoma is *adductor insertion avulsive syndrome*, which is an overuse syndrome analogous to shin splints, but in the thighs (Figures 59.6 and 59.7).

### Imaging Strategy and Findings
### Radiography and Computed Tomography
- Destructive lesion with wide zone of transition
- Lamellated (onion skinning) and spiculated patterns

### Magnetic Resonance Imaging
Refer to Figure 59. 8.

- In greater than 90% of cases, there is bone marrow replacement with intermediate T1 signal and variable T2 signal, ranging from low to high.
- Cortical destruction is visualized.
- Soft tissue mass is seen.

### Nuclear Imaging
- FDG-PET and CT—increased metabolic activity in primary lesion, high accuracy for staging
- Bone scan—increased radiotracer uptake

### Treatment Options
- Systemic chemotherapy
- Surgery and/or radiation for local control

## Langerhans Cell Histiocytosis

### Pathophysiology and Clinical Findings
Langerhans cell histiocytosis (LCH) is in the family of histiocytoses (also see Chapter 77, "Histiocytoses") and is now

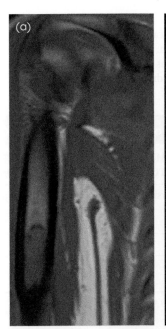
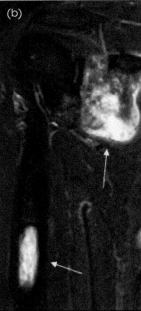

**Figure 59.7.** (*A*) Coronal T1W and (*B*) STIR MR images of the right shoulder show lesions in the scapula and proximal humerus consistent with metastatic disease, in this case because of Ewing sarcoma (*arrows*). Note the bone destruction in the scapular lesion. In the humeral lesion, note the circumscribed, rounded T1 hypointense signal, characteristic of a marrow replacing malignant lesion, in contrast to Figure 59.6.

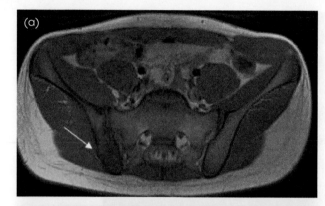

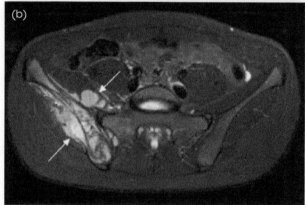

**Figure 59.8.** Ewing sarcoma. (*A*) Axial T1W and (*B*) STIR MR images of the pelvis in a 13-year-old girl with newly diagnosed Ewing sarcoma of the right ilium. Extraosseous soft tissue masses are best seen on the STIR image (*arrows* in *B*). In (*A*), the bone marrow signal is T1 hypointense, compatible with marrow replacement because of the tumor (*arrow*).

classified as a neoplasm, technically a malignancy, but there is a variable disease manifestation. Langerhans cells can deposit in many different organ systems or present as a solitary bone lesion. LCH mainly affects children but is also seen in adults.

The annual incidence is 3-5 per million children. Younger children are more likely to have multiorgan involvement, and it can be a lethal disease. If high-risk organs, including liver, spleen, and bone marrow are involved, the prognosis is poorer, but the overall survival rate with 12 months of chemotherapy is 84%. With involvement limited to bone, survival rates are near 100%.

When bones are affected, the calvarium is the most common site. In the spine, a destructive lesion resulting in a vertebra plana is a classic imaging appearance. When presenting in the pelvis or extremities as a solitary bone lesion, LCH can pose a diagnostic dilemma (Table 59.2). Partly because of its aggressive appearance, LCH is often misdiagnosed as a sarcoma or osteomyelitis. The clinical presentation of LCH overlaps with infection, as CRP and ESR can be elevated in both.

### Imaging Strategy and Findings
### Radiography and Computed Tomography
- A geographic lytic lesion without sclerotic borders is seen; classically, a lytic lesion with beveled edge in the calvarium. When adjacent to a tooth, it can produce the appearance of a *floating* tooth because of the surrounding lucency.
- Periosteal reaction is usually not aggressive.

Magnetic Resonance Imaging
Refer to Figure 59.9.
- Very reactive lesion—perilesional bone marrow and soft tissue edema
  - Endosteal scalloping, periosteal reaction
  - Can have an associated soft tissue mass

### Nuclear Imaging
- PET and CT can be used to monitor treatment response by identifying metabolically active sites.

### Treatment Options
- Varies depending on extent of involvement

| Table 59.2. Comparison of Select Aggressive Bone Conditions in the Pelvis and Extremities | | | | |
|---|---|---|---|---|
| | **OSTEOMYELITIS (HEMATOGENOUS)** | **LANGERHANS CELL HISTIOCYTOSIS (LCH)** | **EWING SARCOMA** | **OSTEOSARCOMA** |
| Location | Metaphysis Pelvis | Metaphysis/Diaphysis > Epiphysis Pelvis | Diaphysis Metadiaphysis Pelvis | Metaphysis Pelvis |
| Size | ++ | +++ | ++++++ | ++++++ |
| Surrounding Reaction | ++++++ | ++++++ | +++ | +++ |
| X-ray | Normal→Aggressive | Geographic Lytic Nonaggressive periosteal reaction | Destructive/Lytic Wide zone Aggressive periosteal reaction | Osteoid matrix Aggressive periosteal reaction |
| Soft tissue mass | N/A | ++ | ++++++ | ++++++ |

Abbreviations: N/A, not applicable.

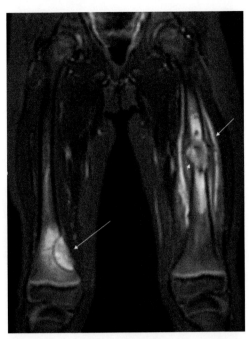

**Figure 59.9.** LCH. Coronal STIR MR image of the femurs in a 4-year-old girl with 2 LCH bone lesions. Both lesions show extensive perilesional BME, characteristic of LCH. The left femoral lesion has an extraosseous soft tissue mass (*short arrow*) component and periosteal reaction (*medium arrow*).

- Ranges from observation (some isolated bone lesions) to chemotherapy
- Image-guided percutaneous intralesional steroid injection

## Key Points

- Focal and diffuse malignant bone marrow diseases demonstrate significant T1 hypointense signal on MRI.
- Fat-containing bone marrow signal abnormalities are unlikely to be malignant, especially when there is macroscopic fat.

- Multiple myeloma and neuroblastoma may produce focal lesions or diffuse marrow infiltration and/or replacement on MRI.
- Leukemia typically produces diffuse marrow replacement with T1 hypointense and T2 hyperintense signal.
- Ewing sarcoma has a permeative pattern on radiography, and there is usually an associated soft tissue mass best seen on MRI.
- Clinical and radiologic features of LCH overlap with infection and malignancy.
- Consider LCH in the differential diagnosis for an aggressive bone lesion, even in the presence of an associated soft tissue mass.

## Recommended Reading

Murphey MD, Senchak LT, Mambalam PK, Logie CI, Klassen-Fischer MK, Kransdorf MJ. From the radiologic pathology archives: Ewing sarcoma family of tumors: radiologic-pathologic correlation. *Radiographics*. 2013;33(3):803–31.

Samet J, Weinstein J, Fayad LM. MRI and clinical features of Langerhans cell histiocytosis (LCH) in the pelvis and extremities: can LCH really look like anything?. *Skeletal Radiol*. 2016;45(5):607–13.

## References

1. Angtuaco EJ, Fassas AB, Walker R, Sethi R, Barlogie B. Multiple myeloma: clinical review and diagnostic imaging. *Radiology*. 2004;231(1):11–23.
2. Carroll KW, Feller JF, Tirman PF. Useful internal standards for distinguishing infiltrative marrow pathology from hematopoietic marrow at MRI. *J Magn Reson Imaging*. 1997;7(2):394–98.
3. Dreizin D, Ahlawat S, Del Grande F, Fayad LM. Gradient-echo in-phase and opposed-phase chemical shift imaging: role in evaluating bone marrow. *Clin Radiol*. 2014;69(6):648–57.
4. Ruzek KA, Wenger DE. The multiple faces of lymphoma of the musculoskeletal system. *Skeletal Radiol*. 2004;33(1):1–8.

# Vascular Bone Tumors

# CHAPTER 60

# Benign Vascular Bone Tumors

G. Scott Stacy

## Introduction

Vascular tumors of bone have been characterized as a spectrum of benign and malignant lesions that arise from endothelial cells. Although malignant lesions are uncommon, benign lesions are much more commonly seen and may be incidentally detected on imaging studies. WHO recognizes 2 benign vascular tumors of bone: *hemangioma* and *epithelioid hemangioma*.

## Hemangioma

### Pathophysiology and Clinical Findings

The term *hemangioma* is widely applied to a common and typically characteristic lesion of bone that is composed of anomalous blood vessels; however, this term is controversial, and in most cases such lesions are perhaps better classified as slow-flow vascular malformations according to the system proposed by the International Society for the Study of Vascular Anomalies (Box 60.1). For this chapter, the traditional, although perhaps less accurate term—hemangioma—is adopted. Hemangiomas occur at any age and may be congenital, although most are identified between the fourth and fifth decades of life.

Hemangiomas are most common in the vertebral bodies, where they occur in approximately 10% of the adult population, followed by the skull. They are rare in other axial and appendicular bones. Most vertebral body and skull hemangiomas are asymptomatic incidental findings detected on imaging studies. Rarely, however, larger vertebral hemangiomas can cause pain and neurologic symptoms from spinal cord and nerve root compression related to encroachment on the central spinal canal and neural foramina. This may occur, for example, during pregnancy, usually in the third trimester, and most commonly in the thoracic spine. Hemangiomas within the appendicular skeleton are often symptomatic at presentation with localized swelling, pain, or a palpable mass. The tibia and femur are the most common sites of hemangioma of long bone, which tends to involve the metaphysis. Rarely, diaphyseal, cortical, or periosteal lesions are encountered. Macroscopically, hemangiomas appear as dark red masses; blood-filled cavities may be separated by thick bony trabeculae. Histologic features are variable, and hemangiomas may be of cavernous, capillary, or venous types. They are composed of thin-walled vessels, lined by a single layer of endothelial cells, permeating the marrow.

When hemangiomas involve a large localized region or spread throughout the skeleton, the term *angiomatosis* is applied. *Cystic angiomatosis* is a term used to describe a rare disease of multifocal hemangiomatous and/or lymphangiomatous lesions of the skeleton, with occasional visceral involvement. *Gorham-Stout disease* is a rare, more aggressive form of angiomatosis, characterized by massive osteolysis associated with adjacent localized proliferation of vascular or lymphatic channels.

### Imaging Strategy

Most hemangiomas arising in the spine are incidental findings on imaging studies and do not require additional workup. Radiographs remain the primary technique for detecting and characterizing bone tumors. MRI is generally the preferred imaging method for staging and preoperative planning of bone tumors.

### Imaging Findings

Spinal hemangiomas classically have a characteristic imaging appearance (Figures 60.1 and 60.2).

#### Radiography

- Imaging shows well-marginated, geographic lucent lesion with vertically oriented thickened trabeculae (*corduroy* pattern). These thickened trabeculae are also apparent on CT and MRI examinations. The hemangioma may replace the vertebral body, but enlargement of the bone is atypical.

#### Computed Tomography

- On transverse images, a *polka dot* pattern reflects the thickened trabeculae in cross section with interposed low-density fat, indicating an indolent lesion. Rarely, a purely osteolytic or finely reticulated "honeycomb" pattern may be found in symptomatic lesions.

#### Magnetic Resonance Imaging

- Most hemangiomas show high signal intensity on T1W images (because of the presence of fat in the lesion) as well as on T2W images without fat suppression.
- Most lesions demonstrate enhancement on contrast-enhanced sequences.
- Symptomatic tumors often show loss of fat and therefore show low signal intensity on T1W images.
- *Atypical hemangiomas* have imaging features that differ from classical descriptions and can mimic other, more aggressive lesions. Although the imaging findings vary they may present with low signal on T1W imaging and bright signal on fluid-sensitive sequences.

**Box 60.1** Simplified International Society for the Study of Vascular Anomalies Classification of Vascular Lesions

- Vascular tumors
  - Benign
    - Infantile hemangioma
  - Locally aggressive
    - Kaposiform hemangioendothelioma
  - Malignant
    - Angiosarcoma
- Vascular malformations
  - Slow flow
    - Capillary malformations (CM)
    - Venous malformations (VM)
    - Lymphatic malformations (LM)
  - High flow
    - Arteriovenous malformations (AVM)

### Nuclear Imaging

- Normal or decreased uptake on bone scintigraphy is typically demonstrated, although some larger lesions have been shown to have atypical increased radiotracer uptake.

Extraspinal hemangiomas have a less characteristic imaging appearance (Figures 60.3 and 60.4).

### Radiography

- In flat bones, such as the calvarium, expansile remodeling may be seen, as well as a *sunburst* pattern of radiating trabeculae.
- In the extremities, hemangioma may present as a nonspecific, well-marginated, geographic, lucent lesion that is typically lobulated with sclerotic margins. A coarse linear, radiating or weblike trabecular pattern may suggest the diagnosis. Cortical breach is atypical but can occur.

**Magnetic Resonance Imaging**

- Hemangiomas of the appendicular long bones have variable imaging characteristics. Heterogeneous hyperintensity on T2W images is most common. On T1W images, the lesions are typically similar in signal intensity to skeletal muscle, although they may be hypointense or hyperintense. Most lesions will have a hypointense margin, and a coarse trabecular pattern may provide a clue to the diagnosis. Often, however, the diagnosis is only able to be achieved histologically.

**Treatment Options**

- Indolent hemangiomas require no treatment.
- Symptomatic hemangiomas can be treated with arterial embolization, surgical decompression and curettage, and vertebroplasty, depending on the patient's symptoms.

### Epithelioid Hemangioma

**Pathophysiology and Clinical Findings**

In contrast to hemangioma, epithelioid hemangioma of bone is rare. It is a controversial entity largely because of features that overlap with malignant vascular neoplasms (ie, hemangioendothelioma). It is composed of epithelioid endothelial cells that form vascular lumina or solid sheets.

Epithelioid hemangiomas can be encountered in patients ranging in age from the first to ninth decades of life, with most occurring in adults at a mean age of approximately 35 years. These lesions are most commonly identified within the long bones of the appendicular skeleton (40%, usually metadiaphyseal) followed by the small bones of the feet, flat bones, vertebrae, and small bones of the hands. Although most are solitary, up to 25% are multifocal, typically in a regional distribution. Even though these lesions can rarely be asymptomatic at presentation, and thus identified incidentally, they most commonly present with pain localized to the involved bone(s). Although the lesion is benign, it can

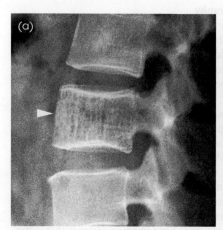
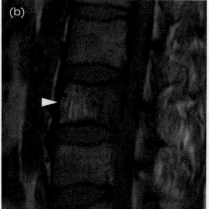
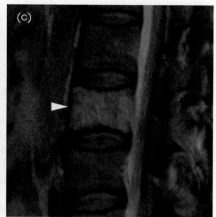

**Figure 60.1.** Hemangioma of the vertebral body. A 38-year-old woman with lower back pain incidentally found to have an L3 vertebral body hemangioma. Lateral radiograph of lumbar spine (*A*) demonstrates vertically oriented thickened trabeculae affecting the L3 vertebral body (*arrowhead*). Sagittal T1W MR image (*B*) also shows vertically oriented thickened trabeculae, as well as increased signal intensity in the anterior half of the vertebral body (*arrowhead*) caused by increased fat content. Sagittal T2W MR image (*C*) demonstrates generalized increased signal intensity and thickened trabeculae in the same vertebral body (*arrowhead*). The constellation of imaging findings is typical of a benign vertebral hemangioma.

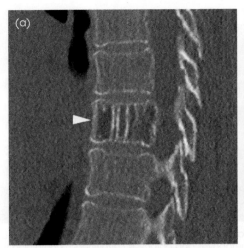
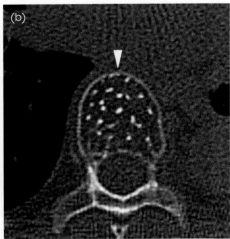

**Figure 60.2.** Hemangioma of the vertebral body. A 90-year-old woman who underwent CT examination to evaluate sternotomy healing. (*A*) Sagittal reformatted CT image of the thoracic spine demonstrates classic corduroy appearance of a hemangioma in the T9 vertebral body (*arrowhead*) caused by low-density fat interspersed between vertically oriented thickened trabeculae. (*B*) Axial CT image demonstrates polka dot appearance characteristic of a hemangioma, also caused by thickened trabeculae within the same vertebral body (*arrowhead*).

be locally aggressive, and there are rare reports of metastasis caused by lymphatic spread. Epithelioid hemangioma grossly appears as a soft red-brown tumor with hemorrhagic contents. Histologic examination displays a lobulated architecture with the center of the lobule containing epithelioid cells and the periphery containing arteriolar-like vessels lined by flat endothelial cells.

Epithelioid hemangiomas lack characteristic imaging features to allow definitive diagnosis; multiplicity may be the only clue that these osseous lesions are of vascular origin (Figures 60.5 and 60.6).

### Imaging Findings
#### Radiography and Computed Tomography
- A well-defined, geographic lucent lesion is seen, occasionally with septation and expansile remodeling. Focal

cortical destruction may be associated with thick periosteal new bone and extension of tumor into the soft tissue.

#### Magnetic Resonance Imaging
- Nonspecific features are shown on MRI, but lesions typically demonstrate heterogeneous low signal intensity on T1W images, intermediate-to-high signal intensity on T2W images, and heterogeneous enhancement on contrast-enhanced sequences.

#### Treatment Options
- Treatment of epithelioid hemangioma is controversial. Once a histologic diagnosis is achieved, some lesions can be treated conservatively, but the preferred method of treatment for most is intralesional curettage.

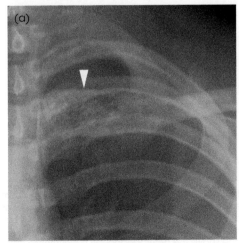
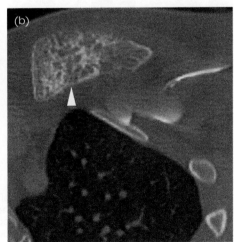

**Figure 60.3.** Hemangioma of the clavicle. A 24-year-old woman with left medial clavicle mass. (*A*) AP radiograph and (*B*) axial CT image of the left clavicle demonstrate a lesion with weblike thickened trabecular pattern involving the medial end of the clavicle (*arrowheads*). Histologic analysis following biopsy confirmed diagnosis of a hemangioma.

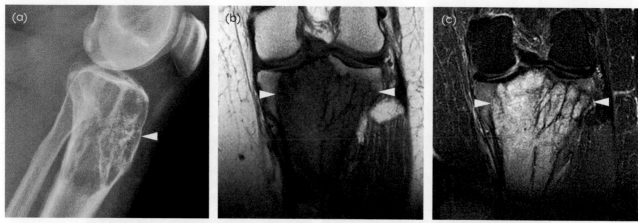

**Figure 60.4.** Hemangioma of the proximal tibia. A 63-year-old woman with left knee pain. (*A*) Lateral radiograph demonstrates a well-marginated geographic lucent lesion in the proximal tibial metaphysis and epiphysis (*arrowhead*) containing thickened, predominantly vertically oriented trabeculae. (*B*) T1W coronal MR image shows the lesion (*arrowheads*) to be predominantly isointense to skeletal muscle, with vertically oriented thickened hypointense trabeculae. (*C*) T2W FS coronal MR image shows hyperintensity of the lesion (*arrowheads*) with hypointense trabeculae. Histologic analysis following biopsy confirmed diagnosis of a hemangioma.

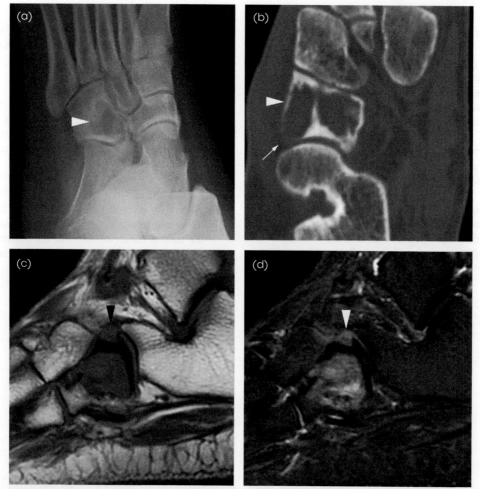

**Figure 60.5.** Epithelioid hemangioma. A 38-year-old woman with left foot pain for several months. (*A*) Oblique radiograph of the left foot demonstrates a well-defined geographic lucent lesion (*arrowhead*) within the cuboid bone with internal septation. (*B*) Axial CT image shows the lucent lesion (*arrowhead*) with septation and focal cortical destruction medially along the dorsal and proximal aspect of the cuboid bone (*arrow*). (*C*) T1W sagittal MR image shows the lesion to be predominantly isointense to skeletal muscle, with focal cortical penetration (*arrowhead*). (*D*) Sagittal STIR MR image shows the heterogeneously hyperintense lesion with focal cortical penetration (*arrowhead*). Histologic analysis following biopsy revealed the diagnosis of epithelioid hemangioma.

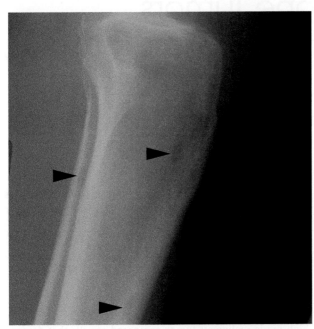

**Figure 60.6.** Multifocal epithelioid hemangioma. A 33-year-old woman with left knee pain. Lateral radiograph of the proximal leg shows multiple small lucent lesions (*arrowheads*) clustered within the proximal tibia and fibula. Histologic analysis following biopsy revealed the diagnosis of multifocal epithelioid hemangioma.

## Key Points

- Benign vascular bone tumors are osseous lesions composed of vascular spaces and blood vessels with no malignant potential.
- Spinal hemangiomas are common and typically asymptomatic, requiring no treatment. The presence of fat and vertically oriented thickened trabeculae help make the diagnosis on imaging studies.
- Calvarial hemangiomas may show a sunburst pattern of radiating trabeculae.
- Hemangiomas of the extremities are rare, typically symptomatic, and have less characteristic imaging findings, often necessitating biopsy.
- Epithelioid hemangioma is a controversial entity, and much less commonly encountered than the traditional hemangioma of bone. It usually presents as a painful mass with nonspecific imaging characteristics, although in up to 25% cases it can be multifocal, typically with a regional distribution. Its prognosis is excellent.

## Recommended Reading

Errani C, Vanel D, Gambarotti M, et al. Vascular bone tumors: a proposal of a classification based on clinicopathological, radiographic and genetic features. *Skeletal Radiol.* 2012;41(12):1495–507.

## References

1. Abrahams TG, Bula W, Jones M. Epithelioid hemangioendothelioma of bone. A report of two cases and review of the literature. *Skeletal Radiol.* 1992;21:509–13.
2. Aksu G, Fayda M, Saynak M, Karadeniz A. Spinal cord compression due to vertebral hemangioma. *Orthopedics.* 2008;31(2):169.
3. Errani C, Zhang L, Panicek DM, Healey JH, Antonescu CR. Epithelioid hemangioma of bone and soft tissue: a re-appraisal of a controversial entity. *Clin Orthop Relat Res.* 2012;470(5):1498–506.
4. Fletcher CDM, Bridge JA, Hogendoorn PCW, Mertens F, eds. *WHO Classification of Tumours of Soft Tissue and Bone.* 4th ed. Lyon, France: IARC Press; 2013.
5. Kadlub N, Dainese L, Coulomb-L'Hermine A, et al. Intraosseous hemangioma: semantic and medical confusion. *Int J Oral Maxillofacial Surgery.* 2015;44:718–24.
6. Lomasney LM, Martinez S, Demos TC, Harrelson JM. Multifocal vascular lesions of bone: imaging characteristics. *Skeletal Radiol.* 1996;25(3):255–61.
7. Lowe LH, Marchant TC, Rivard DC, Scherbel AJ. Vascular malformations: classification and terminology the radiologist needs to know. *Semin Roentgenol.* 2012;47:106–17.
8. Marcucci G, Masi L, Carossino AM, et al. Cystic bone angiomatosis: a case report treated with aminobisphosphonates and review of the literature. *Calcif Tissue Int.* 2013;93:462–71.
9. McAllister VL, Kendall BE, Bull JW. Symptomatic vertebral haemangiomas. *Brain.* 1975;98(1):71–80.
10. Moles A, Hamel O, Perret C, Bord E, Robert R, Buffenoir K. Symptomatic vertebral hemangiomas during pregnancy. *J Neurosurg Spine.* 2014;20:585–91.
11. Murphey MD, Fairbairn KJ, Parman LM, Baxter KG, Parsa MB, Smith WS. From the archives of the AFIP. Musculoskeletal angiomatous lesions: radiologic-pathologic correlation. *Radiographics.* 1995;15(4):893–917.
12. Nielsen GP, Srivastava A, Kattapuram S, et al. Epithelioid hemangioma of bone revisited: a study of 50 cases. *Am J Surg Pathol.* 2009;33(2):270–77.
13. O'Connell JX, Kattapuram SV, Mankin HJ, Bhan AK, Rosenberg AE. Epithelioid hemangioma of bone: a tumor often mistaken for low-grade angiosarcoma or malignant hemangioendothelioma. *Am J Surg Pathol.* 1993;17:610–17.
14. Ozeki M, Fujino A, Matsuoka K, Nosaka S, Kuroda T, Fukao T. Clinical features and prognosis of generalized lymphatic anomaly, kaposiform lymphangiomatosis, and Gorham-Stout disease. *Pediatr Blood Cancer.* 2016;63(5):832–38.
15. Rigopoulou A, Saifuddin A. Intraosseous hemangioma of the appendicular skeleton: imaging features of 15 cases, and a review of the literature. *Skeletal Radiol.* 2012;41(12):1525–36.
16. Sherman RS, Wilner D. The roentgen diagnosis of hemangioma of bone. *Am J Roentgenol Radium Ther Nucl Med.* 1961;86:1146–59.
17. Verbeke SLJ, Bovee JVMG. Primary vascular tumors of bone: a spectrum of entities? *Int J Clin Exp Pathol.* 2011;4:541–51.
18. Vilanova JC, Barceló J, Smirniotopoulos JG. Hemangioma from head to toe: MR imaging with pathologic correlation. *Radiographics.* 2004;24(2):367–85.

# CHAPTER 61

# Malignant Vascular Bone Tumors

G. Scott Stacy

## Introduction

Malignant vascular bone tumors have elicited much controversy and debate. The terms *hemangioendothelioma* and *angiosarcoma* historically have been used both synonymously and to indicate different tumors. Currently, the term angiosarcoma is generally used to describe a high-grade malignant vascular neoplasm, whereas hemangioendothelioma is a more nebulous term that refers to a vascular tumor of *intermediate aggressiveness* (with a range of behavior from benign to low-grade malignant) and various described histological subtypes. Some investigators have proposed that many tumors designated as hemangioendothelioma are equivalent to the *epithelioid hemangioma* described in Chapter 60, "Benign Vascular Bone Tumors." In 1982, epithelioid hemangioendothelioma (EHE) was initially described as a unique soft tissue tumor, but has since been shown to occur in bone, leading some to question whether a low-grade hemangioendothelioma other than EHE even exists. Furthermore, because of its variable histologic appearance, *hemangioendothelioma of bone* is felt by some to be a diagnosis that should be avoided whenever possible. Of note, the term *hemangiopericytoma* was used in the past to describe a vascular tumor of intermediate aggressiveness that could occur in bone. This is now considered to be an obsolete term, with most cases representing extrapleural solitary fibrous tumors.

## Epithelioid Hemangioendothelioma

### Pathophysiology and Clinical Findings
EHE is recognized by WHO as a malignant neoplasm of low-to-intermediate grade, composed of neoplastic cells that have an endothelial phenotype and epithelioid morphology. It is rare, with a broad age range between the first and eighth decades, peaking during the second and third decades of life. The majority (>60%) arise in the lower extremity, with fewer arising in the upper extremity, vertebrae, pelvis, scapulae, clavicles, and ribs. EHE is a multicentric process in approximately 50% of cases, either within a single bone or multiple bones, tending to cluster in an anatomic region. Skeletal involvement may also be a component of multiorgan disease (eg, liver, lung, soft tissue). Common symptoms include local pain and swelling, although lesions are occasionally asymptomatic. Grossly, the tumor is a soft, tan or red hemorrhagic mass. In most cases, well-formed blood vessels are not prominent histologically, and instead the tumor cells are arranged in solid nests and cords embedded in a myxohyaline stroma.

Mitotic activity is usually low. Approximately 20-30% of cases present with distant metastatic disease and the reported 5-year survival rate is approximately 33%.

## Angiosarcoma of Bone

### Pathophysiology and Clinical Findings
Angiosarcoma of bone is recognized by WHO. It is a rare, high-grade malignant tumor composed of cells that demonstrate endothelial differentiation. Angiosarcoma can occur at any age, but has a peak incidence in the third and fourth decades of life. It occurs most commonly in the long bones, followed by the pelvis and axial skeleton. Approximately one-third of cases are multifocal, usually affecting contiguous bones. Patients most commonly present with pain localized to the involved bone(s) as well as soft tissue swelling. Most tumors arise de novo in bone, although angiosarcoma may arise in association with bone infarction or previous radiation. On gross pathology, angiosarcoma is usually a soft, red, bloody mass with irregular margins. It is characterized histologically by pleomorphic endothelial cells that may be spindled or epithelioid in appearance (*epithelioid angiosarcoma*). Lack of a myxohyaline background, high-grade cytologic atypia, and a high mitotic count distinguish angiosarcoma from EHE. The prognosis of angiosarcoma is poor compared to other vascular bone tumors because of its aggressive characteristics and high frequency of distant metastasis at presentation, with an overall 5-year survival rate of 20% that plummets to 0% when there are distant metastases.

### Imaging Strategy for Malignant Vascular Lesions of the Bone
Radiographs remain the primary technique for detecting and characterizing bone tumors. MRI is generally the preferred technique for staging and preoperative planning of bone tumors. Unlike hemangiomas, which often have a characteristic radiologic appearance, malignant vascular tumors of bone typically require histologic sampling to arrive at a definitive diagnosis (Figures 61.1–61.4).

### Imaging Findings
#### Radiography
- Most malignant vascular tumors are purely or predominantly osteolytic, often demonstrating a honeycombing (hole-within-hole) appearance, although hemangioendotheliomas may present as mixed lytic/sclerotic lesions.

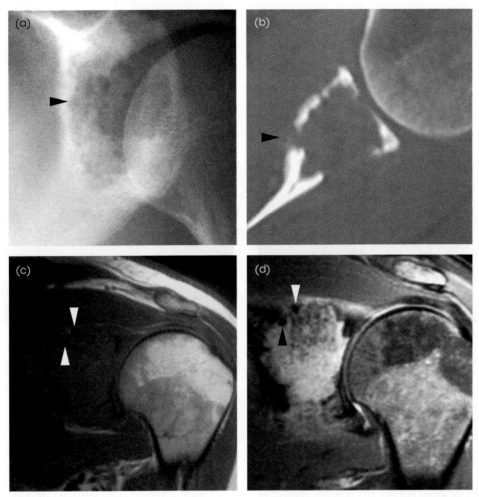

**Figure 61.1.** EHE of the scapula. A 37-year-old woman with left shoulder pain for 6 months. AP radiograph of the shoulder (*A*) shows geographic lucent lesion involving the glenoid (*arrowhead*). (*B*) Axial CT image shows a lucent lesion with areas of cortical destruction (*arrowhead*). (*C*) T1W coronal-oblique MR image shows the lesion to be isointense to skeletal muscle, with cortical destruction. Small round hypointense foci (*arrowheads*) represent flow voids related to vessels. (*D*) PDW FS coronal-oblique MR image shows hyperintensity of the lesion as well as flow voids (*arrowheads*). Histologic analysis following biopsy revealed the diagnosis of EHE.

- EHEs can show well- or poorly circumscribed margins with variable degrees of peripheral sclerosis. Although usually centered in the medullary cavity and confined to bone, they can show expansile remodeling of bone and areas of cortical destruction, with a small soft tissue component seen in approximately 40% of cases. Matrix mineralization is uncommon, and periosteal reaction is rare.

- Although angiosarcomas may have well-defined margins, they are usually poorly marginated osteolytic bone lesions that commonly result in cortical destruction and extension into the soft tissues. Periosteal reaction is usually absent.

- Reactive sclerosis surrounding angiosarcoma lesions is uncommon; however, it may be more commonly associated with angiosarcomas than metastatic disease or multiple myeloma.

- The feature that most commonly allows one to suggest the diagnosis of a vascular bone tumor is the presence of multifocal disease.

**Computed Tomography and Magnetic Resonance Imaging**

- Although CT and MRI provide useful information regarding the extent and pattern of malignant vascular bone tumors, there are no characteristic features that would obviate the need for biopsy.

- Marrow involvement is nonspecific (unless multifocal), with intermediate signal intensity on T1W images, high signal intensity on T2W images, and enhancement following IV gadolinium-based contrast administration. There may be soft tissue extension.

- High-blood-flow serpentine vessels and fluid-fluid levels may be seen.

- Unlike hemangiomas, there is an absence of fat overgrowth.

**Nuclear Imaging**

- Bone scintigraphy may be used to define the total extent of disease and exclude the possibility of multifocal lesions. These lesions will show nonspecific increased radiotracer uptake on scintigraphic examination.

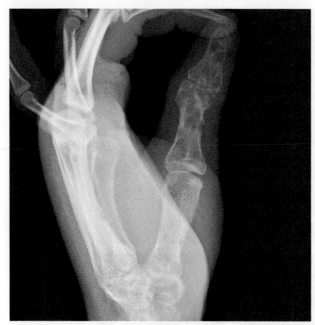

**Figure 61.2.** EHE. An 18-year-old man with left thumb mass. Thumb radiograph demonstrates multiple geographic lucent lesions within the phalanges and first metacarpal. Histologic analysis following biopsy revealed the diagnosis of EHE.

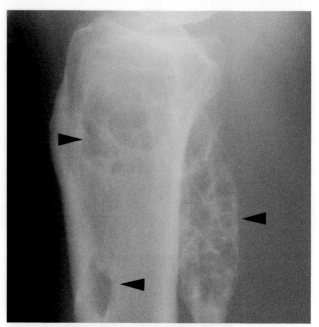

**Figure 61.4.** Multifocal angiosarcoma. A 69-year-old man with right knee pain and swelling. Lateral radiograph of the knee shows multiple geographic lucent lesions in the proximal tibia and fibula (*arrowheads*), with that in the fibula resulting in expansile remodeling. Histologic analysis following biopsy revealed the diagnosis of angiosarcoma.

### Treatment Options

- Treatment of malignant vascular bone tumors is tailored to the individual patient, based largely on the location and extent of disease.
- Surgery represents the cornerstone of treatment for patients with localized disease, and typically consists of

wide resection, although intralesional surgery can be considered for some hemangioendotheliomas.
- Radiation can be used as adjuvant treatment, or may be used alone for unresectable tumors or for multifocal disease. Chemotherapy regimens are under investigation.

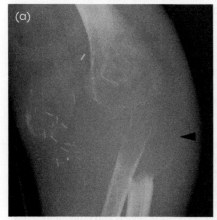
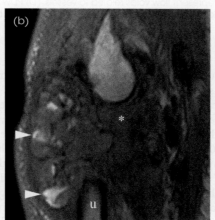
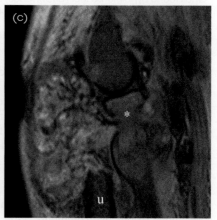

**Figure 61.3.** Multifocal angiosarcoma. A 63-year-old man with elbow mass and pain. (*A*) Lateral elbow radiograph shows a poorly defined destructive lytic lesion of the proximal ulna (*arrowhead*) as well as hyperlucent proximal radius and distal humerus. Surgical clips and calcification in the volar soft tissues reflect a dialysis shunt. (*B*) T1W sagittal MR image shows a destructive mass arising from the proximal ulna (*u*) with involvement of the adjacent proximal radius (*asterisk*). Areas of increased signal intensity within the mass represent hemorrhagic foci (*arrowheads*). (*C*) T2W FS sagittal MR image redemonstrates the destructive mass arising from the proximal ulna (*u*) and involvement of the proximal radius (*asterisk*). A small focus of BME in the posterior capitellum likely represents reactive BME rather than an additional focus of tumor. Histologic analysis following biopsy revealed the diagnosis of angiosarcoma.

## Key Points

- Malignant vascular bone tumors have elicited much controversy and debate. Angiosarcoma (including epithelioid angiosarcoma) is a rare, high-grade malignant neoplasm, whereas hemangioendothelioma (including EHE) is a low-grade tumor.
- The feature that most commonly allows the diagnosis of a malignant vascular bone tumor to be suggested is the presence of multifocal disease; however, there are no characteristic imaging features that would obviate the need for biopsy.

## Recommended Reading

Errani C, Vanel D, Gambarotti M, et al. Vascular bone tumors: a proposal of a classification based on clinicopathological, radiographic and genetic features. *Skeletal Radiol.* 2012;41:1495–507.

## References

1. Abraham JA, Hornicek FJ, Kaufman AM, et al: Treatment and outcome of 82 patients with angiosarcoma. *Ann Surg Oncol.* 2007;14(6):1953–67.
2. Abrahams TG, Bula W, Jones M. Epithelioid hemangioendothelioma of bone. A report of two cases and review of the literature. *Skeletal Radiol.* 1992;21:509–13.
3. Aksu G, Fayda M, Saynak M, Karadeniz A. Spinal cord compression due to vertebral hemangioma. *Orthopedics.* 2008;31(2):169.
4. Choi JJ, Murphey MD. Angiomatous skeletal lesions. *Semin Musculoskelet Radiol.* 2000;4:103–12.
5. Deshpande V, Rosenberg AE, O'Connell JX, Nielsen GP. Epithelioid angiosarcoma of the bone: a series of 10 cases. *Am J Surg Pathol.* 2003;27(6):709–16.
6. Evans HL, Raymond AK, Ayala AG. Vascular tumors of bone: a study of 17 cases other than ordinary hemangioma, with an evaluation of the relationship of hemangioendothelioma of bone to epithelioid hemangioma, epithelioid hemangioendothelioma, and high-grade angiosarcoma. *Hum Pathol.* 2003;34:680–89.
7. Fletcher CDM, Bridge JA, Hogendoorn PCW, Mertens F, eds. *WHO Classification of Tumours of Soft Tissue and Bone.* 4th ed. Lyon, France: IARC Press; 2013.
8. Lomasney LM, Martinez S, Demos TC, Harrelson JM. Multifocal vascular lesions of bone: imaging characteristics. *Skeletal Radiol.* 1996;25(3):255–61.
9. Murphey MD, Fairbairn KJ, Parman LM, Baxter KG, Parsa MB, Smith WS. From the archives of the AFIP. Musculoskeletal angiomatous lesions: radiologic-pathologic correlation. *Radiographics.* 1995;15(4):893–917.
10. Nielsen GP, Srivastava A, Kattapuram S, et al. Epithelioid hemangioma of bone revisited: a study of 50 cases. *Am J Surg Pathol.* 2009;33(2):270–77.
11. O'Connell JX, Kattapuram SV, Mankin HJ, Bhan AK, Rosenberg AE. Epithelioid hemangioma of bone: a tumor often mistaken for low-grade angiosarcoma or malignant hemangioendothelioma. *Am J Surg Pathol.* 1993;17:610–17.
12. Sherman RS, Wilner D. The roentgen diagnosis of hemangioma of bone. *Am J Roentgenol Radium Ther Nucl Med.* 1961;86:1146–59.
13. Verbeke SLJ, Bovée JVMG. Primary vascular tumors of bone: a spectrum of entities? *Int J Clin Exp Pathol.* 2011;4:541–51.
14. Vilanova JC, Barceló J, Smirniotopoulos JG. Hemangioma from head to toe: MR imaging with pathologic correlation. *Radiographics.* 2004;24(2):367–85.
15. Weissferdt A, Moran CA. Epithelioid hemangioendothelioma of the bone: a review and update. *Adv Anat Pathol.* 2014;21:254–59.
16. Wenger DE, Wold LE. Malignant vascular lesions of bone: radiologic and pathologic features. *Skeletal Radiol.* 2000;29(11):619–31.

# Other Bone Tumors

# CHAPTER 62

# Miscellaneous Tumors and Tumorlike Conditions

John Meyer and Nabeel Anwar

## Introduction

A number of commonly encountered benign and malignant skeletal lesions, including cystlike and lipomatous lesions, do not fall within the histological categories noted in other chapters. These lesions often occur in particular groups of patients or in typical locations and may have characteristic features on imaging studies. Therefore, clinical history and imaging findings may help significantly limit the differential diagnosis, and in some cases, may be diagnostic. This can be useful to prevent unnecessary tissue sampling or guide patient management.

## Cystlike Lesions of Bone

Intraosseous cystlike lesions, including unicameral bone cysts, ABCs, and intraosseous ganglia, are commonly encountered lucent lesions. These lesions are not true cysts because they lack an epithelial lining. However, they share many imaging features with cysts, including sharp margins with narrow zones of transition and central fluid contents. Unicameral bone cysts and intraosseous ganglia typically have nonaggressive imaging findings, whereas ABCs can look quite expansile and aggressive. Most of the lesions can be diagnosed on radiography. However, cross-sectional imaging may be needed in indeterminate cases, to guide tissue sampling if necessary or to detect areas of malignant transformation when appropriate.

## Unicameral Bone Cyst (Solitary Bone Cyst)

### Pathophysiology and Clinical Findings

A unicameral bone cyst (UBC) is a benign, fluid-filled lesion that is composed of a single cavity or contains a few small septations. The etiology is uncertain, although some authors have suggested it arises in the setting of increased intramedullary pressure caused by venous obstruction. It generally presents in patients younger than age 30, and most often in patients between ages 10 and 20. UBCs are most commonly located in the metaphyses of long bones, such as the humerus and femur, but may be seen in other bones. They may enlarge while the patient is skeletally immature. However, with skeletal maturation they may migrate to the diaphysis, and they often spontaneously regress after skeletal maturity. These lesions are rare after the age of 30. UBCs are painless unless there is pathologic fracture. In rare instances, patients may experience growth disturbances if the lesion involves the growth plate.

### Imaging Strategy

Most UBCs are well-diagnosed on radiography. CT may help determine the wall thickness to assess risk for the development of pathologic fracture and to detect radiographically occult fractures. MRI is rarely used to diagnose UBCs but can be helpful to confirm fluid contents or to evaluate for complications. In indeterminate cases, IV contrast can be helpful to look for solid elements, which would suggest another diagnosis.

### Imaging Findings
#### Radiography

- Imaging shows well-marginated lucent and mildly expansile lesion with cortical thinning and a thin sclerotic margin (Figure 62.1).
- No periosteal reaction is seen unless there is a pathologic fracture.
- *Fallen fragment sign* is indicative of dependent, displaced fracture fragment through a pathologic fracture, which is essentially pathognomonic of UBC.

#### Computed Tomography

- Mirrors radiographic findings with a fluid-filled cavity (0-20 HU), and occasional fluid-fluid levels especially in the setting of prior fracture
- No enhancement on postcontrast images

#### Magnetic Resonance Imaging

- Imaging shows typical signal characteristics of fluid, including low to intermediate T1W and high T2W signal intensity (Figure 62.2).
- Occasional partial septations and fluid-fluid levels are seen.
- There is no internal enhancement, which helps differentiate it from a solid lesion. However, they may have thin, smooth peripheral enhancement.

### Differential Diagnosis

- ABC is the main differential consideration. Other entities include FD, enchondroma, or Langerhans cell histiocytosis.

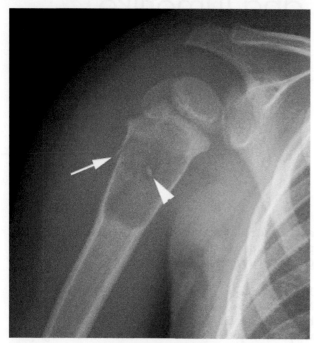

**Figure 62.1.** UBC on radiography. Grashey radiograph of the right shoulder demonstrates a lucent, expansile lesion in the proximal right humerus with a narrow zone of transition, consistent with a UBC. There is a pathologic fracture (*arrow*) along with a fallen fragment sign (*arrowhead*).

### Treatment Strategies
- Intracyst irrigation and curettage
- Can perform image-guided percutaneous intracyst injections of steroid, doxycycline, or bone marrow

---

## Aneurysmal Bone Cyst

### Pathophysiology and Clinical Findings
ABCs are expansile lesions with multiple cystlike cavities that are lined by fibroblasts and multinucleated giant cells. Lesions may be primary or secondary. Secondary ABCs make up approximately one-third of all cases and can be associated with other lesions (ie, giant cell tumor [GCT], osteoblastoma, chondroblastoma, FD, etc). The exact etiology for primary ABCs is unknown, although some authors have suggested they might be related to increased intraosseous venous pressure. Some ABCs are felt to represent a primary neoplasm. The vast majority of patients are younger than age 30, and 80% of ABCs are seen in patients younger than age 20. These occur slightly more commonly in women. They can occur in any bone but are classically observed in long bones and vertebral bodies. When they arise in long bones, they are most commonly eccentrically located in the metaphysis, but they can occur in the diaphysis and epiphysis. ABCs are benign but can be locally aggressive. Patients present with pain and swelling, and pathologic fractures are uncommon.

### Imaging Strategy and Findings
- Different modalities demonstrate a balloonlike expansile lesion with blood-filled spaces.

### Radiography
- Eccentric, lytic, expansile lesion and narrow zone of transition (Figure 62.3)
- Marked cortical thinning, which may appear absent on radiographs
- May be associated with periosteal reaction

### Computed Tomography
- Can see fluid-fluid levels from blood products (better seen on MRI)
- Thin cortical rim better visualized compared to radiography

### Magnetic Resonance Imaging
- Imaging shows multiple fluid- and/or blood-filled cysts of varying sizes with fluid-fluid levels, and different signal intensities from blood products of varying ages.
- Septa separating blood-filled spaces is seen (Figure 62.4). Septa may enhance, but cystic components will not.
- Rarely, ABCs may be more solid with fewer hemorrhagic cavities.

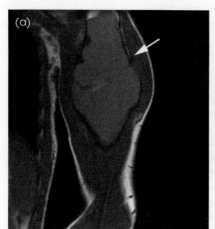
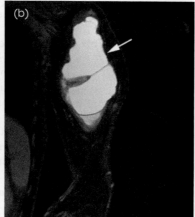
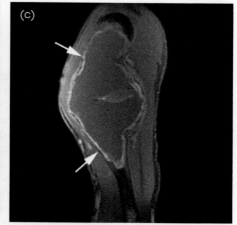

**Figure 62.2.** UBC on MRI. (*A*) Coronal T1W and (*B*) STIR images show a septated, well-circumscribed fluid-filled, expansile lesion (*arrow*). (*C*) On a T1W postcontrast image, there is peripheral (*arrows*) and linear septal enhancement but no internal nodular enhancement.

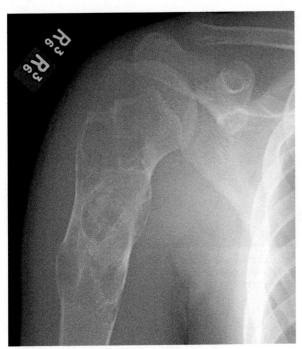

**Figure 62.3.** ABC on radiography. AP radiograph of the right shoulder demonstrates an expansile, lucent lesion in the proximal humerus with a narrow zone of transition, typical of an ABC. It should be remembered that ABCs may occasionally arise from other lesions, such as FD, chondroblastoma, or GCT.

**Angiography**
- Hypervascular, predominantly along the periphery of the lesion

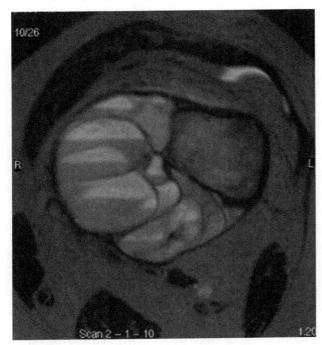

**Figure 62.4.** ABC on MRI. T2W axial images of knee show a multiseptated lesion containing fluid-fluid levels, common in ABCs.

**Nuclear Imaging**
- Increased radiotracer uptake on triple phase bone scintigraphy

**Differential Diagnosis**
- UBC, GCT, NOF
- Telangiectatic osteosarcoma (most worrisome differential)
  - ABCs will have narrow zone of transition.
  - Any area with wide zone of transition, solid enhancing component, or cortical breakthrough necessitates further investigation to exclude telangiectatic osteosarcoma.

**Treatment Options**
- Surgical resection with wide margins is recommended.
  - Preoperative embolization may be helpful to control bleeding during surgery.
- Radiation therapy can be helpful.
- Percutaneous intralesional absolute alcohol injection is another option.

## Intraosseous Ganglion

**Pathophysiology and Clinical Findings**
Intraosseous ganglia are benign, well-marginated, uniloculated or multiloculated, epiphyseal lucent lesions with gelatinous content that generally occur in the subchondral region of long bones. The etiology of these lesions is thought to be either related to intraosseous extension of an extraosseous ganglion or mucoid degeneration of intraosseous connective tissue. These usually occur in middle-aged patients and are asymptomatic. Rarely, they may be associated with pain. Intraosseous ganglia are frequently seen as incidental findings on imaging studies and are generally not treated.

**Imaging Findings**
**Radiography and Computed Tomography**
- Nonaggressive appearing, well-circumscribed, lucent lesion usually with a thin sclerotic rim

**Magnetic Resonance Imaging**
- Signal intensity of fluid with low T1W signal and high T2W signal intensity (Figure 62.5)
- May have thin peripheral enhancement without internal enhancement following IV contrast

## Giant Cell Tumor of Bone

**Pathophysiology and Clinical Findings**
GCTs are usually lesions composed of multinucleated giant cells that may arise from osteoclasts. They are often locally aggressive and can occasionally metastasize to the lungs. GCTs usually occur in younger skeletally mature patients, and 80% arise in patients between ages 20 and 50. They are most common in long bones, particularly the distal femur, proximal tibia, and distal radius. However, they can also occur in the sacrum and vertebrae. Although they originate in the metaphysis, they

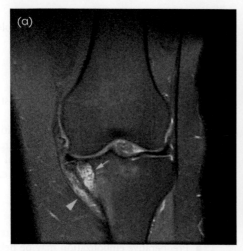
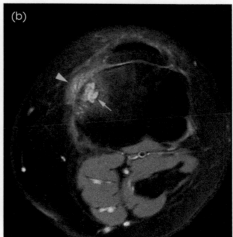

**Figure 62.5.** Intraosseous ganglion. T2W FS (*A*) coronal and (*B*) axial images of the knee depict a well-defined, mildly heterogeneous high signal intensity lesion in the medial proximal tibial epiphysis (*arrow*) with surrounding reactive BME in the tibia. The superficial bundle of the MCL is thickened and demonstrates high signal (*arrowhead*), suggesting an extraosseous component.

often extend to the epiphysis and subchondral bone and can be considered in the differential diagnosis of lesions that are predominantly located in the epiphysis. They infrequently invade the articular cartilage and joint space. Patients present with pain and swelling. They can also cause decreased range of motion and may present with pathologic fracture. Rarely, GCT may undergo malignant transformation.

### Imaging Strategy and Findings
#### Radiography
Refer to Figure 62.6.

- Eccentric intramedullary lesions involving the metaphysis and epiphysis

- Expansile, lobulated lesions with marked cortical thinning (Figure 62.6)
- Entirely lytic in majority of cases without sclerotic rim

#### Computed Tomography
- The findings are similar to radiography.
- Chest CT is useful in cases of malignant GCT with metastasis, where there may be peripheral ossification of lung metastasis

#### Magnetic Resonance Imaging
- Imaging shows inhomogenous low to intermediate T1W signal and inhomogeneous low to high T2W signal. Areas of low signal are often the result of susceptibility

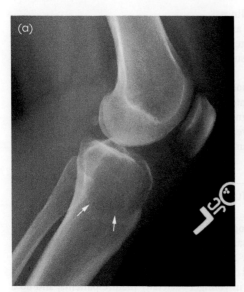
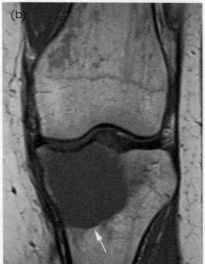
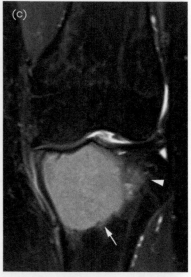

**Figure 62.6.** GCT of bone in a 33-year-old woman. (*A*) Lateral radiograph of the knee demonstrates a lucent lesion in the metaphysis of the proximal tibia extending to subchondral bone and the epiphysis (*arrows*). Note the lack of a sclerotic rim, a common finding in GCTs of bone. (*B*) Coronal T1W MR image of the knee depicts a lesion in the proximal tibia that is hypointense relative to the surrounding normal bone marrow and extends into the epiphysis (*arrow*). (*C*) Coronal T2W MR image demonstrates uniformly bright signal intensity relative to the surrounding bone marrow (*arrow*). Note the surrounding high signal BME in the tibia (*arrowhead*).

artifact in areas of hemosiderin deposition following localized hemorrhage.

- Inhomogeneous enhancement after IV gadolinium administration is seen.
- There may be ABC components (fluid-fluid levels).
- MRI can be used to evaluate for intraarticular extension and to monitor patients following resection for signs of local recurrence.

**Differential Diagnosis**
- The most common differential consideration is ABC. Chondroblastoma, clear cell chondrosarcoma, brown tumors, and telangiectatic osteosarcoma can also be considered.

**Treatment Options**
- Surgical resection is the standard of care. However, there is a high rate of local recurrence.
- Intralesional curettage followed by bone grafting may preserve the most function but is associated with higher rates of recurrence.
- Resection with wide margins may reduce risk of local recurrence but may have greater effect on function.
- Radiation therapy may be used when surgical resection is contraindicated or if the lesion is more aggressive.
- Percutaneous transcatheter embolization prior to surgery can be considered.

## Lipomatous Lesions

### Lipoma

**Pathophysiology and Clinical Findings**
Intraosseous lipomas are the most common lipomatous lesions of bone and contain mature adipose tissue with a few interspersed osseous trabeculae. The vast majority occur in the femur, particularly the intertrochanteric region. However, they can also be seen in the ilium, calcaneus, humerus, and ribs. There is no age predilection although most lesions are diagnosed in the fourth decade of life. They are usually asymptomatic and diagnosed as incidental findings; however, mild pain has been reported in some patients.

**Imaging Findings**
- Radiography and CT
  - Imaging shows a lucent, intramedullary lesion, usually with a thin rim of sclerosis.
  - Fat density lesion on CT (less than −50 HU) is seen.
  - They may have central or diffuse calcification related to fat necrosis (*cockade sign* in the calcaneus).
- MRI
  - Mostly mature fat on MRI that is isointense to subcutaneous fat (high T1W and T2W signal)
  - Fat-suppression technique nulls signal
  - Calcifications are low on T1W and T2W sequences
  - Low signal rim corresponding to sclerosis
  - Can be associated with cystic degeneration and resemble a UBC

**Differential Diagnosis**
- UBC (especially in calcaneus), GCT

**Treatment Options**
- Curettage and bone grafting for symptomatic lesions

### Liposclerosing Myxofibrous Tumor
**Pathophysiology and Clinical Findings**
Liposclerosing myxofibrous tumor (LSMFT) is a benign fibroosseous lesion that contains a mix of materials, including fatty, fibrous, and myxomatous tissue, along with fat necrosis and cystic degeneration. They are usually discovered in patients in the fourth decade. Approximately half of the cases present with pain, although these lesions are also commonly incidentally noted on imaging studies. Almost 90% occur in the intertrochanteric region of the femur. Pathologic fractures may occur but are rare. Although the lesion is benign, approximately 10% will undergo malignant transformation to osteosarcoma or pleomorphic sarcoma.

**Imaging Strategy and Findings**
Refer to Figure 62.7.

- Radiography and CT
  - Geographic lucent lesion with sclerotic margin may be mildly expansile.
  - CT findings mirror radiographic findings.
  - Multiple types of tissue are contained, so these lesions can have varying densities depending on composition.
  - Most contain matrix and can be globular, linear, or ringlike densities,
  - Fat density usually not seen.
- MRI
  - Sclerotic rim and matrix are low signal.
  - Variable T2W signal intensity depending on tissue type, and T1W signal is isointense to muscle.
  - Fat signal is unlikely to be seen.

Because of the risk of malignant transformation serial follow-up imaging may be needed to detect the development of aggressive bone destruction and extraosseous soft tissue.

**Differential Diagnosis**
- Intraosseous lipoma, FD

**Treatment Options**
- Curettage and bone grafting for symptomatic lesions
- Surgical fixation or arthroplasty if there is a pathologic fracture

## Miscellaneous Lesions

### Chordoma

**Pathophysiology and Clinical Findings**
Chordomas are slowly growing, locally aggressive, low- to intermediate-grade malignant lesions that develop in the midline of the axial skeleton from notochordal remnants. Patients are usually older than age 30. They occur most

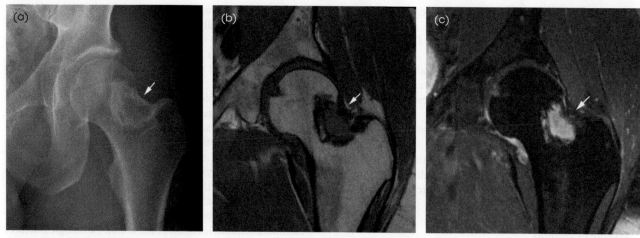

**Figure 62.7.** LSMFT incidentally noted in a 45-year-old man. (*A*) AP radiograph of the left hip demonstrates a mildly expansile femoral neck lucent lesion with a thick, irregular sclerotic rim (*arrow*). No frank cortical osteolysis is seen. (*B*) Coronal T1W MR image of the pelvis demonstrates an intermediate signal intensity lesion although no macroscopic fat is seen (*arrow*). (*C*) Coronal T1W FS postcontrast MR image demonstrates diffuse enhancement (*arrow*).

frequently in the sacrum, and approximately 40% of sacral tumors are chordomas. These lesions are also commonly noted in the sphenooccipital region, particularly in the clivus. C2 lesions are the next most common location but are unusual.

### Imaging Findings
- Radiography and CT
  - Lytic, destructive lesion with lobulated margins that may contain peripheral calcifications
  - Usually slow-growing so may have nonaggressive features, including narrow zone of transition, no periosteal reaction, and incomplete sclerotic rim

- Can have extraosseous soft tissue mass that may displace bowel and/or bladder on radiographs
- MRI
  - Low and isointense T1W and high T2W signal compared to skeletal muscle; may be inhomogeneous; calcifications low signal on all pulse sequences (Figure 62.8)
  - Enhances on postcontrast imaging
- Nuclear imaging
  - FDG avid on PET scan

### Differential Diagnosis
- GCT, plasmacytoma, metastasis

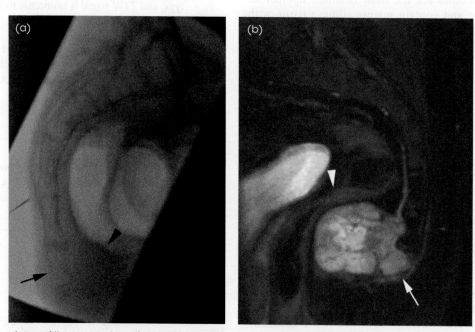

**Figure 62.8.** Chordoma of the sacrum in a 62-year-old man. (*A*) Lateral spot fluoroscopic image of the sacrum and coccyx demonstrates an indistinct appearance of the first coccygeal segment cortex (*arrow*) with a soft tissue mass extending into the presacral region (*arrowhead*). (*B*) On sagittal T2W MR image of the pelvis there is a high signal intensity mass arising from the coccyx (*arrow*) and exerting mass effect on the rectum (*arrowhead*). Subsequent biopsy was diagnostic of a chordoma.

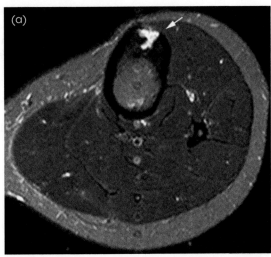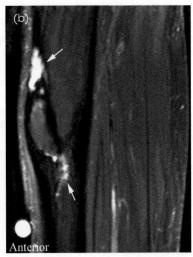

**Figure 62.9.** Osteofibrous dysplasia spectrum. (*A*) Axial STIR image of the mid tibial diaphysis in a 33-year-old woman with anterior lower leg swelling shows a lobulated, expansile lesion arising in the anterior tibial diaphyseal cortex (*arrow*) with surrounding cortical thickening. (*B*) Sagittal T1W FS postcontrast image demonstrates areas of enhancement within the lesion (*arrows*). Subsequent biopsy revealed osteofibrous dysplasia.

### Treatment Options

- En bloc surgical resection is treatment of choice. However, local recurrence and functional impairment is common.
- Additional targeted radiation therapy may be helpful to decrease risk of local recurrence.

### Adamantinoma (Osteofibrous Dysplasia Spectrum)

### Pathophysiology and Clinical Findings

Adamantinoma is a low-grade malignant lesion that usually presents in the second and third decades of life and 85-90% of cases present in the anterior tibia, particularly in the distal meta-diaphysis. These lesions metastasize in approximately 20% of cases, most commonly to the lungs and regional lymph nodes. Osteofibrous dysplasia is a benign condition that also has a predilection for the anterior tibial cortex. It has been suggested that adamantinoma and osteofibrous dysplasia are lesions within the same spectrum. Differentiating these conditions may be difficult by imaging alone, and establishing the diagnosis usually requires tissue sampling.

### Imaging Findings

- Radiography and CT
    - Imaging shows cortical, expansile, lytic lesion, classically within the anterior cortex of the mid to distal tibia.
    - Adamantinoma may appear nonaggressive initially but can present with cortical osteolysis later.
    - Chest CT may be needed to detect pulmonary metastases.
- MRI (Figure 62.9)
    - Multiloculated, cortically based lesion with possible extraosseous soft tissue mass breaking through cortex
    - Isointense to mildly hyperintense to muscle on T1W imaging and hyperintense on T2W sequences
    - Enhances following IV contrast administration
    - May identify radiographically occult daughter lesions

### Differential Diagnosis

- Osteofibrous dysplasia, FD, ABC

### Treatment Options

- Wide surgical excision is the treatment of choice.

### Key Points

- UBCs are mildly expansile lucent lesions, either with a single cavity or a few internal septations, usually seen in patients younger than age 30 .
- ABCs are markedly expansile lesions with numerous septations and fluid-fluid levels, also usually seen in patients younger than age 30.
- ABCs can either be primary or may arise from other lesions, such as chondroblastomas, FD, and GCTs.
- ABCs can either arise from telangiectatic osteosarcomas or can mimic them on imaging. In these cases, targeted tissue sampling of either solid or nodular areas or areas of aggressive-appearing bone destruction may confirm the presence of malignancy.
- GCT of bone is an expansile, locally aggressive lesion most commonly located in the metaphysis and epiphysis of long bones (especially around the knee). Occasional pulmonary metastases have been reported.
- Chordomas arise in the midline of the axial skeleton from notochordal remnants and are most common in the sacrum and clivus.
- Adamantinomas are a malignant lesion arising in the anterior tibial diaphyseal cortex. These probably represent a spectrum with osteofibrous dysplasia.

### Recommended Reading

Mascard E, Gomez-Brouchet A, Lambot K. Bone cysts: unicameral and aneurysmal bone cyst. *Orthop Traumatol Surg Res.* 2015;101(1 suppl):S119–27.

Murphey MD, Carroll JF, Flemming DJ, Pope TL, Gannon FH, Kransdorf MJ. From the archives of the AFIP: benign musculoskeletal lipomatous lesions. *Radiographics*. 2004;24(5):1433–66.

## References

1. Chugh R, Tawbi H, Lucas DR, Biermann JS, Schuetze SM, Baker LH. Chordoma: the nonsarcoma primary bone tumor. *Oncologist*. 2007;12(11):1344–50.
2. Hakim DN, Pelly T, Kulendran M, Caris JA. Benign tumours of the bone: a review. *J Bone Oncol*. 2015;4(2):37–41.
3. Hatori M, Watanabe M, Hosaka M, Sasano H, Narita M, Kokubun S. A classic adamantinoma arising from osteofibrous dysplasia-like adamantinoma in the lower leg: a case report and review of the literature. *Tohoku J Exp Med*. 2006;209(1):53–59.
4. Park HY, Yang SK, Sheppard WL, et al. Current management of aneurysmal bone cysts. *Curr Rev Musculoskelet Med*. 2016;9(4):435–44.
5. Yazdi HR, Rasouli B, Borhani A, Noorollahi MM. Intraosseous lipoma of the femur: image findings. *J Orthop Case Rep*. 2014;4(1):35–38.

# Secondary Bone Tumors and Radiation Changes

# CHAPTER 63

# Metastatic Disease

Stephanie McCann and Stephen Thomas

## Introduction

Metastatic disease from carcinomas accounts for approximately 70% of malignant tumors involving the skeleton. Notable high incidences are found in patients with breast, lung, prostate, and renal cell carcinoma, with some having specific imaging features. Patients with metastatic bone lesions may be asymptomatic or may present with localized bone pain, pathologic fracture, neurologic impingement, or an associated soft tissue mass. Imaging plays an important role in detection, diagnosis, prognosis, planning, and treatment response of metastatic bone lesions. Modalities available for imaging skeletal metastases include radiography, MRI, bone scintigraphy, CT, and hybrid fusion techniques such as PET/CT and PET/MRI, which offer the most sensitive and specific evaluation of metastatic bone lesions.

## Pathophysiology

The most common mechanism of metastatic tumor spread is via hematogenous spread of tumor emboli. The distribution pattern of cancer cells to the bone is believed to be caused by venous flow from breast and prostate toward the vena cava and into the vertebral venous plexus. The hematogenous tumor emboli initially seed the vascular-rich red marrow of the bones, and the entry of cancer cells into the venous circulation of the bone marrow is facilitated by the slow blood flow and particular anatomy of the venous sinusoids.

The cytokines involved in normal bone turnover provide a rich microenvironment to support cancer cells once they have reached the bone. The tumor cells interrupt normal bone cell turnover by releasing local cytokines and growth factors. Certain cytokines, such as parathyroid hormone-related protein and tumor necrosis factor $\alpha$ or $\beta$, may directly upregulate osteoclast activity, whereas interleukin-1 and interleukin-6 may indirectly promote osteoclast activity and osteolysis by inducing chronic inflammation. Depending on the rate of osteoclastic and osteoblastic activity, bone metastases can be osteoblastic (bone forming) or osteolytic (bone destructive). Metastases from kidney, thyroid, and lung tend to be osteolytic, whereas prostate and breast carcinoma metastases are frequently osteoblastic (Figure 63.1). However, there is often a combination of both processes in most metastases. Osteolytic lesions tend to be more aggressive and result in pathologic fractures, whereas sclerotic metastases typically have slower progression.

## Distribution of Skeletal Metastatic Disease

Metastatic disease to the spine, pelvis, ribs, and the ends of long bones are preferred sites of metastasis as they are rich in red marrow. Within the spine, the lumbar spine has the highest rate of metastatic disease (53%), followed by the thoracic spine (36%) and the cervical spine (12%) (Figure 63.2). Within the vertebrae, the lesions prefer the posterior part of the vertebral body and pedicles. Acral metastases (beyond the elbows and knees) can be seen in lung, breast, and renal cancer (Figure 63.3). These lesions can be asymptomatic and may not be imaged on skeletal surveys. Most metastases are located in the medullary (marrow) cavity. However, certain metastases from lung, breast, and renal carcinomas can be purely cortical.

## Pathologic Fractures

Fractures that occur through weakened segments of bones, often with low-energy trauma, are called *pathologic fractures*. A wide variety of conditions can weaken bones, including osteogenesis imperfecta, renal osteodystrophy, Paget disease of the bone, and FD, among other etiologies. Skeletal neoplasms, particularly metastases, are one of the most common causes of pathologic fractures. Although both osteoblastic and osteolytic lesions can predispose patients to develop fractures, lytic lesions are much more commonly associated with fractures. Other factors, such as lesion size and location, and depth of cortical involvement, may also increase the risk of pathologic fracture. Lesions in the lower extremity, particularly those in the proximal femur, are at higher risk of pathologic fracture because of the stress of weight-bearing. Additionally, lesions associated with deeper cortical destruction also have a higher risk of pathologic fracture. Two systems, the *Mirels scoring system* (Table 63.1) and *Harrington criteria* (Table 63.2), have been developed to help assess risk of pathologic fracture in order to determine whether a particular lesion needs to be prophylactically surgically stabilized. Because most of the criteria are well-assessed on imaging studies, radiologists can provide a valuable role in determining risk of pathologic fractures.

## Imaging Strategy and Findings
### Radiography

- This is often the initial diagnostic test in the evaluation of bone pain as it is widely available and cost-effective.
- Used to assess bone structures and mechanical alignment, however, radiographs are not recommended as a screening tool because of poor sensitivity in detecting bone changes.
- Osteolytic lesions are not detected on radiography until there is 25-50% of bone mineral loss.
  - Such osteolytic activity can place patients at increased risk for fracture (Figure 63.4).
- Osteolytic lesions appear as areas of faint trabecular thinning, lucent foci, and can have a permeative appearance as the tumor spreads in the medullary space

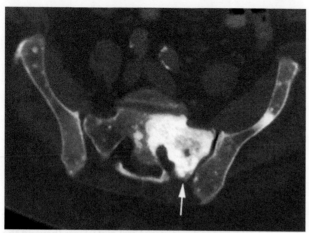

**Figure 63.1.** Osteoblastic metastasis of prostate carcinoma. Axial CT image demonstrates numerous sclerotic lesions in the pelvis in a 70-year-old male patient with prostate carcinoma, the largest of which involves the left sacral ala (*arrow*).

and creates pressure within the marrow, resorption of trabeculae, and outward growth to cause destruction of the cortex (Figure 63.5).

- Aggressive osteolytic lesions tend to have a wide zone of transition and irregular borders.
- Osteoblastic (sclerotic) lesions tend to be nodular, rounded, have a narrower zone of transition, and can have a well-circumscribed border.
- With treatment, osteolytic skeletal metastases tend to form new reactive bone and become sclerotic.
  - The sclerosis extends from the periphery to the center of the lesion over time.

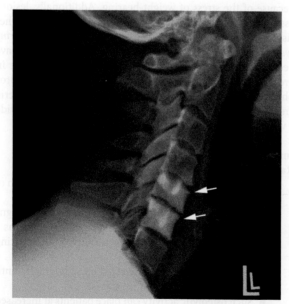

**Figure 63.2.** Vertebral osteoblastic metastasis. Lateral radiograph of the cervical spine in a 56-year-old male patient with known lung carcinoma shows diffuse sclerosis of the C5 and C6 vertebral bodies (*arrows*), known as the *ivory vertebral body sign*.

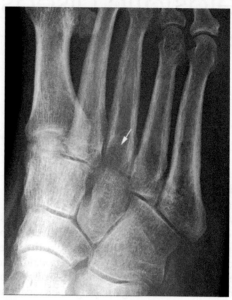

**Figure 63.3.** Acral osteolytic metastasis. AP radiograph of the right midfoot of a 55-year-old male patient with lung carcinoma shows a subtle acral lytic metastatic lesion in the base of the third metatarsal (*arrow*).

- Worsening osteolysis, within sclerotic or mixed lesions, or progressive enlargement of an existing lesion, are indicators of disease progression.

**Nuclear Imaging**
- The most sensitive and cost-effective whole body examination for identifying lytic and sclerotic lesions is a radionuclide bone scan with technetium 99m methylene diphosphonate ($^{99m}$Tc-MDP).

| **Table 63.1. Mirels Scoring System for Pathologic Fracture** |
|---|
| ■ Patients are assigned points based on 4 criteria:<br>1. Location of lesion—upper limb, lower limb, peritrochanteric<br>2. Size of lesion measured as a percentage of involvement of the diameter of the bone—<1/3, between 1/3 and 2/3, >2/3<br>3. Type of lesion—blastic, mixed, lytic<br>4. Pain—mild, moderate, severe<br>■ Imaging is required for 3 of 4 categories.<br>■ Within each criterion, the first element gets 1 point, the second gets 2 points, and the third element gets 3 points. For example, if a patient has mild pain, 1 point is awarded; for severe pain, 3 points are awarded.<br>■ Points are added. If the score is <7, there is a low risk of pathologic fracture; if >8, there is a high risk of fracture and prophylactic surgical stabilization should be considered.<br>■ Although radiographs may be sufficient, MRI or CT can be helpful to make an accurate determination of depth of cortical involvement. |

## Table 63.2. Harrington Criteria—4 Criteria for Pathologic Fracture

1. >50% cortical destruction
2. Lesions size >2.5 cm
3. Proximal femoral lesions with lesser trochanteric avulsion
4. Persistent pain during weight-bearing despite irradiation

- Bone scans have been found to detect metastatic lesions up to 18 months earlier than radiographs.
- The overall sensitivity for detecting bony metastases is 95%, with a false-negative rate of 2-5%.
- Most malignant lesions demonstrate increased radiotracer uptake (Figure 63.6), whereas some aggressive lytic lesions may demonstrate a photopenic defect (occasionally called a *cold defect*).
- Renal cell carcinoma and slow-growing tumors, such as thyroid carcinoma, can present as photopenic defects on a bone scan.
- Diffuse osseous metastases can result in a superscan, or symmetric activity in the bones with decreased renal and soft tissue activity. Metastases result in increased osteoid and immature woven bone production.
- Bone scintigraphy is not specific for neoplasia, and there is a broad differential diagnosis for areas of increased radiotracer uptake:
  - Benign etiologies that should not be confused with metastatic lesions include Paget disease, FD, fracture, benign osseous tumors, arthritis, osteomyelitis, and ON.
  - Therefore, skeletal structures with increased radiotracer uptake on bone scan are usually further evaluated and characterized with radiography and subsequently, if needed, with MRI or CT.

### Positron Emission Tomography/Computed Tomography
- PET/CT imaging of the whole body using 18F-fluorodeoxyglucose is very sensitive in detecting bone metastases that have high metabolic activity.
- PET/CT is 94% sensitive and 97% specific in detecting and characterizing metastatic disease (Figure 63.7).

### Computed Tomography
- CT is not a useful screening tool for skeletal metastasis as it is only sensitive for lesions involving cortical bone and less so for tumors restricted to the marrow space, because they must be very extensive to be detectable.
- CT has a sensitivity of 73% and a pooled specificity of 95%.
- CT is often used to better characterize lesions detected on radiography or bone scan.
- CT is an excellent modality for guiding percutaneous biopsies or targeted treatments, such as ablations, particularly in the spine and pelvis (Figure 63.8).

### Magnetic Resonance Imaging
- Excellent contrast resolution enables better evaluation of the bone marrow and soft tissues compared to the

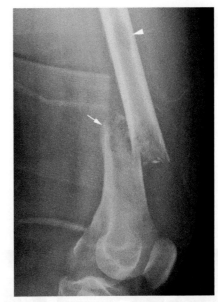

**Figure 63.4.** Osteolytic metastasis with pathologic fracture in a 67-year-old male patient with multiple myeloma. Lateral radiograph of the right femur shows a pathologic fracture (*arrow*) through a lytic lesion with permeative destruction in the femoral diaphysis with displacement. A second, more proximal lesion with mild endosteal scalloping is seen (*arrowhead*).

other imaging modalities; in addition to imaging the affected region, whole body MRI can be performed.

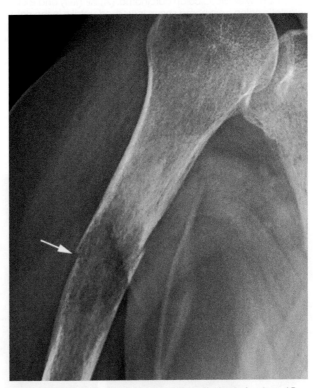

**Figure 63.5.** Osteolytic metastasis with pathologic fracture. AP radiograph of the shoulder in a 65-year-old male patient with metastatic hepatocellular carcinoma shows a permeative lytic lesion with cortical thinning in the humeral shaft with a pathologic fracture (*arrow*).

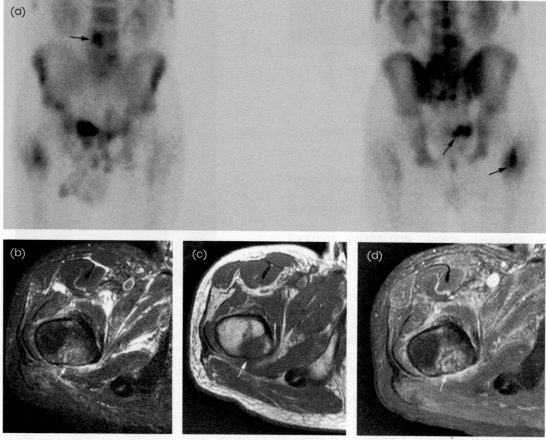

**Figure 63.6.** Metastatic colon carcinoma. (*A*) AP (*left*) and PA (*right*) views of a radionuclide bone scan of the pelvis in a patient with metastatic colon carcinoma shows increased uptake in the right anterior pubic ramus, posterior proximal right femur, and lumbar spine (*arrows*). (*B*) Axial T2W FS, (*C*) axial T1W precontrast, and (*D*) axial T1W postcontrast MR images through the proximal right femur demonstrates a heterogeneous T2 hyperintense, T1 hypointense, heterogeneously enhancing metastatic lesion (*arrows*) along the posterior proximal femur with cortical thinning and mild adjacent soft tissue edema.

- In cases with poor renal function, noncontrast MRI with T1W and fluid-sensitive sequences can be performed to detect metastatic disease.

- On a per-patient basis, MRI is 91% sensitive and 95% specific and is thus superior to both CT and planar skeletal scintigraphy.

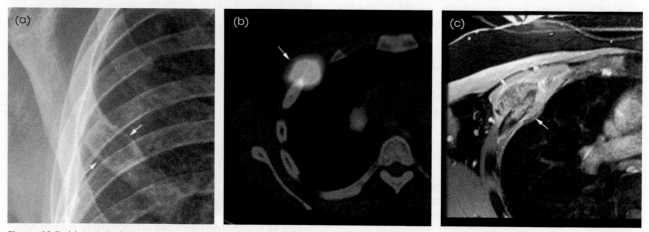

**Figure 63.7.** Metastatic lesion of the rib in a 23-year-old female patient with lymphoma. (*A*) AP radiograph shows an expansile lytic lesion in an anterolateral right rib (*between arrows*). (*B*) Axial fused PET/CT image demonstrates a hypermetabolic focus involving the same rib. Also note the additional hypermetabolic focus in a right hilar lymph node. (*C*) Axial T1W postcontrast MR image of the chest shows destruction of the affected rib with an associated, heterogeneously enhancing mass (*between arrows*).

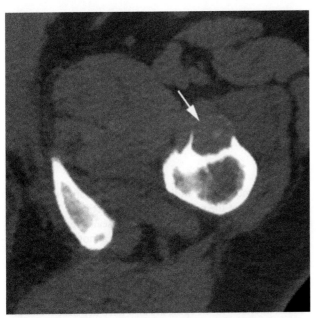

**Figure 63.8.** Cortical osteolytic metastasis of the proximal femur. Axial CT image (during bone biopsy) demonstrates a cortically based metastatic lesion with soft tissue component involving the anterior proximal left femur (*arrow*). Biopsy confirmed metastatic lung carcinoma.

- Most metastatic lesions are hypointense on T1 and hyperintense on T2W or STIR imaging.
  - Lesions have variable enhancement depending on their vascularity.
- MRI is particularly helpful in characterizing extraosseous soft tissue extension and to determine whether a lesion involves surrounding structures, such as neurovascular bundles. This may impact therapeutic options.

## Treatment Options
- Treatment of underlying primary malignancy, including chemotherapy, immunotherapy, and hormonal therapy, is the first goal of therapy if possible.
- Tailored chemotherapy is used to treat systemic disease.
- For lesions that may predispose to or have already sustained pathologic fracture, surgical stabilization should be considered.
- For painful metastases, radiation therapy and image-guided percutaneous ablation with cementoplasty can be considered.

- Pharmacologic pain control can also be achieved with NSAIDs and opioid medications.

## Key Points
- Metastatic carcinomas represent 70% of malignant tumors involving bone.
- The spine, pelvis, and ribs are the most common sites of metastatic disease.
- Cortical metastasis can occur from lung, breast, and renal carcinomas.
- $^{99m}$Tc-MDP whole body bone scan and 18F-fluorodeoxyglucose PET/CT are the most sensitive whole body modalities to detect bone metastasis.
- MRI is a sensitive modality to detect bone metastasis and is helpful in characterizing extraosseous soft tissue extension.
- The Mirels criteria provides a scoring system to identify bones that are at risk of pathologic fracture.

## References
1. Brenner AI, Koshy J, Morey J, Lin C, DiPoce J. The bone scan. *Semin Nucl Med.* 2012;42(1):11–26.
2. Bussard KM, Gay CV, Mastro AM. The bone microenvironment in metastasis; what is special about bone? *Cancer Metastasis Rev.* 2008;27(1):41–55.
3. Miric A, Banks M, Allen D, et al. Cortical metastatic lesions of the appendicular skeleton from tumors of known primary origin. *J Surg Oncol.* 1998;67(4):255–60.
4. O'Sullivan GJ, Carty FL, Cronin CG. Imaging of bone metastasis: an update. *World J Radiol.* 2015;7(8):202–11.
5. Roberts CC, Daffner RH, Weissman BN, et al. ACR appropriateness criteria on metastatic bone disease. *J Am Coll Radiol.* 2010;7(6):400–409.
6. Talbot JN, Paycha F, Balogova S. Diagnosis of bone metastasis: recent comparative studies of imaging modalities. *Q J Nucl Med Mol Imaging.* 2011;55(4):374–410.
7. Walton ZJ, Holmes RE, Chapin RW, Lindsey KG, Leddy LR. Bronchogenic squamous cell carcinoma with soft-tissue metastasis to the hand: an unusual case presentation and review of the literature. *Am J Orthop (Belle Mead NJ).* 2014;43(12):E324–27.
8. Yang HL, Liu T, Wang XM, Xu Y, Deng SM. Diagnosis of bone metastases: a meta-analysis comparing 18FDG PET, CT, MRI and bone scintigraphy. *Eur Radiol.* 2011;21(12):2604–17.
9. Yu HH, Tsai YY, Hoffe SE. Overview of diagnosis and management of metastatic disease to bone. *Cancer Control.* 2012;19(2):84–91.

# CHAPTER 64

# Radiation Changes

Stephen Thomas and Stephanie McCann

## Introduction

Radiation therapy (RT) is very effective in treating soft tissue masses and primary and secondary bone tumors. It may be aimed at cure, as adjuvant therapy, or for palliation. RT of bone pathology is primarily administered as external beam with the goals of decreasing tumor size, pain relief, preservation of function, and maintenance of skeletal integrity. Imaging is frequently used for bone tumor localization, treatment planning, evaluating response to RT, and for potential post-RT complications. Side effects and complications from RT depend on skeletal maturity, duration of therapy, and radiation dose. When the radiation target is nonosseous, osseous structures within the radiation field may be affected. Irradiation of immature long bones produces limb shortening, overtubulation, sclerosis, and bowing of the irradiated bone. Radiation changes in mature bone include replacement of the hematopoietic cellular elements, sclerosis, osteoradionecrosis, pathologic fracture, and after a latency period, radiation-induced neoplasms.

## Radiation Changes Specific to the Immature Skeleton

### Bone Density Changes

RT can induce osteopenia in children. The risk is between 8% and 23% at doses above 20 Gy and is seen 30 weeks postirradiation. Associated risk of pathologic fracture, however, is unclear.

### Appendicular Skeleton

Radiation effects in growing bone primarily arises in the radiosensitive chondrocytes in the epiphyseal growth plate. However, the effects are dose dependent. There are few long-lasting effects for radiation doses less than 10 Gy. Radiation doses between 10 and 20 Gy produce partial growth arrest, whereas doses in excess of 20 Gy result in complete long bone growth arrest and limb shortening in patients. Radiation to the immature hip joint can result in capital femoral epiphyseal slippage when exposed to doses in excess of 25 Gy. Skeletally immature patients who receive hip radiation are at increased risk of developing ON of the femoral epiphysis, which primarily occurs at radiation doses of 20 Gy and likely results from the radiation damage to the blood supply of the femoral epiphysis. The addition of corticosteroids causes a synergistic effect. When a joint is radiated, the radiation causes premature bone differentiation of the articular cartilage and chondrocyte senescence, which can lead to premature OA.

In the metaphysis, radiation results in deficient absorptive processes of the calcified bone and cartilage. This causes bowing, fraying, and bandlike metaphyseal sclerosis (Figure 64.1). In the diaphysis, radiation causes abnormal periosteal activity, resulting in bone remodeling that causes narrowing of the diaphyseal diameter or overtubulation.

### Axial Skeleton

Radiation effects to the spine are also dose dependent and are seen at doses greater than 10 Gy. Vertebral bodies show subcortical lucent zones within a year after the end of RT. The subcortical lucent zones progress over the next 1–2 years to form growth arrest lines, which parallel the epiphysis of the vertebral body. The transverse lines in the vertebral bodies can produce a bone-in-bone appearance on radiography. Scalloping of the cartilage plates can occur. At higher radiation doses, growth arrest of the vertebral bodies is accelerated (Figure 64.2). If the radiation involves a portion of the vertebral body, scoliosis concave to the radiation portal can develop from hypoplasia of the segment in up to 80% of patients with approximately 40% of patients developing greater than 20 degrees of scoliosis.

Pelvic radiation exposure at sufficient doses can result in hypoplasia of a hemi-pelvis or ilium (Figure 64.3), acetabular dysplasia, or coxa valga or vara. In the thorax, rib hypoplasia occurs for ribs included in the radiation field.

## Radiation Changes in the Mature Skeleton

The appearance of bone marrow on MRI after the initiation of RT depends on the therapy duration and dose. BME and necrosis can be seen on STIR images as early as 7 days after initiation of therapy. Additionally, postcontrast T1W images show enhancement during the same period. As early as 3-6 weeks after the start of treatment, T1W images of the marrow demonstrate increased and heterogeneous signal intensity, which is postulated to be caused by fatty replacement of the marrow (Figure 64.4). Fatty conversion has been found to be irreversible after irradiation higher than 40 Gy. The reversibility time of fatty conversion at doses lower than 40 Gy is variable because of numerous factors including anatomic location, concurrent chemotherapy, and granulocyte-stimulating agents.

### Osteonecrosis

In the mature bone, radiation changes manifest as abnormal bone repair because of inhibition of osteoblast function, resulting in bone death and ON. Radiation necrosis is dose dependent with potentially reversible changes occurring at less

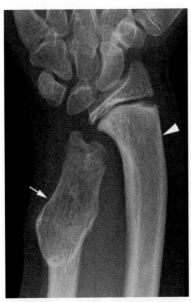

**Figure 64.1.** Postradiation deformity of the long bones in a 17-year-old skeletally immature patient with prior radiation to the distal ulna for metastatic neuroblastoma. PA radiograph of the left wrist shows the effects of radiation-produced shortened ulna (*arrow*) and bowing of the distal radial metaphysis (*arrowhead*).

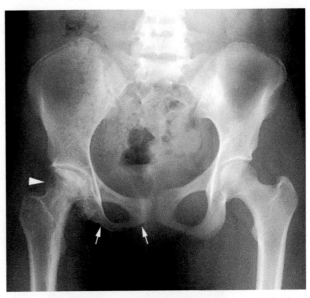

**Figure 64.3.** Postradiation innominate bone hypoplasia. Pelvic radiograph of an 18-year-old patient with prior RT for a right pelvic sarcoma shows hypoplasia of the right ilium, ischium, and pubis (*arrows*). Radiation to the right femoral head resulted in ON with collapse (*arrowhead*).

than 30 Gy, which is termed *radiation osteitis*. Cell death and bone devascularization occurs in treatment doses higher than 50 Gy. The terms radiation osteitis and *osteoradionecrosis* are often used interchangeably in the literature.

Radiographically, ON is seen as an initial decrease in bone density with subsequent development of a mixed radiolucent and sclerotic appearance with coarse trabeculae

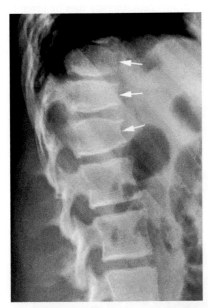

**Figure 64.2.** Postradiation deformity of the spine in a skeletally immature patient. Lateral radiograph of the lumbar spine of a 19-year-old patient with prior abdominal RT shows hypoplastic T10 to L1 vertebral bodies (*arrows*), with scalloping of the anterior aspect of the endplates, which resulted in a focal kyphosis.

(Figure 64.5). This occurs from attempts at osseous repair as a result of deposition of new bone on ischemic trabeculae. ON is thought to occur at higher radiation doses and may constitute the extreme of the continuum (Figure 64.6). The mandible is particularly prone to osteoradionecrosis as it is a superficial structure, which exposes it to high radiation doses needed to treat oropharyngeal carcinoma, and it has a poor blood supply. Osteoradionecrosis usually occurs within a year of completing RT.

The differential diagnosis for osteoradionecrosis is recurrent malignancy, radiation-induced malignancy, and infection. Unlike the other entities, radiation-induced ON is confined to the radiation portal.

### Fractures

Treatment-induced ON produces structurally weak bone that can easily fracture as the RT inhibits bone repair. Sites prone to fractures include the femoral neck, ilium, pubis, and sacrum (Figure 64.7).

### Radiation-Induced Tumors
### Benign

Osteochondromas are the most common benign radiation-induced tumor. These appear to be particularly common in patients who receive total body irradiation before bone marrow transplantation at an early age and occur after a shorter latency period than malignant sarcomas. They are histologically identical to spontaneously arising lesions. The dose of radiation required to induce osteochondroma development varies between 15 and 50 Gy.

### Malignant

Radiation-induced sarcoma (RIS) is a rare complication of radiation that typically occurs several years after the end of RT (Figure 64.8). The minimum radiation dose for RIS is usually

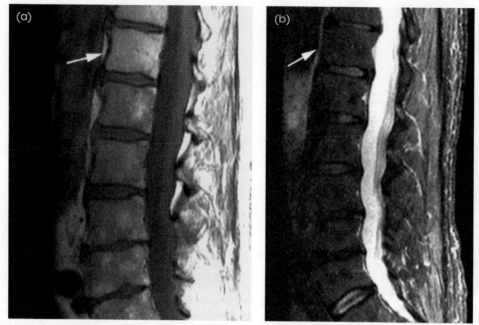

**Figure 64.4.** Fatty marrow replacement at the site of prior radiation portal in a 65-year-old man with prior history of thoracic spine radiation for metastasis. (*A*) Sagittal T1W MR image of the lumbar spine demonstrates fatty bone marrow replacement in the visualized lower thoracic spine with normal red marrow in the lumbar spine (*arrow*). (*B*) Sagittal STIR MR image shows homogenous fat suppression of the bone marrow signal (*arrow*).

30 Gy. The criteria for RIS that has been used are (1) latent period of 3-4 or more years, (2) malignancy arising within the irradiated field, (3) sarcomatous change at pathology, and (4) the RIS must differ from the original lesion. Most second malignancies that arise in bone are osteosarcomas, although fibrosarcomas, MFHs, and other sarcomas may occur.

**Treatment Options**

- When treating long bones with RT, internal orthopedic stabilization is frequently required in addition to radiation to treat or minimize risk of fracture. Common appendicular sites are the humerus and femur, which are fixed with long intramedullary nails. When there is no intent for cure, the potential spread of tumor cells by intramedullary nailing is acceptable.
- For RIS, the goal of surgical treatment is wide excision with tumor-free margins. This may include amputation when necessary.
- Neoadjuvant chemotherapy may be given to control disease prior to surgery.
- Occasionally, additional RT may be helpful as well. However, this may be limited by cumulative dose.

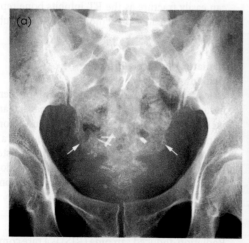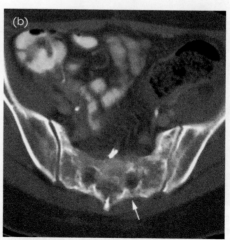

**Figure 64.5.** Radiation-related osteosclerosis in a 67-year-old woman with prior pelvic radiation for colorectal carcinoma. (*A*) AP pelvic radiograph demonstrates patchy sclerosis of the bony trabeculae in the sacrum (*arrow*). (*B*) Axial CT image of the pelvis better demonstrates coarsened bony trabeculae without cortical thickening in the same region (*arrow*).

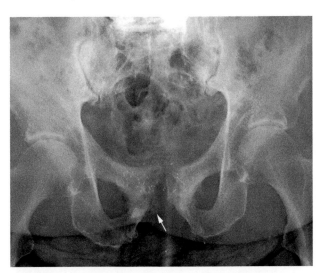

**Figure 64.6.** Radiation-induced ON in a 75-year-old man with prior pelvic radiation for prostate carcinoma. AP pelvic radiograph demonstrates sclerosis and poorly defined cortical margins of the symphysis pubis (*arrow*).

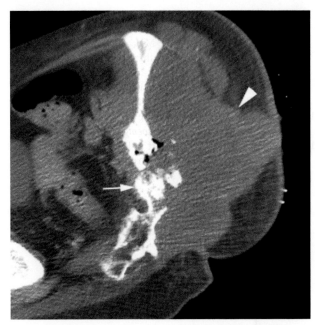

**Figure 64.8.** RIS in a 67-year-old woman with history of left pelvis radiation for breast metastasis 10 years prior. The patient presented with a left pelvic mass. Axial CT image of the pelvis demonstrates sclerosis and bone destruction of the left ilium (*arrow*) with a large associated soft tissue mass (*arrowhead*) that was a biopsy proven sarcoma. Foci of gas are likely related to recent biopsy.

## Key Points

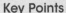

- Radiation changes in bone are dose dependent.
- Radiation can induce osteopenia and in severe cases, ON, leading to fractures.
- Bone deformities, such as growth arrest and bowing deformities, are some of the side effects in the immature skeleton.
- Osteochondromas are the most common benign radiation-induced bone tumor.
- RISs can rarely occur several years after irradiation.

## Recommended Reading

Mitchell MJ, Logan PM. Radiation-induced changes in bone. *Radiographics*. 1998;18(5):1125–36.

## References

1. Bluemke DA, Fishman EK, Scott WW, Jr. Skeletal complications of radiation therapy. *Radiographics*. 1994;14(1):111–21.

2. Daldrup-Link HE, Henning T, Link TM. MR imaging of therapy-induced changes of bone marrow. *Eur Radiol*. 2007;17(3):743–61.

3. Eastley N, Newey M, Ashford RU. Skeletal metastases—the role of the orthopaedic and spinal surgeon. *Surg Oncol*. 2012;21(3):216–22.

4. Hopewell JW. Radiation-therapy effects on bone density. *Med Pediatr Oncol*. 2003;41(3):208–11.

5. Jereczek-Fossa BA, Orecchia R. Radiotherapy-induced mandibular bone complications. *Cancer Treat Rev*. 2002;28(1):65–74.

6. Libshitz HI, Edeiken BS. Radiotherapy changes of the pediatric hip. *AJR Am J Roentgenol*. 1981;137(3):585–88.

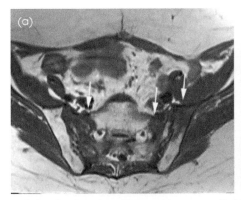
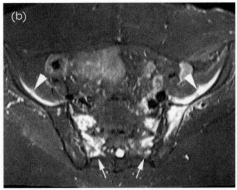

**Figure 64.7.** Postradiation fractures in a 68-year-old woman with history of pelvic radiation for gynecologic malignancy who presented with pelvic pain. (*A*) Axial T1W image of the pelvis demonstrates bilateral low signal stress fracture lines in the sacral alae and left ilium (*arrows*). Note radiation-induced fatty replacement of the background bone marrow. (*B*) Axial STIR MR image shows BME at the fracture sites (*arrows*). Note a small amount of fluid in the left greater than right iliopsoas bursae (*arrowheads*).

7. Mitchell MJ, Logan PM. Radiation-induced changes in bone. *Radiographics*. 1998;18(5):1125–1136; quiz 242–43.

8. Neuhauser EB, Wittenborg MH, Berman CZ, Cohen J. Irradiation effects of roentgen therapy on the growing spine. *Radiology*. 1952;59(5):637–50.

9. Roebuck DJ. Skeletal complications in pediatric oncology patients. *Radiographics*. 1999;19(4):873–85.

10. Rutherford H, Dodd GD. Complications of radiation therapy: growing bone. *Semin Roentgenol*. 1974;9(1):15–27.

11. Saintigny Y, Cruet-Hennequart S, Hamdi DH, Chevalier F, Lefaix JL. Impact of therapeutic irradiation on healthy articular cartilage. *Radiat Res*. 2015;183(2):135–46.

12. Schriock EA, Schell MJ, Carter M, Hustu O, Ochs JJ. Abnormal growth patterns and adult short stature in 115 long-term survivors of childhood leukemia. *J Clin Oncol*. 1991;9(3):400–405.

13. Silverman CL, Thomas PR, McAlister WH, Walker S, Whiteside LA. Slipped femoral capital epiphyses in irradiated children: dose, volume and age relationships. *Int J Radiat Oncol Biol Phys*. 1981;7(10):1357–63.

14. Stevens SK, Moore SG, Kaplan ID. Early and late bone-marrow changes after irradiation: MR evaluation. *AJR Am J Roentgenol*. 1990;154(4):745–50.

# Soft Tissue Tumors

# CHAPTER 65

# Benign Soft Tissue Masses

Kevin J. Blount

## Introduction

Soft tissue masses can arise from any of the mesenchymal elements including fat, skeletal muscle, nerves, vascular structures, or fibrous tissue. The 12 categories of soft tissue tumors according to WHO are adipocytic, fibroblastic/myofibroblastic, so-called fibrohistiocytic, smooth muscle, pericytic (perivascular), skeletal muscle, vascular, chondroosseous, gastrointestinal stromal tumors, nerve sheath tumors, tumors of uncertain differentiation, and undifferentiated/unclassified sarcomas.

The clinical presentation of soft tissue masses may be important in determining the appropriate approach to diagnosis and management. Most soft tissue masses are painless and present as palpable lesions, although some masses result in pain or neurologic symptoms caused by mass effect on adjacent structures. A history of recent trauma to the area should be considered because hematoma or myositis ossificans can appear as soft tissue masses. A history of familial syndrome, genetic or systemic disorders may be relevant, especially in the setting of multiple soft tissue tumors, such as neurofibromatosis in cases of multiple nerve sheath tumors, or Mazabraud syndrome in the setting of multiple soft tissue myxomas and FD. Additionally, some soft tissue masses have a predilection for specific locations in the body, and location can be diagnostic when certain lesions have a classic presentation. For example, Morton neuroma presents along the plantar aspect of the foot, usually within the second and third web spaces; elastofibroma is seen along the inferomedial border of the scapula; and glomus tumor is most common in the nail bed of the finger. In these situations, the imaging features and location can provide a high likelihood of diagnosis and obviate the need for percutaneous biopsy.

## Imaging Strategy

The primary imaging modalities for evaluation of soft tissue masses are radiography, US, and MRI. CT offers limited information regarding the internal contents of soft tissue masses, and MRI is the preferable cross-sectional imaging modality in most situations.

When evaluating a soft tissue mass, it is important to consider the size of the lesion, homogeneity and heterogeneity of its internal contents, and tumor margins; however, these features cannot reliably indicate benign or malignant origin. Many benign lesions are small with well-defined margins, homogeneous internal contents, and a superficial location. Nonetheless, if the imaging features are not entirely classic for a specific diagnosis, biopsy should be performed.

## Radiography

- Radiography is usually the first step in evaluating soft tissue masses.
- It can assess for underlying skeletal deformity and bone involvement, including osseous invasion or destruction.
- It can help determine the presence or absence of soft tissue calcifications within the mass, such as phleboliths within a hemangioma.
- The possibility that the soft tissue mass is arising from a bone tumor should be considered.

## Magnetic Resonance Imaging

- Because of superior soft tissue detail and multiplanar capabilities, MRI is the most comprehensive imaging modality.
- To define the anatomic location of the lesion and relationship to adjacent structures, axial plane and at least 1 longitudinal plane are usually imaged.
- A combination of T1W nonfat-suppressed and fluid-sensitive sequences in at least 2 planes is used.
- The internal architecture of a mass is well evaluated by MRI.
    - May indicate cellular origin and presence or absence of internal necrosis
- MRI is also helpful for defining extent of a lesion, its relationship to surrounding structures, degree of perilesional edema, and associated lymphadenopathy.
- Postcontrast images are useful:
    - They are most helpful for differentiating solid versus cystic lesions and areas of central necrosis.
    - Comparing precontrast with postcontrast images may distinguish true enhancement from hemorrhage or proteinaceous fluid, which may be hyperintense on T1W images.
- Internal complexity, such as septation or solid component, can be demonstrated.

## Ultrasound

- This modality is useful for defining the internal composition of masses, particularly differentiating cystic versus solid lesions, and also evaluating the degree of vascularity with Doppler flow.
- US can evaluate for internal septations or solid components.
- US is reliable for measuring size of soft tissue masses and relationships to neurovascular structures.
- US-guided biopsy is the preferred method for sampling most soft tissue masses.

- US is most helpful in very superficial lesions or lesions in the extremities with characteristic locations, such as lipoma, glomus tumor, plantar fibroma, and Baker cyst.

## Specific Diagnoses

There are certain soft tissue masses with imaging and clinical characteristics that are diagnostic and thus obviate the need for biopsy. Although this is not a comprehensive list of benign soft tissue masses, familiarity with these common benign soft tissue lesions can guide appropriate treatment.

## Lipoma

### Pathophysiology and Clinical Presentation

Lipomas are benign mesenchymal tumors of adipose tissue and are the most common soft tissue neoplasm with an approximate incidence of 2.1 per 100 people (Figure 65.1). They occur in a wide age range but are most frequent between the fifth and seventh decades of life. Lipomas are divided into superficial and deep lesions. Superficial lipomas are most commonly soft, mobile, and measure less than 5 cm. Deep lipomas are often intramuscular and can be much larger in size, measuring up to 20 cm. They occur most often around the back, neck, and proximal extremities. Although they tend to be asymptomatic and are detected on palpation, they can occasionally be associated with pain and tenderness. Because these lesions are usually soft, they uncommonly produce mass effect on adjacent structures, such as underlying nerves. Although many lipomas have a fibrous capsule, some subcutaneous lipomas may be unencapsulated, and the internal adipose tissue blends with the surrounding normal subcutaneous fat. The lack of an apparent capsule can make detection of these lesions on imaging difficult. The main diagnostic dilemma is distinguishing these lesions from low-grade liposarcomas, which can have similar imaging features.

### Imaging Strategy and Findings

- Well-differentiated liposarcoma is the primarily differential consideration for benign lipoma because both entities have a predominant fat component:
  - Lesion size greater than 10 cm, internal septations greater than 2 mm in thickness, or solid nonfatty components are features that suggest liposarcoma.
  - Biopsy of suspected well-differentiated liposarcoma can be helpful if the nonfatty elements are targeted, however, there is potential for sampling error.

### Radiography and Computed Tomography

- When larger, these lesions may present on radiographs as radiolucent foci within the soft tissues.
- On CT, the lesions are usually homogeneously lucent, with Hounsfield units measuring between –60 and –120.
- Lipoma can present with internal mineralization, which may represent areas of fat necrosis.

### Magnetic Resonance Imaging

- Lipomas are characterized by signal isointense to fat on all sequences.
- Lipomas can have a few thin and delicate internal vessels.
  - They can have internal septations that are thin and smooth.
  - Presence of internal, nonadipose soft tissue elements, or thickened and/or irregular septations should prompt tissue sampling.
- Margins can be difficult to differentiate from surrounding subcutaneous tissues.

### Ultrasound

- Wide variety of appearances are visualized:
  - May be echogenic or hypoechoic depending on the number of internal reflectors with a given lesion
- Internal complexity or significant internal vascularity on Doppler imaging may prompt close follow-up or tissue sampling.

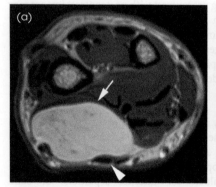 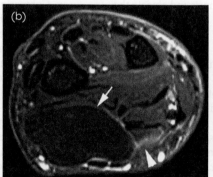 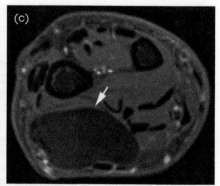

**Figure 65.1.** Soft tissue lipoma in a 67-year-old woman. (*A*) Axial T1W and (*B*) STIR MR images of the forearm show a well-circumscribed mass in the forearm deep to the palmaris longus (*arrowhead*) and flexor carpi ulnaris tendons and overlying the remaining flexor musculature that follows fat signal on all pulse sequences, including fat suppression on STIR imaging (*arrows*). On the STIR image, the median nerve is mildly radially displaced (*arrowhead*). No nonfatty internal nodularity is seen. Although this region of the lesion did not have internal septations, lipomas can have a few smooth, thin septations. (*C*) On axial T1W FS postcontrast MR imaging, the lesion (*arrow*) shows no internal enhancement that would suggest a nonfatty soft tissue component and would raise concern for liposarcoma.

### Treatment Options
- Depend on symptoms
    - If asymptomatic, usually no treatment is required.
    - For symptomatic lesions, surgical resection may be advised.
        - Lipomas can occasionally recur if entire lesion is not resected.

## Myxoma

### Pathophysiology and Clinical Presentation
Myxomas are benign lesions of mesenchymal origin characterized by myxoid matrix and are typically intramuscular (Figure 65.2). They generally arise in patients between the fifth and seventh decades of life, and the lesion has a female predilection. They are most commonly seen in the thigh, upper arm, calf, or gluteal region. Multiple myxomas are associated with monostotic or polyostotic FD (Mazabraud syndrome).

### Imaging Strategy and Findings
- Biopsy is often requested to confirm the diagnosis of myxoma, even if the imaging features are classic. Otherwise, myxomas should be followed by imaging to confirm stability.

### Magnetic Resonance Imaging
- Imaging demonstrates homogeneous high signal intensity on T2W sequences and low or intermediate signal on T1W images.
- Myxomas can mimic cystic lesions on fluid-sensitive sequences. Therefore, postcontrast imaging is critical to confirm the solid nature of the lesion.
    - Myxomas typically show mild or moderate degree of enhancement after IV administration of gadolinium.
    - Occasionally, they may demonstrate peripheral enhancement only and mimic a cystic lesion.

### Differential Diagnosis
- Cystic lesions, such as ganglion cysts

- Myxoma variants including myxoid liposarcoma, myxofibrosarcoma, and myxoid chondrosarcoma
    - Internal complexity within the lesion may suggest myxoma variant, such as the presence of lacy or amorphous fat in the setting of myxoid liposarcoma.

### Treatment Options
- Surgical excision is curative.
- Local recurrence is rare. When they occur, the recurrence is indolent.

## Peripheral Nerve Sheath Tumors

### Pathophysiology and Clinical Findings
Peripheral nerve sheath tumors are commonly encountered soft tissue lesions arising along the courses of peripheral nerves. These are most frequently observed in the fifth and sixth decades of life. The vast majority of the lesions are benign, although malignant peripheral nerve sheath tumors are seen. Benign peripheral nerve sheath tumors include schwannomas and neurofibromas. Schwannomas are typically encapsulated and separable from the adjacent nerve, and nerve function is often preserved after resection. Conversely, neurofibromas cannot be separated from the nerve, and excision may require sacrifice of the nerve. Although distinguishing between these entities is clinically relevant to help guide surgical management, the imaging appearances often significantly overlap and it may not be possible to make the distinction (Figure 65.3).

A small percentage (<5%) of schwannomas occur in the setting of neurofibromatosis type 2. Neurofibromatosis type 1 (NF1) is identified by multiple neurofibromas and often plexiform neurofibromas, which are characterized by involvement of a long segment of nerve, giving a *bag of worms* appearance. Malignant transformation of peripheral nerve sheath tumors is associated with a percentage of NF1 patients, and lifetime risk of malignant transformation has been estimated at approximately 5%.

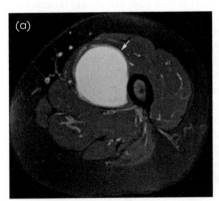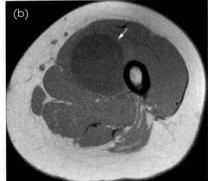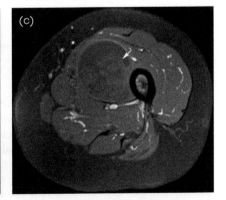

**Figure 65.2.** Intramuscular myxoma in a 48-year-old woman who presented with a palpable abnormality. (*A*) Axial T2W FS image shows a hyperintense, fluid signal intensity lesion within the vastus medialis muscle (*arrow*). (*B*) Axial T1W image demonstrates that the lesion (*arrow*) is hypointense compared to the adjacent skeletal muscle, and (*C*) T1W FS postcontrast image shows mild internal enhancement (*arrow*), consistent with a solid rather than a cystic lesion. There is no internal complexity or nodularity to suggest myxoma variant or malignancy, however, biopsy was performed and confirmed the diagnosis.

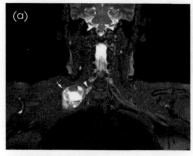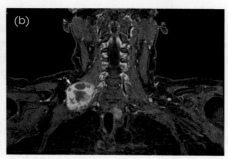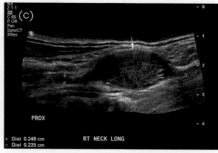

**Figure 65.3.** Peripheral nerve sheath tumor of the brachial plexus in a 41-year-old woman. (*A*) Coronal STIR SPACE (thin-section 3D SE) of the brachial plexus demonstrates a fusiform mass (*arrow*) with an edematous C7 nerve root entering the lesion (*arrowhead*). (*B*) Coronal T1W FS postcontrast image demonstrates heterogeneous enhancement of the mass (*arrow*). (*C*) Long-axis extended FOV US image demonstrates the typical appearance of a peripheral nerve sheath tumor, including the fusiform, hypoechoic mass (*arrow*), and entering and exiting nerve fascicles (*calipers*).

## Imaging Findings
### Magnetic Resonance Imaging and Ultrasound
- Peripheral nerve sheath tumors present as well-circumscribed lesions with fusiform shape in continuity with an entering and exiting nerve, and usually near the expected location of a large nerve.
- T1 and T2 signal characteristics, as well as the enhancement pattern, can vary, therefore the morphology and location of the lesion are most suggestive.
- Occasionally, the lesion may be eccentrically positioned within a nerve and displacing the nerve fascicles, suggesting that it represents a schwannoma rather than a neurofibroma.
- *Target sign.* Imaging shows low to intermediate central T2 MRI signal intensity surrounded by high T2 signal intensity, secondary to fibrous tissue with a high collagen content in the lesion's core, with the peripheral high intensity corresponding to more myxomatous tissue.
- *Split fat sign.* Rim of normal fat around the nerve sheath tumor as it enlarges can be helpful in diagnosis.
- Some lesions may be associated with cystic degeneration.

## Treatment Options
- Surgical excision is curative.
- In cases of malignant transformation, surgical resection with wide margins and regional RT is the most common treatment.

## Superficial Fibromatosis

### Pathophysiology and Clinical Findings
Fibromatoses are a group of benign fibroblastic lesions that are locally infiltrative. These lesions are more common in men than women. They may be either superficial or deep and can demonstrate variable growth. Superficial fibromatoses are almost always seen in white patients, particularly in those from Northern Europe and older than age 65. With progressive collagen deposition, lesions can result in firm palpable abnormalities and contractures. Superficial lesions in adults are divided into palmar (Dupuytren disease) or plantar (Ledderhose disease) fibromatoses and tend to grow more slowly than their deep counterparts. Histologically,

they consist of spindle cells and fibroblastic proliferation with variable collagen deposition that impacts the imaging appearances. Newer lesions tend to be more cellular with less collagen content and have a tendency for growth. More mature lesions may be paucicellular with abundant collagen deposition; these lesions often demonstrate little or no growth. In addition, local recurrence is seen in up to 50% of patients despite surgical excision, which may also be related to the degree of cellular content.

### Imaging Strategy and Findings
- MRI and US are both useful.
  - US is helpful to quickly confirm the diagnosis and characterize the lesion size and whether there are associated additional lesions.
  - Although not always necessary, MRI with IV contrast may be most helpful to assess the extent of microscopic disease at the margins of the lesion.

### Magnetic Resonance Imaging
- Imaging shows palmar location characterized by multiple cordlike nodular masses in the superficial volar aspect of the palm, embedded within the aponeurosis:
  - Lesions tend to taper at the margins and blend with the normal palmar fascia.
  - Low signal on T1W and T2W MR images is caused by a dense collagen matrix.
- Plantar location is characterized by mass lesions within or adjacent to the plantar aponeurosis (Figures 65.4 and 65.5).
  - Isointense or hypointense to muscle on T1W and T2W MR images
- Lesions with low signal on all sequences have low cellularity and dense collagen, whereas lesions with intermediate or high signal have a higher level of cellularity.
  - Lesions with a higher cellularity have been shown to have a higher recurrence rate after excision.
  - Postcontrast MRI also shows greater degree of enhancement of lesions with higher cellularity.
  - Because fibromatoses are locally infiltrative, when determining the size of the lesion, it is important to measure the entire area of enhancement, which may indicate microscopic disease.

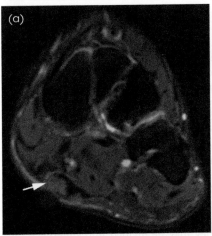 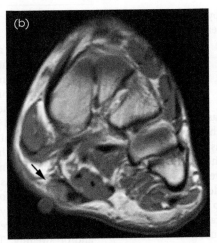 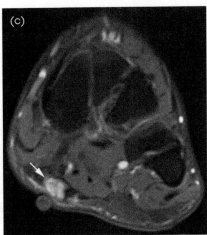

**Figure 65.4.** Plantar fibroma on MRI in a 54-year-old man with palpable abnormality along the sole of the midfoot. (*A*) Coronal T2W FS and (*B*) coronal PDW NFS images of the midfoot demonstrate a lobulated lesion arising from the superficial surface of the central plantar fascial cord (*arrows*). The lesion is hyperintense on T2W imaging and intermediate in signal on PDW imaging, and there are areas of dark signal that represent more densely packed collagen fibers. (*C*) Postcontrast T1W FS imaging shows pronounced enhancement of the lesion (*arrow*) consistent with a more cellular lesion that could grow or recur if the lesion were resected. A vitamin E capsule indicates the site of the patient's palpable lesion.

### Treatment Options
- Lesions can rarely spontaneously regress.
- Surgical excision is treatment of choice; however, local recurrence is common.

## Deep Fibromatosis

### Pathophysiology and Clinical Findings
In adults, deep fibromatosis is divided into intraabdominal, abdominal, and extraabdominal fibromatosis.

- Intraabdominal fibromatosis occurs in the setting of Gardner syndrome (familial adenomatous polyposis, multiple osteomas) with mesenteric, pelvic, or retroperitoneal mass lesions.

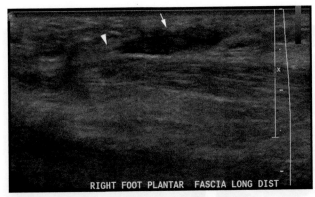

**Figure 65.5.** Plantar fibroma on US in a 63-year-old woman with palpable abnormality along the sole of the midfoot. Long-axis US image shows a predominantly hypoechoic fusiform lesion along the plantar aspect of the midfoot (*arrow*) corresponding to the patient's palpable abnormality. The lesion is continuous with the plantar fascia (*arrowhead*), which has a uniform, parallel arrangement of collagen fibers.

- Abdominal fibromatosis typically occurs within the musculature of the anterior abdominal wall.
- Extraabdominal fibromatosis most commonly occurs in the upper arm, chest wall, thigh, or head and neck.

Extraabdominal deep fibromatosis is also known as *desmoid-type fibromatosis*. It most commonly occurs between the second and fourth decades of life and has a female predilection, particularly in younger patients. It presents as a firm soft tissue mass that infiltrates the surrounding tissues and can encase neurovascular bundles. This can lead to restriction in range of motion and neurologic deficits. Similar to superficial fibromatosis, these lesions tend to grow and have high rates of recurrence following resection.

### Imaging Findings
**Magnetic Resonance Imaging**
- Ill-defined, infiltrative margins that may taper along fascial planes (*fascial tail sign*)
  - May encase neurovascular structures
- Usually present as larger lesions, between 5 and 10 cm
- May be multifocal
- Variable signal characteristics on MRI, similar to those of superficial fibromatosis
  - Most lesions demonstrate significant enhancement on postcontrast imaging.
  - Greater enhancement suggests higher degree of cellularity.
  - Following chemotherapy, there is often progressive dark signal related to decreasing cellularity and increasing collagen deposition.

### Treatment Options
- Resection with wide margin when possible is recommended.
- If it encases vital structures, the lesion may only be able to be debulked.

- Chemotherapy and immunotherapy agents have been helpful to stabilize disease and decrease growth.

## Nodular Fasciitis

### Pathophysiology and Clinical Findings
Nodular fasciitis is a benign fibrous mass most commonly occurring in the subcutaneous tissues of the upper extremities (especially the volar aspect of the forearms), head and neck, or trunk. Less commonly, it can be seen in the lower extremities. It presents as a rapidly growing nodule over a 2-4 week period and is often associated with pain and tenderness. Most lesions measure less than 4 cm but can grow up to 10 cm. Nodular fasciitis typically originates from the surface of the fascia and extends into the subcutaneous tissues. Subcutaneous lesions are much more common than fascial or intramuscular ones.

### Imaging Findings
#### Magnetic Resonance Imaging
- Imaging shows homogenous hypointense or isointense mass on T1W images, heterogeneous intermediate-to-high on T2W MRI images.
- Enhancement pattern is variable, however linear extension along the fascia (fascial tail sign) may aid in the diagnosis.

#### Ultrasound
- Hypoechoic nodule, sometimes with internal hyperechoic foci; occasional perilesional hyperechogenicity or peripheral hyperechoic nodules

### Treatment Options
- Lesions are often self-limited and spontaneously regress after several weeks.
- Percutaneous biopsy and possible excision should be considered in lesions that do not regress.
- Intralesional steroid injections may be helpful to induce regression of lesions.

## Hemangioma

### Pathophysiology and Clinical Findings
Vascular soft tissue lesions are divided into high-flow lesions, such as arteriovenous malformations, and low-flow lesions, such as hemangiomas. Hemangiomas are the most common vascular soft tissue lesion; however, there is overlap between hemangioma and other vascular malformations. They often contain disorganized vascular and nonvascular elements, particularly fat, the presence of which can aid in the diagnosis. Hemangiomas are further subdivided based on the predominant vessel type, with capillary hemangioma the most common, followed by cavernous hemangioma. They usually occur in young adults (younger than 30 years old), have a female predilection, and present with chronic pain and/or swelling. They may be divided into superficial and deep lesions. Superficial lesions result in blue skin discoloration; however, deep lesions are intramuscular and not clinically visible. Hemangiomas may enlarge in pregnant women because of hormonal influences.

### Imaging Features
#### Radiography and Computed Tomography
- May show phleboliths
- Can result in pressure remodeling of adjacent bone

#### Magnetic Resonance Imaging
Refer to Figure 65.6.

- Imaging shows intermediate to low signal on T1W images and high T2 signal vascular elements, which are serpentine in morphology. There may be high T1W fat signal interspersed within the lesion.
- Lesions may be associated with adjacent muscle atrophy related to ischemia from steal phenomenon.
- Prominent enhancement on postcontrast imaging, sometimes with feeding vessels, is seen.

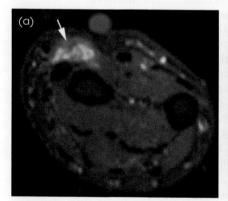 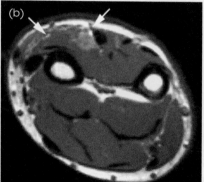 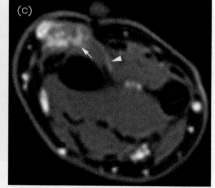

**Figure 65.6.** Soft tissue hemangioma in a 47-year-old man with palpable forearm abnormality. (A) Axial STIR image of the mid forearm shows a lobulated hyperintense lesion deep to the vitamin E capsule that was placed at the site of the patient's palpable abnormality (*arrow*). (B) Axial T1W image demonstrates a few small areas of internal fat (*arrows*). The lesion is slightly hyperintense to the adjacent skeletal muscle. (C) Early postcontrast T1W FS image shows heterogeneous enhancement with tortuous blood pool spaces (*arrow*) as well as at least 1 supplying vessel (*arrowhead*).

## Glomus Tumor

### Pathophysiology and Clinical Findings

Glomus tumors are an uncommon benign vascular tumor that arises from the glomus body, which is a dermal appendage that helps regulate temperature. Because glomus bodies are most commonly found in the fingers and toes, glomus tumors are also most common in the digits, particularly deep to the nails. They usually present in the fourth and fifth decades of life. Subungual lesions are more common in women. Glomus tumors are generally solitary and associated with pain, especially when subjected to hot or cold temperatures. When close to the skin surface, the skin may have a bluish discoloration.

### Imaging Features
### Radiography

- The lesion itself is usually small and not detectable on radiographs. However, it commonly produces pressure erosion on the underlying bone, with a scalloped cortical margin and smooth rim of thin sclerosis.

### Magnetic Resonance Imaging

- The lesion is bright on fluid-sensitive sequences and intermediate on T1W imaging.
- Because lesions are typically small, they may be difficult to see on routine imaging.
- Avid, uniform enhancement following IV gadolinium-based contrast administration often makes lesions more conspicuous.

### Ultrasound

Refer to Figure 65.7.

- Small, hypoechoic nodules corresponding to a palpable abnormality or site of pain
- Intense vascularity on Doppler US
- Pressure erosion of underlying bone

### Treatment Options

- Surgical excision and nail bed repair if subungual

## Myositis Ossificans

### Pathophysiology and Clinical Findings

Myositis ossificans (MO) is a benign soft tissue lesion most commonly occurring in skeletal muscle, characterized by heterotopic bone formation. It usually occurs in young adults. Three subgroups of MO have been described: nontraumatic MO, which is developed in the absence of any trauma; *myositis ossificans circumscripta*, which is secondary to direct trauma, and *myositis ossificans progressiva*. The imaging appearances of MO vary depending on the age of the lesion, and MO can be difficult to differentiate from malignancy (pseudosarcomatous appearance). Therefore it is important to keep this diagnosis in mind when assessing partially mineralized soft tissue masses.

MO progressiva, also known as *fibrodysplasia ossificans progressiva*, is an uncommon disorder characterized by progressive ectopic soft tissue ossification that results in significant deformity and limited range of motion at affected joints.

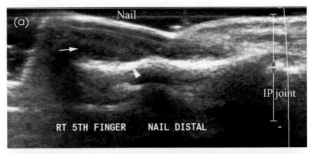

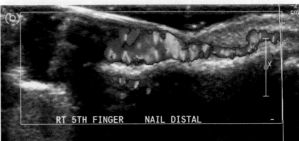

**Figure 65.7.** Glomus tumor in a 47-year-old woman with a painful mass in the nail bed of the fifth finger. (*A*) Long-axis US of the nail bed demonstrates a hypoechoic solid lesion (*arrow*) with pressure erosion of the underlying distal phalanx (*arrowhead*). The nail is elevated away from the bone. (*B*) Color Doppler image in long axis shows significant blood flow in and around this lesion. The imaging features and location provide a high likelihood of diagnosis, and biopsy is not necessary.

It has an autosomal dominant inheritance pattern and may arise sporadically. Symptoms usually begin in early childhood, between 2 and 5 years. Patients may present with other skeletal deformities, most commonly involving the toes and fingers, such as shortening of the great toe or interphalangeal ankylosis.

### Imaging Features
### Radiography and Computed Tomography

Refer to Figure 65.8.

- *Zonal pattern* is the most important diagnostic feature, with central nonossified cellular focus and peripheral rim of mature lamellar bone. It is critical to identify the zonal pattern as soon as possible because biopsy during

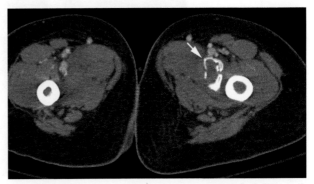

**Figure 65.8.** MO in an 18-year-old woman. Axial CT of the pelvis demonstrates a left distal iliopsoas muscle lesion with developing peripheral calcification (*arrow*) that represents zonal phenomenon seen in maturing MO.

the early stage prior to zonal pattern may lead to misdiagnosis of sarcoma.

- Radiography may be normal, especially early in the development of the lesion.
- CT is the most useful imaging modality for demonstrating peripheral mature ossification.
- Later in the process, the lesion can resorb or can form an osseous excrescence attached to the underlying bone.

### Magnetic Resonance Imaging

- MO is classified into 3 stages (early, intermediate, and late) which correlates with the clinical and imaging appearance.
  - Early or acute MO lasts approximately 1 week and consists of fibroblasts and myofibroblasts, which can mimic soft tissue sarcoma. During this phase, there may be faint calcification on CT imaging, and high T1 signal, marked enhancement, and extensive edema on MRI.
  - Intermediate or subacute MO lasts approximately 10 days and is characterized by a shell of maturing lamellar bone. The lesion begins to show zonal phenomenon on CT imaging with a rim of calcification at the periphery. There is more inhomogeneous signal on T1W and T2W images.
  - Late or maturation stage begins between the second and fifth weeks of evolution of MO, with bone production at the periphery of the lesion on CT and signal characteristics following bone marrow on MRI. During this phase biopsy will reveal the characteristic zonal pattern.

### Treatment Options

- Usually conservative
- Surgical resection occasionally needed for patients with limitation in movement or mass effect on underlying structures

## Soft Tissue Ganglion Cysts

### Pathophysiology and Clinical Findings

Ganglion cysts, or ganglia, are fluid-filled structures with a fibrous shell that likely arise in areas of weakness in synovial-lined structures, such as joint capsules and tendon sheaths. Thus, they are commonly seen around joints and tendons in areas of repetitive stress, such as the dorsum of the wrist. Unlike true synovial cysts, ganglia are not lined by synovium.

### Imaging Features
### Magnetic Resonance Imaging
Refer to Figure 65.9.

- Commonly, lobulated fluid signal intensity structures on T2W and STIR pulse sequences are seen.
- Usually hypointense to skeletal muscle on T1W imaging, however, if the fluid is proteinaceous or if there has been internal bleeding it may be hyperintense.
- Ganglion cysts may contain fine internal septations.
- A small neck between the ganglion and the structure of origin is often seen, which confirms the diagnosis.
- Mild thin peripheral and/or septal enhancement may be demonstrated or there is no significant enhancement following IV gadolinium administration.

### Treatment Options

- The cyst can be compressed until it ruptures and fluid resorbs.
- Blind or US-guided cyst fenestration and aspiration may also help to decompress the lesion.
- Intralesional steroid may have little benefit.
- Open resection is definitive treatment although ganglia may recur unless the neck is also resected.

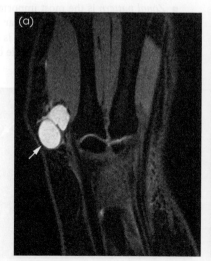
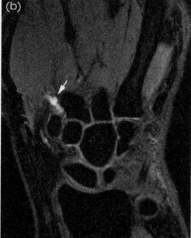

**Figure 65.9.** Soft tissue ganglion cyst in a 41-year-old woman with dorsal wrist pain and palpable abnormality. Two images from a coronal heavily T2W FS thin-section GRE image of the wrist demonstrate on (*A*), a bilobed fluid signal intensity structure (*arrow*) overlying the dorsum of the radiocarpal joint, and on (*B*), a fluid signal neck arising from the dorsal articulation between the second metacarpal and trapezium (*arrow*). The identification of the neck confirms the diagnosis and site of origin of the ganglion.

## Key Points

- Benign soft tissue masses are much more common than malignant lesions, however, some lesions have features that are indeterminate and necessitate biopsy.
- Some soft tissue masses, such as lipoma, peripheral nerve sheath tumor, fibromatosis, hemangioma, and glomus tumor, have imaging and clinical characteristics that are diagnostic and thus obviate the need for biopsy.
- Because of superior soft tissue detail, MRI is the most comprehensive imaging modality. US can play a role in evaluation of soft tissue masses, particularly those in superficial locations, or for biopsy guidance. Radiographs provide an initial assessment of bone involvement or presence of soft tissue calcification.
- Clinical history is important with specific attention to history of recent trauma, known familial syndromes, and rate of growth of the lesion.

## Recommended Reading

Kransdorf MJ, Murphey MD. Imaging of soft-tissue musculoskeletal masses: fundamental concepts. *Radiographics*. 2016;36(6):1931–48.

Manaster BJ. Soft-tissue masses: optimal imaging protocol and reporting. *AJR Am J Roentgenol*. 2013;201(3):505–14.

## References

1. Bancroft LW, Pettis C, Wasyliw C. Imaging of benign soft tissue tumors. *Semin Musculoskelet Radiol*. 2013;17(2):156–67.
2. Goodwin RW, O'Donnell P, Saifuddin A. MRI appearances of common benign soft-tissue tumours. *Clin Radiol*. 2007;62(9):843–53.
3. Murphey MD, Carroll JF, Flemming DJ, Pope TL, Gannon FH, Kransdorf MJ. From the archives of the AFIP: benign musculoskeletal lipomatous lesions. *Radiographics*. 2004;24(5):1433–66.
4. Walker EA, Fenton ME, Salesky JS, Murphey MD. Magnetic resonance imaging of benign soft tissue neoplasms in adults. *Radiol Clin North Am*. 2011;49(6):1197–217.
5. Wu JS, Hochman MG. Soft-tissue tumors and tumorlike lesions: a systematic imaging approach. *Radiology*. 2009;253(2):297–316.
6. Zhuang KD, Tandon AA, Ho BC. MRI features of soft-tissue lumps and bumps. *Clin Radiol*. 2014;69(12):e568–83.

# CHAPTER 66

# Malignant Soft Tissue Masses

Kevin J. Blount

## Introduction

Although imaging features of some soft tissue masses are diagnostic of benign lesions, most lesions have indeterminate imaging findings with more aggressive behavior that warrants tissue sampling or at least closer follow-up. Certain clinical and imaging factors may be helpful in suggesting that a particular lesion is more likely malignant and limiting differential considerations. For example, the rate of growth of a mass is critical, as a rapidly enlarging mass is highly concerning for malignancy, although a benign mass with active hemorrhage can also result in rapid enlargement. Furthermore, some malignant soft tissue tumors have distinct age distributions: Rhabdomyosarcoma is more common in children and young adults, synovial sarcoma is typically found in young adults, and undifferentiated high-grade pleomorphic sarcoma and liposarcoma usually present in older adults. A known history of malignancy and radiation can be relevant when there is a possibility of metastatic disease or RIS. Lymphoma, multiple myeloma, and some carcinomas can present as soft tissue masses. Finally, history of familial syndrome or other systemic disorder should be considered. For example, larger heterogeneous soft tissue lesions may represent malignant peripheral nerve sheath tumors in patients with neurofibromatosis. The role of imaging is often to better define the size, location, and bone and soft tissue involvement of these lesions, and to help detect distant metastases to guide subsequent management. After initial radiographs MRI is considered the best imaging modality to characterize malignant soft tissue lesions. The following chapter discusses general imaging approaches to malignant soft tissue lesions and briefly summarizes some of the most salient features of commonly encountered lesions.

## Imaging Strategy and Findings
### Radiography
- Typically performed first to define the site of the lesion, origin from bone or soft tissue (or both), size of the lesion, presence of bone destruction, and internal calcification or ossification

### Magnetic Resonance Imaging
- This is the most comprehensive imaging modality because of superior soft tissue resolution and multiplanar capabilities.
  - MRI features of different tumors overlap and often prevent making a diagnosis without tissue sampling.
  - Usually T1W nonfat-suppressed and fluid-sensitive sequences in the axial plane and at least 1 longitudinal plane are performed to define the anatomic location of the lesion and relationship to adjacent structures.
- The internal architecture of a mass is well evaluated by MRI:
  - May indicate cellular origin and presence or absence of internal necrosis
  - Can help define a target for biopsy, particularly if there is a solid or enhancing component, which is more suggestive of malignancy
- MRI is also helpful for defining the extent of the lesion, its relationship to surrounding structures, degree of perilesional edema, and associated lymphadenopathy.
- Postcontrast images can aid diagnosis:
  - They are most helpful for differentiating solid versus cystic lesions.
  - Comparing precontrast with postcontrast images may distinguish true enhancement from hemorrhage or proteinaceous fluid, which may be hyperintense on T1W images but does not enhance.
  - Internal complexity, such as septations or solid components, can be demonstrated.
  - Malignant lesions typically show more avid enhancement; however, degree of enhancement is not a reliable distinguishing feature of benign or malignant origin.
  - It is helpful to determine whether there is internal necrosis, which can be used to look for therapeutic response on serial examinations.
  - Dynamic contrast-enhanced MRI is performed in some institutions to detect viable tumor prior to tissue sampling or to determine treatment response.
- Although still under investigation, functional imaging, such as diffusion-weighted imaging (DWI), has shown promise in helping to distinguish benign versus malignant nature of some soft tissue masses. On DWI, apparent diffusion coefficient (ADC) values less than 1.1 are more commonly seen in malignant lesions, whereas values greater than 2.5 have been associated with cystic lesions.

### Computed Tomography
- MRI is preferable for soft tissue detail; however, CT may be warranted if MRI is unavailable.
- CT has greater sensitivity for calcification than MRI and may provide useful information in the setting of chondroid lesions or possibly MO.
- Because of fine bony detail, CT is helpful for evaluating cortical breakthrough and pathologic fracture.

## Nuclear Imaging

- PET/CT has been shown to improve preoperative staging.
- Nuclear imaging is also used for the detection of tumor recurrence, particularly for metabolically active tumors:
    - PET/CT is not sensitive for detecting tumors with low metabolic activity, such as low-grade liposarcoma.

## Soft Tissue Sarcomas

### Pathophysiology and Clinical Findings

Soft tissue sarcomas represent a variety of malignant neoplasms originating from different mesenchymal cell types. Overall, these lesions develop in patients of all ages and have a slight male predominance. Most commonly, they present in the lower extremity followed by the trunk and upper extremity. Taken as a whole, the 5-year survival rate for soft tissue sarcomas is approximately 50%. However, lesions deep to the fascia and larger than 5 cm carry a worse prognosis.

If a lesion is considered indeterminate by clinical and/or imaging data, then biopsy is indicated. Biopsy can be performed via percutaneous or open route. The biopsy approach should be carefully chosen because of the possible spread of malignant cells along the biopsy tract, which may be resected if a limb-sparing procedure is performed.

## Undifferentiated High-Grade Pleomorphic Sarcoma

### Pathophysiology and Clinical Findings

Formerly known as *malignant fibrous histiocytoma* (MFH), undifferentiated high-grade pleomorphic sarcoma is the most common soft tissue sarcoma of adults, typically presenting between ages 50 and 70 years. These tumors usually present in the extremities and trunk but can arise in visceral organs, as well as bone (discussed in Chapter 57, "Malignant Fibrous Lesions of the Bone"). Patients usually present with a painless, enlarging intramuscular mass and constitutional symptoms, such as fever and unexpected weight loss. Occasionally they may be seen after prior radiation exposure. The 5-year survival rate varies between 40 and 60%.

### Imaging Findings
#### Magnetic Resonance Imaging
Refer to Figure 66.1.

- Imaging shows heterogenous intramuscular soft tissue mass with variable enhancement depending on the presence of hemorrhage or necrosis.
- High-grade pleomorphic sarcoma can invade and destroy adjacent bone.
- These tumors can hemorrhage internally; therefore, all hematomas and hemorrhagic lesions should be carefully evaluated for presence of an underlying lesion. Solid or nodular enhancing components suggest presence of a mass rather than hematoma or traumatic fluid collection.
- Internal calcifications are present in 10-15% of cases.

### Treatment Options
- Surgery with wide excision and radiation, or amputation are the treatments of choice.

## Fibrosarcoma

### Pathophysiology and Clinical Findings

Fibrosarcoma is a malignant tumor with fibrous matrix, which typically develops in older, male patients (40-70 years old). It presents as a painless, slowly enlarging mass in the deep soft

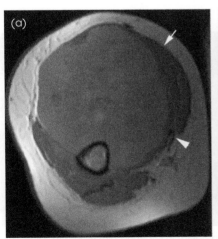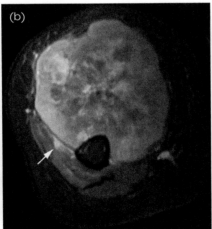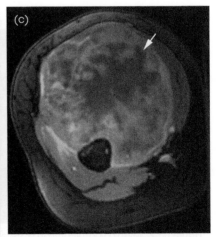

**Figure 66.1.** Pleomorphic undifferentiated high-grade sarcoma of the arm in a 43-year-old woman. (*A*) Axial PDW MR image of the arm shows a large, complex, heterogeneous solid mass that is mildly hyperintense compared to skeletal muscle involving the anterior muscular compartment. The mass arises from the brachialis muscle and has mass effect on the overlying biceps muscle (*arrow*) as well as the brachial neurovascular bundle (*arrowhead*). (*B*) The lesion is heterogeneous and hyperintense on the T2W FS MR image and is associated with mild triceps muscle edema (*arrow*) that could be reactive or caused by localized muscle invasion. (*C*) Axial T1W FS postcontrast MR image shows heterogeneous but predominantly peripheral and nodular enhancement. Nonenhancing areas (*arrow*) may be related to central necrosis. Biopsy was performed confirming undifferentiated high-grade pleomorphic sarcoma (formerly known as MFH).

tissues of the extremities and trunk and may also arise from bone (discussed in Chapter 57).

## Imaging Findings
### Magnetic Resonance Imaging
- Low signal on T1W images and hyperintense on T2W images with areas of enhancement

---

## Liposarcoma

### Pathophysiology and Clinical Findings
Liposarcomas are malignant neoplasms that develop from adipose tissue and most commonly occur between the fifth and seventh decades of life. They can develop anywhere in the body and may contain variable amounts of fat. Lesions with abundant mature-appearing fat may be difficult to differentiate from benign lipomas, although some imaging features are considered more worrisome for malignancy. For example, a deeper location of the tumor, such as location in the retroperitoneum, is considered suspicious for liposarcoma. There are 5 histologic subtypes of liposarcoma: *well-differentiated, dedifferentiated, myxoid, pleomorphic,* and *mixed* types.

### Well-Differentiated Liposarcoma
- This is a low-grade, slow-growing malignancy that does not metastasize.
- It is the most common subtype of liposarcoma, accounting for 50% of all liposarcomas.
- Twenty-five to forty percent of lesions progress to dedifferentiation.
- *Imaging findings* (Figure 66.2)
  - A well-differentiated lipoma is composed of greater than 75% fat with thickened septae or nodular components less than 2 cm in size.
  - Lower percentage of fat in the lesion, size larger than 10 cm, septae greater than 2 mm thick, or

nonlipomatous nodular or globular foci favor well-differentiated liposarcoma over lipomas.
  - Nodular areas of nonfatty soft tissue and nodular enhancement may indicate regions of dedifferentiation.

### Myxoid Liposarcoma
- The second most common subtype of liposarcoma, accounting for 20-50% of liposarcomas
- Often metastasizes to extrapulmonary locations

## Imaging Findings
### Magnetic Resonance Imaging
- Present as large, fluid signal intensity masses, usually containing some fat that is less than 10% of the overall lesion
- Usually demonstrates nodular or diffuse heterogeneous enhancement, which helps to differentiate from a cystic lesion

### Pleomorphic and Dedifferentiated Subtypes
- Aggressive and can metastasize
  - The 5-year survival rate is 30%.
- Imaging findings
  - It may not contain visible fat, and if fat is present, it can be lacy, amorphous, or linear.

### Dedifferentiated Subtype
- Most common in the retroperitoneum

### Treatment Options
- Surgical resection with wide margins is the treatment of choice.
- Radiation and chemotherapy can be considered in patients with metastatic disease.
- Myxoid liposarcoma is much more radiosensitive and chemosensitive than other subtypes.

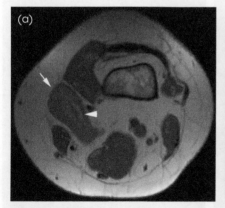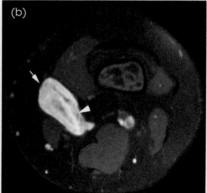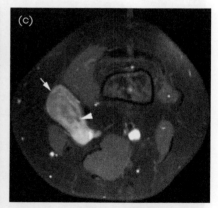

**Figure 66.2.** Myxoid liposarcoma in a 35-year-old woman with a well-marginated medial distal thigh intermuscular mass. (*A*) Axial PDW MR image of the right thigh without FS shows a well-circumscribed mass (*arrow*) arising between the vastus medialis and the sartorius muscles. There are areas of internal hyperintense signal (*arrowhead*) that follow fat signal intensity on all pulse sequences. Corresponding T1W imaging without FS also showed bright signal in these regions (*not shown*). (*B*) Axial T2W FS imaging demonstrates that the mass is largely hyperintense (*arrow*), indicating a high water content and consistent with a myxoid lesion. However, the areas of bright signal on the nonfat-suppressed sequences lose signal on fat-suppressed imaging (*arrowhead*), indicating the presence of internal fatty elements. (*C*) Postcontrast T1W FS axial image of the lesion demonstrates avid enhancement (*arrow*) with relative sparing of the fatty elements (*arrowhead*). It should be noted that myxoid liposarcomas often do not have areas of macroscopic fat on MRI. However, the presence of demonstrable fat can allow diagnosis prior to tissue sampling.

## Synovial Sarcoma

### Pathophysiology and Clinical Findings

Synovial sarcoma generally occurs in young adults between ages 15 and 35 years. It usually develops in the extremities in an extraarticular location within 5 cm from a joint. Sixty to seventy percent occur in the lower limb and the popliteal fossa is the most common site. The lesion demonstrates aggressive behavior with metastasis, particularly to the lung, or recurrence in 80% of patients.

### Imaging Strategy and Findings
**Magnetic Resonance Imaging**
Refer to Figure 66.3.

- Imaging shows a heterogenous multilocular mass, often hyperintense on T2W imaging, with heterogeneous or nodular enhancement.
- Synovial sarcoma contains amorphous, scattered, or coarse calcifications in approximately 30% of cases.

### Treatment Options
- Surgical excision with wide margins and either adjuvant or neoadjuvant RT is treatment of choice.

## Dermatofibrosarcoma Protuberans

### Pathophysiology and Clinical Findings

Dermatofibrosarcoma protuberans is an intermediate-grade tumor that usually presents in the third to fifth decades of life in the trunk, head and neck, upper extremity, or lower extremity. It presents as a slow-growing skin lesion, sometimes brown or blue in color, involving the subcutaneous adipose tissue. In some instances, it may be several lesions that coalesce to form a plaque. Tumor cells can extend far from the center of the tumor via fingerlike projections into the subcutaneous tissue and superficial fascia. Thus, despite wide local resection, the tumor can recur locally. In rare cases, it can metastasize and should be considered to have malignant potential.

### Imaging Strategy and Findings
- MRI is helpful to evaluate the extent and depth of the lesion.
  - Imaging typically shows high signal on fluid-sensitive images with postcontrast enhancement.
  - Measurement of the entire area of enhancement may be helpful to identify foci of tumor that extend away from the lesion.

### Treatment Options
- Surgical resection with wide margins is the treatment of choice.

## Malignant Peripheral Nerve Sheath Tumors

### Pathophysiology and Clinical Findings

Malignant peripheral nerve sheath tumors are rare neoplasms that dedifferentiate from peripheral nerve sheath tumors, such as benign plexiform neurofibromas, or are associated with neurofibromatosis type 1 (NF1). Between 25% and 70% of cases are seen in patients with NF1, and these lesions most commonly present between the ages of 20 to 40 years. Approximately 10% of patients with NF1 will develop a malignant peripheral nerve sheath tumor, and these patients present with new or worsening pain referable to a specific lesion. There is often rapid enlargement of a previously stable benign peripheral nerve sheath tumor. These lesions are usually larger than 5 cm in size and associated with medium to large nerves (sciatic nerve, brachial plexus, and sacral plexus).

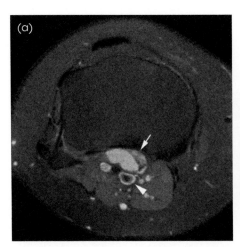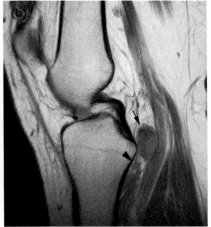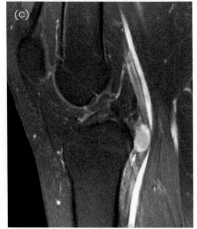

**Figure 66.3.** Synovial sarcoma of the knee in an 18-year-old woman. (*A*) Axial PDW FS and (*B*) sagittal PDW NFS images of the knee show a well-circumscribed near fluid signal intensity soft tissue lesion posterior to the tibial epiphysis. On the axial image, there is slightly darker tissue along the medial border of the lesion, indicating lesion complexity (*arrow*), and the lesion exerts mass effect on the popliteal neurovascular bundle (*arrowhead*). On the sagittal image, the inferior margin of the lesion abuts the popliteus muscle (*arrowhead*). Many synovial sarcomas exhibit bright signal on fluid-sensitive sequences and can mimic cystic lesions, such as ganglia. (*C*) However, sagittal T1 FS postcontrast image demonstrates avid enhancement of the lesion, consistent with a solid mass (*arrow*). The mass was confirmed as a synovial sarcoma on subsequent biopsy.

### Imaging Findings
**Magnetic Resonance Imaging**
- Central necrosis and lesion heterogeneity are more common in malignant nerve sheath tumors compared to benign lesions.

### Nuclear Imaging
- On PET/CT, areas of greater fluorodeoxyglucose (FDG) avidity and metabolic activity in a peripheral nerve sheath tumor may be associated with malignant transformation.

### Treatment Options
- Complete surgical resection with wide margins is treatment of choice.
- Adjuvant radiation, if the lesion is larger than 5 cm, may be helpful to prevent local recurrence.

---

## Leiomyosarcoma

### Pathophysiology and Clinical Findings
Leiomyosarcoma is a high-grade smooth muscle tumor that can metastasize. It may arise in the retroperitoneum, from larger blood vessels. When it develops in the extremities, it presents as a slowly enlarging mass, typically the thigh.

### Imaging Findings
- Imaging findings are nonspecific; the lesion is usually heterogeneous because of hemorrhage, necrosis, and/or cystic degeneration.

### Key Points
- Malignant soft tissue tumors have a wide range of clinical and imaging presentations and may relate to a known history of malignancy or metastatic disease. If a particular mass does not demonstrate typical features of benign lesions, biopsy should be performed.

- Undifferentiated pleomorphic sarcoma is the most common type of primary soft tissue sarcoma. Fibrosarcoma, liposarcoma, and synovial sarcoma are less common with distinct age predilections.
- A history of familial syndrome or systemic disorder may be relevant if there is malignant transformation of a previously benign process (ie, neurofibromatosis).
- MRI is the most comprehensive imaging modality for workup of malignant soft tissue lesions, and can often help define a target for biopsy, particularly if there is a solid or enhancing component.

### Recommended Reading
Kransdorf MJ, Murphey MD. Imaging of soft-tissue musculoskeletal masses: fundamental concepts. *Radiographics*. 2016;36(6):1931–48.

Manaster BJ. Soft-tissue masses: optimal imaging protocol and reporting. *AJR Am J Roentgenol*. 2013;201(3):505–14.

### References
1. Amini B, Jessop AC, Ganeshan DM, Tseng WW, Madewell JE. Contemporary imaging of soft tissue sarcomas. *J Surg Oncol*. 2015;111(5):496–503.
2. Baheti AD, O'Malley RB, Kim S, et al. Soft-tissue sarcomas: an update for radiologists based on the revised 2013 World Health Organization Classification. *AJR Am J Roentgenol*. 2016;206(5):924–32.
3. Morley N, Omar I. Imaging evaluation of musculoskeletal tumors. *Cancer Treat Res*. 2014;162:9–29.
4. Torreggiani WC, Al-Ismail K, Munk PL, Nicolaou S, O'Connell JX, Knowling MA. Dermatofibrosarcoma protuberans: MR imaging features *AJR Am J Roentgenol*. 2002;178(4):989–93.
5. Walker EA, Salesky JS, Fenton ME, Murphey MD. Magnetic resonance imaging of malignant soft tissue neoplasms in the adult. *Radiol Clin North Am*. 2011;49(6):1219–34.

# Articular Tumorlike Diseases

# CHAPTER 67

# Synovial Chondromatosis

Winnie A. Mar

## Introduction

Synovial chondromatosis is divided into primary and secondary forms. Primary synovial chondromatosis is an uncommon benign neoplastic process that affects joints, bursae, and tendon sheaths (Figures 67.1 and 67.2). This chapter focuses on primary synovial chondromatosis rather than secondary synovial chondromatosis where intraarticular bodies are caused by OA. Although the term *synovial osteochondromatosis* is used to refer to calcified disease, the more general term, *synovial chondromatosis* (which includes both mineralized and nonmineralized disease), is preferred. Pathologically, there is subsynovial hypertrophy with cartilaginous nodules. These cartilaginous bodies can detach and may calcify and ossify.

## Primary Synovial Chondromatosis

### Pathophysiology and Clinical Findings

This disease can occur in any age group. However, it most commonly occurs in people between ages 20 and 40 years with normal joints. It has a male predominance. Symptoms include joint pain, swelling, decreased range of motion, and mechanical symptoms, such as locking. The knee and hip joints are most commonly involved. The diagnosis is best made radiologically, because this can mimic low-grade chondrosarcoma on histology. Complications include secondary OA caused by mechanical effect from the joint bodies.

### Imaging Strategy

Radiographs are the initial test of choice to detect mineralized intraarticular bodies. Nonmineralized synovial chondromatosis may mimic PVNS on radiographs, however, the difference is well depicted on MRI. Cross-sectional imaging, preferably MRI, can be performed if the diagnosis is not clear on radiographs, or for presurgical planning. IV contrast is not usually needed, unless the diagnosis is unclear, such as in nonmineralized synovial chondromatosis. Fusion of the chondral bodies may occur, giving the appearance of a mass. It is important to note if intraarticular disease extends into a bursa or tendon sheath, as this may affect surgical management (Figures 67.3 and 67.4).

Synovial chondromatosis should be differentiated from intraarticular bodies of OA. The bodies in synovial chondromatosis are typically of uniform size, smaller than those seen in OA and may be loose or attached to the synovium. In contrast to OA, significant degenerative changes are not seen. Occasionally, the mineralized bodies can mimic rice bodies, which are more commonly seen in chronic inflammatory conditions such as tuberculous arthritis or RA.

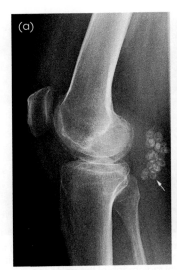 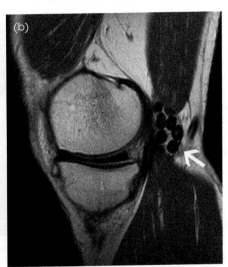

**Figure 67.1.** Synovial chondromatosis of the Baker cyst in a 52-year-old man with longstanding knee pain. (*A*) Lateral radiograph of the knee shows multiple calcified bodies of similar size within the Baker cyst (*arrow*). (*B*) Sagittal PDW MRI of the same knee shows that the calcified bodies (arrows) within the Baker cyst are hypointense.

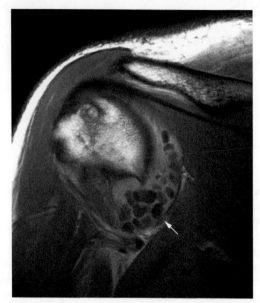

**Figure 67.2.** Synovial chondromatosis of the shoulder joint in a 31-year-old man with shoulder pain for 1-2 years. Coronal T2W NFS MR image of the shoulder shows multiple similarly sized intraarticular hypointense bodies within the axillary pouch of the glenohumeral joint (*arrow*). There is also an erosion of the inferior medial humeral head.

## Imaging Findings
### Radiography
- Imaging shows multiple bodies of similar size within a joint, tendon sheath, or bursa.
- Bodies initially have ring-and-arc mineralization.
- Extrinsic osseous erosions occur in 30% of patients, particularly in joints with a tight capsule such as the hip.
- Joint-space narrowing is not seen unless longstanding.

### Ultrasound
- Effusion
- If noncalcified, hypoechoic mass without Doppler flow
- Calcified nodules echogenic and shadowing; may be mobile

### Computed Tomography
- Calcifications are usually present.
- Nonmineralized synovial chondromatosis is low density with lobular borders caused by hyaline cartilage.
- Extrinsic erosions are well depicted with CT.

### Magnetic Resonance Imaging
- Joint effusion
- Low T1W signal intensity, intermediate to high T2W signal bodies
- Calcified bodies peripherally T1 and T2 hypointense
- Ossified bodies with central fatty marrow

### Magnetic Resonance Arthrography and Computed Tomography Arthrography
- May increase conspicuity of numerous filling defects in cases of noncalcified disease

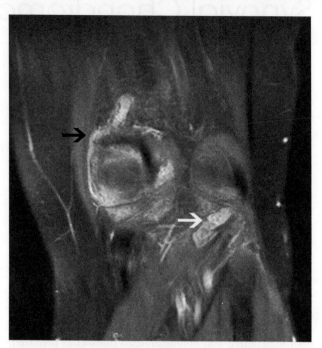

**Figure 67.3.** Noncalcified synovial chondromatosis of the knee in a 59-year-old woman with knee pain. A coronal T2W FS MR image shows multiple T2 hyperintense noncalcified cartilaginous bodies in the knee (*black arrow*) extending into the popliteus tendon sheath (*white arrow*), which can resemble rice bodies seen in other conditions.

### Nuclear Imaging
- Increased uptake on bone scintigraphy caused by increased calcium and phosphate metabolism

### Treatment Options
- Surgery is recommended. It can be arthroscopic or open; arthroscopic surgery cannot be used if there is extraarticular extension.
- Optimal treatment involves the removal of intraarticular bodies and synovectomy.

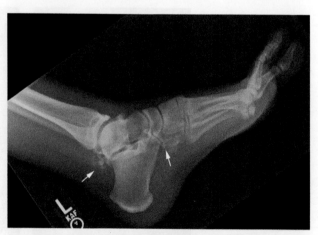

**Figure 67.4.** Flexor hallucis longus (FHL) tendon sheath synovial chondromatosis in a 34-year-old man with a history of trauma. Lateral radiograph of the ankle shows multiple calcified bodies along the course of the FHL tendon sheath extending into the plantar midfoot (*arrows*). Mild tibiotalar OA is also seen, but the number of bodies is out of proportion to the degree of OA.

## Key Points

- Synovial chondromatosis is a benign neoplastic disorder.
- Multiple calcified or noncalcified bodies are seen within a joint, bursa, or tendon sheath.
- Extrinsic osseous erosions can be seen.

## Recommended Reading

Murphey MD, Vidal JA, Fanburg-Smith JC, Gajewski DA. Imaging of synovial chondromatosis with radiologic-pathologic correlation. *Radiographics*. 2007;27:1465–88.

## References

1. McKenzie G, Raby N, Ritchie D. A pictorial review of primary synovial osteochondromatosis. *Eur Radiol*. 2008;18:2662–69.
2. Robinson P, White LM, Kandel R, Bell RS, Wunder JS. Primary synovial osteochondromatosis of the hip: extracapsular patterns of spread. *Skeletal Radiol*. 2004;33:210–15.
3. Walker EA, Murphey MD, Fetsch JF. Imaging characteristics of tenosynovial and bursal chondromatosis. *Skeletal Radiol*. 2011;40:317–25.

# CHAPTER 68

# Pigmented Villonodular Synovitis

Winnie A. Mar

## Introduction

Pigmented villonodular synovitis (PVNS) is a rare benign neoplastic disorder, typically occurring between the ages of 20 and 50 years. The diffuse intraarticular form is referred to as PVNS by WHO. The localized form may be intraarticular or extraarticular, involving tendon sheaths or bursae. The extraarticular localized form is the most common type, and is referred to as *giant cell tumor of the tendon sheath* by WHO.

## Intraarticular Pigmented Villonodular Synovitis

### Pathophysiology and Clinical Findings

Diffuse intraarticular PVNS comprises 23% of PVNS cases, and is evenly distributed between men and women. It is monoarticular, with the knee being the most commonly involved joint (Figure 68.1). The hip, ankle, shoulder, and elbow are the next most commonly involved articulations. The synovial proliferation may result in extrinsic erosions of bone, particularly in joints with a tight capsule such as the hip (Figures 68.2). Clinical symptoms include joint pain and swelling. Hemosiderin is deposited from recurrent episodes of bleeding, resulting in characteristic MRI findings. Localized intraarticular PVNS, also known as *focal nodular synovitis*, almost exclusively occurs in the knee (Figure 68.3). Pathology shows histiocytes, multinucleated giant cells, and hemosiderin. The localized forms have a variable amount of hemosiderin, usually less than diffuse PVNS. Both the localized and generalized forms appear similar histologically. Malignant PVNS is exceedingly rare and can metastasize to the lymph nodes and lung.

### Differential Diagnosis

- Gout, amyloid, hemophilic arthropathy, and synovial chondromatosis
- GCT of the tendon sheath; fibroma of the tendon sheath

### Imaging Strategy

- Imaging should begin with radiographs.
- MRI should be performed next and is most specific. A thorough evaluation before surgery should be performed in order to ensure adequate resection, particularly in the knee, in which disease can localize in joint recesses.

- US can also be performed in evaluation of localized extraarticular PVNS.

## Imaging Findings
### Radiographs

- Imaging may be normal.
- Joint effusion can be of increased density because of hemarthrosis.
- Erosions are most commonly seen in joints with a limited capacity, such as the hip, and are present on both sides of the joint.
- Joint-space narrowing and osteophytes not typically seen, in contrast to OA.

### Computed Tomography

- Hyperdense synovial proliferation or mass because of hemosiderin

### Magnetic Resonance Imaging

- T2 is usually isointense to hypointense, although sometimes heterogeneous and hyperintense.
- T1 is hypointense, with marked hypointensity or *blooming* on GRE because of susceptibility artifact from hemosiderin deposition.
- Focal nodular synovitis may lack susceptibility and demonstrate diffuse high signal on fluid-sensitive sequences.
- It usually enhances following IV contrast.

### Nuclear Imaging

- Uptake is present in fluorine 18-fluorodeoxyglucose ([18]F-FDG) PET and thallium 201.
- Uptake on technetium 99m methylene diphosphonate ([99m]Tc-MDP) bone scan in the blood pool phase is caused by hyperemia of the mass.

## Treatment Options

- If extensive, arthroscopic resection or synovectomy is recommended.
- Recurrence rate for diffuse PVNS is 20-50%, with a very low recurrence rate for localized PVNS.
- Radiotherapy, either intraarticularly injected radioisotopes, or external beam, can be used to treat recurrence, or in initial extensive disease.
- Radiofrequency ablation has been used for localized intraarticular PVNS in areas difficult to access by surgery.
- If refractory, with severe OA, the patient may require arthroplasty or arthrodesis.

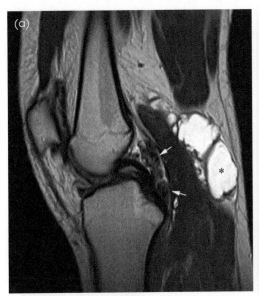
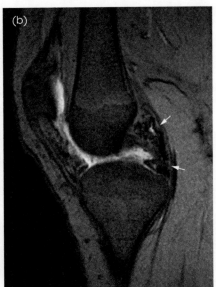

**Figure 68.1.** Diffuse PVNS of the knee joint and Baker cyst. A 15-year-old girl with knee pain. Sagittal T2W (*A*) and sagittal GRE (*B*) MR images the knee show T2 hypointense lesion (*arrows*) in the joint, which becomes more hypointense on GRE (*arrows*) because of blooming from susceptibility artifact. A large amount of fluid (*asterisk*) is also seen in the Baker cyst in (*A*) with T2 hypointense nodularity.

## Giant Cell Tumor of the Tendon Sheath

### Pathophysiology and Clinical Findings
GCT of the tendon sheath most commonly affects women, with 90% of cases involving the finger or hand. The foot and ankle are the next most commonly involved. It usually presents as a painless mass along a tendon.

### Imaging Findings
#### Radiographs
- Soft tissue swelling or mass
- No calcifications
- Possible extrinsic bone erosion

#### Ultrasound
- Hypoechoic, well-defined solid mass closely associated with tendon
- Increased Doppler flow
- Does not move with tendon because of tendon sheath origin

#### Magnetic Resonance Imaging
Refer to Figure 68.4.
- Mass abutting the tendon sheath usually with T1 hypointensity and T2 intermediate signal

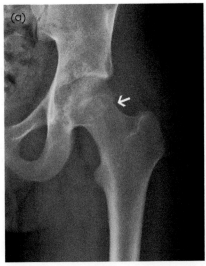
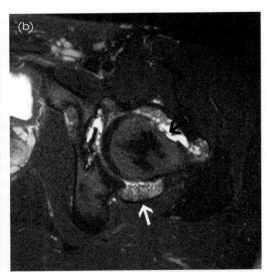

**Figure 68.2.** Diffuse PVNS in a 19-year-old man with chronic hip pain. (*A*) Frontal radiograph of the hip shows acetabular and femoral erosions. There is extrinsic erosion at the proximal lateral aspect of the femoral neck (*arrow*), with additional hip joint narrowing and suggestion of developing secondary OA. (*B*) Axial T2W FS MR image of the same patient shows a joint effusion with T2 hypointense intraarticular bodies (*white arrow*) and erosions of the femoral neck (*black arrow*).

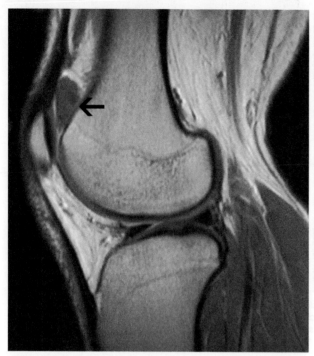

**Figure 68.3.** Focal PVNS in a 23-year-old man with knee pain, clicking and locking, and a palpable mass of the superolateral knee. Sagittal PDW MR image shows a mass in the region of the suprapatellar joint recess (*arrow*). The lesion is relatively uniform and similar in signal intensity, which could reflect a lack of prior hemorrhage and hemosiderin deposition and can be seen with focal nodular synovitis.

intensity or hypointensity; occasionally heterogeneously hyperintense on fluid-sensitive sequences
- Diffuse or heterogeneous enhancement following IV contrast

### Nuclear Imaging
- Often moderate uptake present in [18]F-FDG PET and thallium 201

#### Key Points
- PVNS is currently thought to be a benign neoplastic disorder.
- Joints, tendon sheaths, and bursae may be involved.
- Intraarticular (diffuse and localized) and extraarticular forms exist.
- The knee is the most common location of the intraarticular form.
- GCT of the tendon sheath most commonly occurs in the fingers and hand.

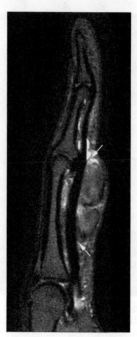

**Figure 68.4.** GCT of the tendon sheath in a 25-year-old woman with a nontender index finger mass. Sagittal T2W FS MR image shows a hypointense lobulated mass abutting the volar aspect of the flexor tendon (*arrows*).

- Characteristic MRI findings of T1 and T2 hypointensity, and blooming on GRE sequences are caused by hemosiderin.

### Recommended Reading
Murphey MD, Rhee JH, Lewis RB, Fanburg-Smith JC, Flemming DJ, Walker EA. Pigmented villonodular synovitis: radiologic-pathologic correlation. *Radiographics*. 2008;28:1493–518.

### References
1. Broski SM, Murdoch NM, Skinner JA, Wenger DE. Pigmented villonodular synovitis: potential pitfall on oncologic 18F-FDG PET/CT. *Clin Nucl Med*. 2016;41:e24–31.
2. Garner HW, Ortiguera CJ, Nakhleh RE. Pigmented villonodular synovitis. *Radiographics*. 2008;28:1519–23.
3. Lalam RK, Cribb GL, Cassar-Pullicino VN, et al. Radiofrequency thermo-ablation of PVNS in the knee: initial results. *Skeletal Radiol*. 2015;44:1777–84.
4. Lynskey SJ, Pianta MJ. MRI and thallium features of pigmented villonodular synovitis and giant cell tumours of tendon sheaths: a retrospective single centre study of imaging and literature review. *Br J Radiol*. 2015;88:20150528.

10

# Miscellaneous

# CHAPTER 69

# Hypertrophic Osteoarthropathy

Noam Belkind and Adam C. Zoga

## Introduction

*Hypertrophic osteoarthropathy* (HOA) is a clinical triad of symptoms distinguished by periostitis, digital clubbing, and painful swollen joints associated with a wide array of disease processes. When the underlying disease pathology is primarily pulmonary, HOA is more specifically termed *hypertrophic pulmonary osteoarthropathy* (HPOA). HPOA was described by Bamberger in 1889 and Marie in 1890, and is alternatively known as Pierre Marie-Bamberger syndrome.

### Pathophysiology and Clinical Findings

HOA can be classified into primary and secondary forms. Primary HOA is an autosomal dominant genetic disorder, also known as *pachydermoperiostosis*, with its clinical presentation typically beginning in childhood. Primary HOA is rare and is responsible for 3-5% of all cases. Secondary HOA is the more common form and is associated with both neoplastic and nonneoplastic diseases of the pulmonary, gastrointestinal, and cardiac systems. The most prevalent etiology of secondary HOA, accounting for approximately 80% of cases, is a paraneoplastic syndrome resulting from either primary or metastatic neoplastic lung disease. Of patients with primary lung malignancy, the incidence of HPOA varies but is typically quoted to be between 1 and 2%, with most of those cases demonstrating non-small cell lung carcinoma on histopathology. Nonneoplastic causes of HPOA include pulmonary fibrosis, pulmonary arteriovenous fistula, and cystic fibrosis. Other nonpulmonary etiologies of secondary HOA include infective endocarditis, congenital cyanotic cardiac disease, cirrhosis, biliary atresia, primary sclerosing cholangitis, inflammatory bowel disease, gastrointestinal polyposis, and thalassemia.

Clinical presentations vary depending on severity of disease, and patients may initially be asymptomatic. In primary HOA, digital clubbing may be the only clinical manifestation of the syndrome. Although they too may initially present without symptoms, with more severe disease, patients with HPOA and periostitis caused by pulmonary malignancy can experience deep bone pain, which is often more pronounced in the lower extremities. On physical examination, the periostitis may be tender to palpation. If the disease process is long-standing, the periostitis and long bone thickening can become clinically apparent in the wrists and ankles. Effusions in the large joints of the extremities are also common, with associated joint pain, tenderness, and swelling. Of note, there is no palpable synovial proliferation on physical examination, and arthrocentesis typically demonstrates a normal leukocyte count. These findings emphasize the noninflammatory nature of joint effusions in HPOA as likely representing a sympathetic response to the adjacent periostitis.

## Imaging Strategy and Findings

The principal imaging findings in HPOA are related to periostitis and periosteal new bone formation affecting the long bones of the appendicular skeleton in a bilateral and symmetric fashion. Early in the disease, a monolayer of new smooth periosteal bone is formed circumferentially around the diaphyses of the long bones, effectively increasing the overall circumference of the bone without altering the overall shape.

### Radiography

- Imaging demonstrates a smooth layer of periosteal new bone involving the long bone diaphyses, most commonly affecting the tibia and fibula (Figure 69.1).
- With progressive disease, the periostitis migrates in a centripetal fashion toward the metaphyses and, in primary HOA, can involve the epiphyses as well.
  - Progressive disease also results in more long bones being affected (Figure 69.2).
- Long-standing disease and worsening disease severity result in the further deposition of periosteal bone formation, which loses its smooth monolayer shape and becomes lamellated and irregular.
- Joint effusions may be evident on radiographs.
- There are no periarticular erosions or periarticular osteopenia, underscoring the underlying pathophysiology of sympathetic response to adjacent periostitis rather than a true inflammatory condition within the joint itself.

### Nuclear Imaging

- Radionuclide bone scintigraphy is effective in detecting early changes of HPOA and HOA, and may demonstrate periostitis before radiographs become positive.
  - Bone scintigraphy with technetium 99m ($^{99m}$Tc)-hydroxymethylene diphosphonate shows a symmetric pattern of diffuse bilateral increased periosteal radiotracer uptake.
  - Typical pattern of linear radiotracer uptake is seen running in parallel to normal cortical bone uptake and is known as the *parallel track* or *double line* sign (Figure 69.3).
  - Blood pool images show hyperemia in the periosteal regions of the affected long bones, with corresponding increased periosteal linear radiotracer uptake on delayed-phase imaging.
    - This is in contradistinction to metastatic bone disease, in which abnormal radiotracer uptake

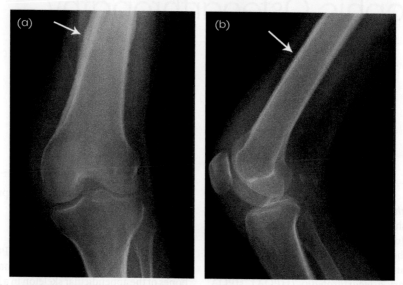

**Figure 69.1.** Radiographic appearance of HOA in the distal femur in a 55-year-old woman who presented to the emergency department with night pain. AP (*A*) and lateral (*B*) radiographs of the knee show no articular abnormality. However, there is periosteal elevation at the distal femur circumferentially (*arrows*).

occurs within the medullary space, and is more asymmetric and irregular in appearance.

- Abnormal radiotracer uptake may be seen predominantly in the symptomatic and affected joint spaces in patients with joint involvement.
- PET/CT demonstrates findings similar to those on bone scintigraphy; PET images show linear areas of increased fluorodeoxyglucose (FDG) uptake in the periosteal regions of the affected long bones corresponding to areas of increased metabolic activity.

**Magnetic Resonance Imaging**

- Periostitis can be best appreciated on STIR imaging as linear foci of hyperintense periosteal signal that parallel the diaphyses and metaphyses of the affected long bones.
- Periosteal STIR hyperintensity may be present prior to the development of abnormalities on radiographs.

- Recent case reports have suggested that HPOA can be associated with soft tissue and muscular edema that is not appreciated on radiographs or nuclear scintigraphy.
- Edema in the surrounding soft tissues and adjacent musculature will be evident as increased signal on T2W sequences.
- MRI can also illustrate synovial fluid associated with HPOA, and is more sensitive for detecting small effusions than other imaging modalities.

**Treatment Options**

- Considering these findings, it is perhaps not surprising that resolution of HPOA related symptoms occurs once the tumor is treated.
- This has been found to be the case whether the tumor is treated with surgical debulking, systemic chemotherapy alone, or chemoradiation:

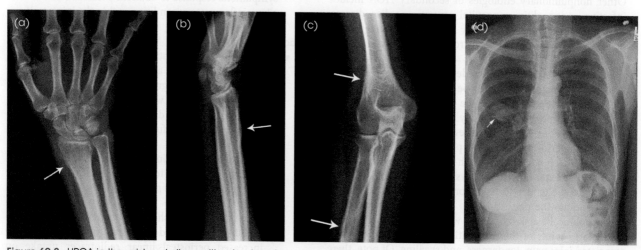

**Figure 69.2.** HPOA in the wrist and elbow without pain or trauma associated with lung carcinoma. AP (*A*) and lateral (*B*) radiographs of the wrist from the same patient show very smooth, corticated periostitis indicating chronicity (*arrows*). A single AP radiograph of the ipsilateral elbow (*C*) shows similar periosteal elevation in long bones (*arrows*). (*D*) A frontal chest radiograph was obtained because of suspicion for HOA. Note a large perihilar mass (*arrow*) that yielded a tissue diagnosis of non-small cell lung cancer.

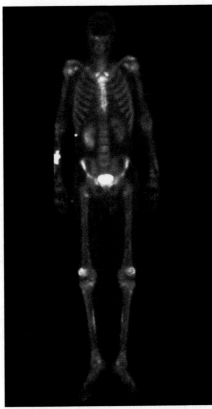

**Figure 69.3.** Bone scintigraphy findings of HPOA in a 67-year-old smoker with known non-small cell lung carcinoma during a staging workup. A frontal scintigraphic view from $^{99m}$Tc-methylene diphosphonate (MDP) bone scan shows increased radiotracer uptake in typical locations at the periosteum of all lower extremity long bones.

- Symptoms can resolve as soon as 24 hours following tumor resection.
- Resolution of imaging findings occurs alongside the resolution of clinical symptoms.
- For patients who are poor surgical candidates, a few symptomatic treatment options exist:
  - Cyclooxygenase-2 inhibitors have been successfully used to treat bone pain refractory to opioid analgesics.
  - Bisphosphonates can also reduce bone pain by interfering with osteoclastic activity, as well as decreasing fracture risk.
  - The somatostatin analog, octreotide, has been shown to provide pain relief in patients failing other analgesic regimens.

## Key Points
- Conventional radiographic evaluation is the primary imaging tool for the diagnosis of HOA, but bone scintigraphy

with $^{99m}$Tc-hydroxymethylene diphosphonate is sensitive and may be positive before radiographic findings.
- In the setting of HPOA, MRI can show periosteal soft tissue and muscle edema along with the radiographic findings of periostitis.
- The most prevalent etiology of secondary HOA is a paraneoplastic syndrome resulting from either primary or metastatic neoplastic lung disease.

### Recommended Reading
Weissman B. *Imaging of Arthritis and Metabolic Bone Disease.* Philadelphia, PA: Saunders Elsevier; 2009.

Pope T, Bloem HL, Beltran J, Morrison WB, Wilson DJ. *Musculoskeletal Imaging.* 2nd ed. Philadelphia, PA: Elsevier Health Sciences; 2014.

### References
1. Armstrong DJ, McCausland EM, Wright GD. Hypertrophic pulmonary osteoarthropathy (HPOA) (Pierre Marie-Bamberger syndrome): two cases presenting as acute inflammatory arthritis. Description and review of the literature. *Rheumatol Int.* 2007;27(4):399–402.
2. Capelastegui A, Astigarraga E, García-Iturraspe C. MR findings in pulmonary hypertrophic osteoarthropathy. *Clin Radiol.* 2000;55(1):72–75.
3. Ito T, Goto K, Yoh K, et al. Hypertrophic pulmonary osteoarthropathy as a paraneoplastic manifestation of lung cancer. *J Thorac Oncol.* 2010;5(7):976–80.
4. Izumi M, Takayama K, Yabuuchi H, Abe K, Nakanishi Y. Incidence of hypertrophic pulmonary osteoarthropathy associated with primary lung cancer. *Respirology.* 2010;15(5):809–12.
5. Makis W, Abikhzer G, Rush C. Hypertrophic pulmonary osteoarthropathy diagnosed by FDG PET-CT in a patient with lung adenocarcinoma. *Clin Nucl Med.* 2009;34(9):625–27.
6. Pineda C, Martínez-Lavín M. Hypertrophic osteoarthropathy: what a rheumatologist should know about this uncommon condition. *Rheum Dis Clin North Am.* 2013;39(2):383–400.
7. Pourmorteza M, Baumrucker SJ, Al-Sheyyab A, Da Silva MA. Hypertrophic pulmonary osteoarthropathy: a rare but treatable condition in palliative medicine. *J Pain Symptom Manage.* 2015;50(2):263–67.
8. Sainani NI, Lawande MA, Parikh VP, Pungavkar SA, Patkar DP, Sase KS. MRI diagnosis of hypertrophic osteoarthropathy from a remote childhood malignancy. *Skeletal Radiol.* 2007;36(suppl 1):S63–66.
9. Strobel K, Schaefer NG, Husarik DB, Hany TF, Steinert H. Pulmonary hypertrophic osteoarthropathy in a patient with nonsmall cell lung cancer: diagnosis with FDG PET/CT. *Clin Nucl Med.* 2006;31(10):624–26.
10. Touraine S, Wybier M, Sibileau E, et al. Non-traumatic calcifications/ossifications of the bone surface and soft tissues of the wrist, hand and fingers: a diagnostic approach. *Diagn Interv Imaging.* 2014;95(11):1035–44.

# CHAPTER 70

# Neuropathic Arthropathy

Vishal Desai and Adam C. Zoga

## Introduction

Neuropathic arthropathy represents a spectrum of destructive, generally monostotic, osseous and joint processes. This was initially described by Jean-Martin Charcot in 1868 in patients with tertiary syphilis, specifically tabes dorsalis, who were found to have severe arthritis in the knees and ankles, earning it the moniker *Charcot joint*. Although the initial cause in this group of patients was theorized by Charcot to be dysregulation of the osseous trophic centers, it was later correctly attributed to damage of the dorsal spinal column.

### Pathophysiology and Clinical Findings

Much research into the etiology of this specific arthropathy spawned 2 supported theories: the *neurotraumatic* and *neurovascular* theories. The common denominator in both is similar, *loss of neural stimulus*. Where the theories differ, however, is the path toward the eventual destructive changes. The neurotraumatic theory suggests that the loss of pain and proprioception leads to muscle imbalance with constant uneven loading, precipitating ligamentous and tendinous injury, microtrauma, and, if untreated, progressive osseous destruction. The neurovascular theory suggests that neural dysfunction causes decreased sympathetic vascular tone, resulting in vascular dilatation and hyperemia. This in turn would lead to subchondral bone resorption, weakening, microtrauma, and ultimately destruction.

Accordingly, neuropathy (central or peripheral) is a necessary component of the underlying disease processes leading to Charcot joint. The most common cause in developed countries by a large margin is diabetes mellitus, as a consequence of both polyneuropathy and microangiopathy. Additional causes are listed in Table 70.1.

The patient demographics for neuropathic arthropathy mirror those of diabetes with prevalence increasing with age and severity of diabetes; there is a 15% prevalence in the high-risk diabetic population and 30% in diabetic patients with peripheral neuropathy. Clinical presentation typically includes insidious onset of a swollen painless joint, often identified incidentally or brought to attention because of deformity. Neuropathic osteoarthropathy is usually unilateral, but it can be bilateral in approximately 20% of cases. In chronic neuropathic arthropathy, the joint is swollen but often demonstrates normal temperature with normal inflammatory markers. Physical examination reveals an insensate foot and instability. In the acute phase, however, the findings can include a warm erythematous extremity with a joint effusion. Complications of skin ulceration are seen in up to 40% of patients, which can complicate the clinical picture.

### Imaging Strategy

- The radiographic findings of neuropathic arthropathy are well-established for both the hypertrophic and atrophic patterns.
- MRI is useful as a problem-solving tool, particularly when the diagnosis is not clear in early disease, to differentiate from infection, to assess for complications such as stress fractures, or to assess for early ligament or cartilage damage.
- The role of CT is further limited and may be used similarly for problem-solving or for surgical planning.
- Nuclear scintigraphy is primarily used for detecting superimposed osteomyelitis.

### Imaging Findings
### Radiography

- Although a mixed pattern is most common, findings can be hypertrophic or atrophic.
- The classic description of a Charcot joint details the hypertrophic form, with findings including destruction, sclerosis, intraarticular bodies, joint distention, dislocation, and disorganization (Box 70.1; Figure 70.1).
  - Most often seen in the lower extremity and spine, although a pure hypertrophic form is uncommon (<20% of cases).
  - Early features can closely mimic OA, however rapid progression, ill-defined osteophytes, and joint destruction are more characteristic of neuropathic arthropathy.
- The purely atrophic form is seen in approximately 40% of cases, commonly in the upper extremity and often caused by syringomyelia (Figure 70.2).
  - Findings include severe periarticular bone resorption with a well-defined, almost surgical-appearing margin.
  - There is a relative lack of osteophytes and sclerosis.
  - Early features, such as periarticular osteopenia, are similar to septic arthritis.
- Additional features in both patterns include large hemorrhagic effusions and osseous debris in the joint.
- Fractures of the weakened underlying bones are commonly missed clinically because of loss of pain perception and can be obscured on radiographs because of the destructive joint changes and disorganization.
  - This often results in bizarre healing with exuberant callus formation.
  - Repetitive uneven loading on the affected joint, particularly in the foot, leads to recurrent ligamentous and tendinous injury, resulting in joint subluxation and propagating joint destruction and disorganization.

## Table 70.1. Causes of Neuropathic Arthropathy

| CAUSES | MNEMONIC (STARTS WITH S) |
|---|---|
| **Diabetes** | Sugar (diabetes) |
| **Syringomyelia** | Syringomyelia |
| Spinal cord injury | Spinal cord injury or |
| Tabes dorsalis | Spastic paraplegia |
| Alcoholism | Syphilis |
| Vitamin B$_{12}$ deficiency | Spirits (alcohol) |
| Intraarticular or systemic steroids | Subacute combined degeneration |
| Multiple sclerosis | Steroids |
| Central or peripheral nerve tumors | |
| Riley-Day syndrome (familial dysautonomia) | |
| Charcot-Marie-Tooth disease | |

## Box 70.1. Classic Features of Neuropathic Arthropathy (mnemonic)

### The Six D's

Destruction
Disorganization
Debris (loose bodies)
Density (sclerosis)
Distention (joint effusion)
Dislocation (dislocation/subluxation)

## Common Clinical Scenarios

### Upper Extremity

Neuropathic arthropathy affects the shoulder and to a much lesser extent, the elbow. This is most commonly caused by a central cord lesion or injury, particularly syringomyelia. As such, cervical spine MRI should be performed in the setting of an unexplained neuropathic shoulder. Clinically, the patients present with a shoulder mass caused by a large joint effusion and distention of the subacromial-subdeltoid bursa. There is a predominantly atrophic pattern with resorption of the humeral head and neck, which can appear surgically resected in advanced cases. The clinical and radiographic diagnosis can sometimes be confused with a lytic mass, particularly when the osseous debris gives a false appearance of chondroid matrix overlying the resorbed humeral head. Although involvement on both sides of the joint points toward neuropathic arthropathy, MRI may be necessary for confirmation.

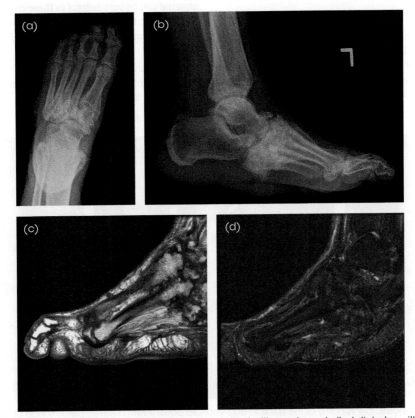

**Figure 70.1.** Hypertrophic neuropathic arthropathy in a 58-year-old patient with poorly controlled diabetes with an insensate arthritis and a shallow plantar ulcer. (*A*) AP and (*B*) lateral radiographs of the foot demonstrate classic hypertrophic changes of neuropathic arthropathy with large osteophytes, sclerosis, disorganization, and destructive changes. This most commonly occurs in the midfoot, as seen in this case. (*C*) T1W and (*D*) STIR sagittal MR images confirm the chronic destructive joint changes of neuropathic arthropathy with a relative lack of BME. No soft tissue sinus tract was seen to indicate osseous infection.

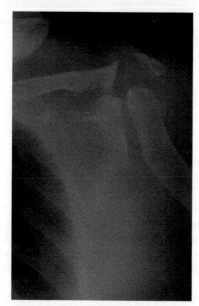

**Figure 70.2.** Atrophic neuropathic arthropathy in a 33-year-old patient with progressive bilateral upper extremity weakness. AP view of the left shoulder demonstrates advanced resorption of the humeral head with surgical-appearing margins with additional destructive changes of the acromion, consistent with the atrophic pattern of neuropathic arthropathy commonly seen in the upper extremity. Note osseous debris about the left shoulder. Syringomyelia is the most common cause (this patient had underlying cervical cord injury).

## Lower Extremity

Neuropathic arthropathy is most prevalent in the foot and ankle, with diabetes as the primary etiology. A mixed atrophic and hypertrophic pattern predominates. Clinical features depend on the chronicity of disease although the joint is usually swollen in the setting of a large joint effusion. The midfoot is most frequently affected, specifically the tarsometatarsal joints followed by the intertarsal articulations. There is often fragmentation and subluxation of the Lisfranc joint in addition to destructive changes and sclerosis in the midfoot. Less commonly, the forefoot is affected with periarticular osteolysis of the metatarsals, or the hindfoot is involved with talar collapse and calcaneal fractures. In advanced disease, there is laxity or collapse of the longitudinal arch leading to an acquired rocker bottom deformity. Because of the altered mechanics in a rocker bottom foot, not only do these patients end up with missed fractures, but they are at increased risk for foot ulcerations and osteomyelitis.

### Diabetic Foot

The diabetic foot predisposes to both neuropathic arthropathy and osteomyelitis, and differentiation by imaging alone is not always possible because of significant overlap in findings. In the acute phase of neuropathic arthropathy, there is joint swelling and erythema, however, the skin is intact and MRI demonstrates subchondral BME in the affected joints, typically in the midfoot. In contrast, osteomyelitis affects the pressure points, more commonly of the forefoot and hindfoot, with overlying ulceration and associated BME. In chronic neuropathic arthropathy, caused by the rocker bottom deformity, the cuboid becomes a primary weight-bearing structure and can serve as a pressure point for ulceration. The presence of a sinus tract, edema beyond the subchondral location, and the extent of T1 marrow hypointensity can suggest concomitant osteomyelitis. Nuclear imaging can be very helpful in these cases with a high sensitivity and specificity with the combined use of a triple-phase bone scan and a tagged white blood cell (WBC) scan.

### Spinal Neuropathic Arthropathy

Spinal neuropathic arthropathy (Figure 70.3) primarily affects the lumbar and lower thoracic spine and is most frequently

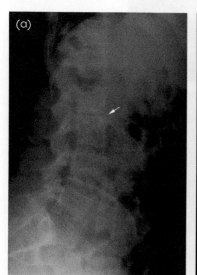
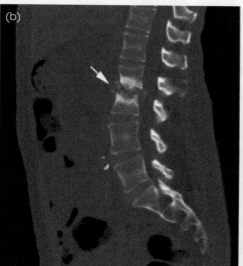
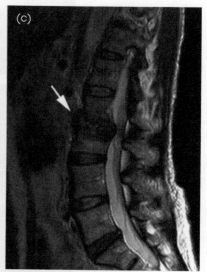

**Figure 70.3.** Mixed neuropathic arthropathy of the spine in a 73-year-old patient with a mixed presentation of lower extremity radiculopathy, pain, and weakness. (A) Lateral radiograph of the lumbar spine demonstrates disc space narrowing, endplate sclerosis, and erosive endplate changes at L2-L3 (arrow). This is indistinguishable from osteomyelitis on radiographs. (B) Sagittal reformatted CT image demonstrates extensive osseous debris and marked endplate sclerosis at the same level (arrow). (C) T2W sagittal MR image confirms a chronic process with minimal edema and involvement of more than 1 spinal column (arrow). This pattern is commonly seen with spinal neuropathic arthropathy. Differentiation from osteomyelitis is important but often difficult.

caused by diabetes or paraplegia from a variety of causes. The findings may be in an atrophic, hypertrophic, or mixed pattern. Radiographs demonstrate lysis or sclerosis of the vertebral bodies, disc space narrowing, large endplate osteophytes, and often a paraspinal soft tissue mass. Subluxation and acute spinal curvature can also be seen. As in the extremities, this raises a diagnostic dilemma, with imaging features similar to discitis/osteomyelitis. The extent of osseous fragmentation is much greater in neuropathic arthropathy and can extend to the spinal musculature or even the spinal canal. There are often calcifications within the paraspinal soft tissue mass in Charcot spine, and the masses are smaller in size and lack the enhancement pattern seen with osteomyelitis. Additionally, neuropathic arthropathy commonly involves all 3 columns of the spine whereas osteomyelitis typically involves only 1. Although CT or MRI can help characterize these findings, diagnosis requires clinical history, blood cultures, and potentially biopsy. Finally, destructive dialysis-related spondyloarthropathy can also mimic neuropathic spondyloarthropathy, and these conditions can be seen in a similar patient population (see Chapter 51, "Amyloidosis").

## Treatment Options
- A majority of cases of neuropathic arthropathy are treated conservatively with short-term immobilization and long-term stress reduction on the affected joint.
- Operative treatment is generally reserved for patients with joint instability or recurrent ulcerations and includes resection of bony prominences, osteotomy and fusion to correct rocker bottom deformity, and arthrodesis as indicated.
- Neuropathic arthropathy is considered a contraindication for arthroplasty.

## Key Points
- The imaging algorithm for a clinical neuropathic arthropathy is radiographic examination followed by MRI.
- With the diabetic foot, a direct sinus tract from a skin defect to bone is the most reliable finding to indicate osteomyelitis and septic arthropathy in the setting of infection superimposed on a Charcot arthropathy.
- Neuropathic spondylopathy, generally involves all 3 columns of the spine whereas osteomyelitis typically involves only 1.
- Neuropathic arthropathy is much less common in the upper extremities, where it is often reflective of a central cord lesion or injury, particularly syringomyelia.

## Recommended Reading
Weissman B. *Imaging of Arthritis and Metabolic Bone Disease.* Philadelphia, PA: Saunders Elsevier; 2009.

Pope T, Bloem HL, Beltran J, Morrison WB, Wilson DJ. *Musculoskeletal Imaging.* 2nd ed. Philadelphia, PA: Elsevier Health Sciences; 2014.

## References
1. Ahmadi ME, Morrison WB, Carrino JA, et al. Neuropathic arthropathy of the foot with and without superimposed osteomyelitis: MR imaging characteristics. *Radiology.* 2006;238 (2): 622–31.
2. Baker JC, Demertzis JL, Rhodes NG, Wessell DE, Rubin DA. Diabetic musculoskeletal complications and their imaging mimics. *Radiographics.* 2012;32(7):1959–74.
3. Jones EA, Manaster BJ, May DA, Disler DG. Neuropathic osteoarthropathy: diagnostic dilemmas and differential diagnosis. *Radiographics.* 2000;20(spec no)S279–293.
4. Ergen FB, Sanverdi SE, Oznur A. Charcot foot in diabetes and an update on imaging. *Diabet Foot Ankle.* 2013;4:10.3402
5. Lacout A, Lebreton C, Mompoint D et al. CT and MRI of spinal neuroarthropathy. *AJR Am J Roentgenol.* 2009;193(6):W505–14.
6. Ledermann HP, Morrison WB. Differential diagnosis of pedal osteomyelitis and diabetic neuroarthropathy: MR Imaging. *Semin Musculoskelet Radiol.* 2005;9(3):272–83.
7. Mautone M, Naidoo P. What the radiologist needs to know about Charcot foot. *J Med Imaging Radiat Oncol.* 2015;59(4):395–402.
8. Morrison WB, Ledermann HP. Work-up of the diabetic foot. *Radiol Clin North Am.* 2002;40:1171–92.
9. Palestro CJ, Mehta HH, Patel M, et al. Marrow versus infection in the Charcot joint: indium-111 leukocyte and technetium-99m sulfur colloid scintigraphy. *J Nucl Med.* 1998;39(2):346–50.
10. Schwarz GS, Berenyi MR, Siegel MW. Atrophic arthropathy and diabetic neuritis. *AJR Am J Roentgenol.* 1969;106:523–29.
11. Sommer TC, Lee TH. Charcot foot: the diagnostic dilemma. *Am Fam Physician.* 2001;64(9):1591–98.
12. Tan PL, Teh J. MRI of the diabetic foot: differentiation of infection from neuropathic change. *Br J Radiol.* 2007;80(959):939–48.
13. Toledano TR, Fatone EA, Weis A, Cotten A, Beltran J. MRI evaluation of bone marrow changes in the diabetic foot: a practical approach. *Semin Musculoskelet Radiol.* 2011;15:257–68.
14. Wagner SC, Schweitzer ME, Morrison WB, et al. Can imaging findings help differentiate spinal neuropathic arthropathy from disk space infection? Initial experience. *Radiology.* 2000;214(3):693–99.
15. Wukich DK, Raspovic KM, Hobizal KB, Rosario B. Radiographic analysis of diabetic midfoot Charcot neuroarthropathy with and without midfoot ulceration. *Foot Ankle Int.* 2014;35(11):1108–15.

# Index